CALL SIGN - DUSTOFF
A HISTORY OF U.S. ARMY AEROMEDICAL EVACUATION FROM CONCEPTION TO HURRICANE KATRINA

by
DARREL WHITCOMB

Borden Institute
Martha K. Lenhart, MD, PhD, FAAOS
Colonel, MC, US Army
Director and Editor in Chief

Editorial Staff: Marcia A. Metzgar
Volume Editor

Douglas Wise
Layout Editor

The opinions or assertions contained herein are the personal views of the authors and are not to be construed as doctrine of the Department of the Army or the Department of Defense.

Published by the Office of The Surgeon General
Borden Institute
Fort Detrick
Frederick, MD 21702

Library of Congress Cataloging-in-Publication Data

Whitcomb, Darrel D., 1947-
  Call sign "Dustoff" : a history of U.S. Army aeromedical evacuation from Conception to Hurricane Katrina / by Darrel Whitcomb.
    p. cm.
  Includes bibliographical references and index.
  Summary: "Explores the conceptualization of the initial attempts to use aircraft for evacuation, reviews its development and maturity through conflicts, and focuses on the history of the MEDEVAC post-Vietnam through Hurricane Katrina"--Provided by publisher.
  1. Helicopter ambulances--United States--History. 2. United States. Army--Transport of sick and wounded--History. 3. United States. Army. Medical Service Corps--History. I. Title.
  UH503.W44 2011
  355.3'45--dc22
                                                                    2011001043

ISBN 978-0-16-087937-1

For sale by the Superintendent of Documents, U.S. Government Publishing Office
Internet: bookstore.gpo.gov Phone: toll free (866) 512-1800; DC area (202) 512-1800
Fax: (202) 512-2104 Mail: Stop IDCC, Washington, DC 20402-0001

ISBN 978-0-16-087937-1

Contents

Foreword

DUSTOFF Medic, SFC Brian "Papa" Brockett, knelt over his patient, doing his normal assessment, checking for unknown wounds and asking "Are you okay?" to check his alertness. The young Marine Infantryman merely wiped the blood from his face, where he had taken a round as he burst through the door of an Iraqi home in search of insurgents. He smiled and replied, "I'm okay. I knew you'd come." As "Papa" retold this story, his eyes filled with tears, and his voice waivered with the return of the emotion of knowing the faith our Warriors place in DUSTOFF crews to be there for them in their time of need. This story was told in 2008; however, it resonates with the same fervor as did Major Charles Kelly's last words of 1 July 1963, "When I have your wounded."

And so it is today. The current DUSTOFF crews run to their aircraft, confident that they can—and will—face the dangers that await them over the next hill and then they go where others dare not. They cross mine fields, face incoming fire from those who would do harm to their comrades in arms, and willingly risk their own lives to medically evacuate others. They are the Warriors of compassion, standing on the shoulders of Soldiers like Charles Kelly, Pat Brady, Mike Novosel, Steve Hook, Tiny Simmons, Charles Allen, John Temperilli, Ernie Sylvester, Doug Moore, Paul Bloomquist, Hank Tuell, and thousands of others who earlier flew the medical evacuation helicopters.

The inevitable consequence of war is the production of casualties. After World War II, visionaries like Spurgeon Neel recognized the efficacy of using helicopters to evacuate casualties from the battlefield. He and others led the fight to develop the MEDEVAC helicopters into the single greatest lifesaving system developed by our Armed Forces. Neel realized that this capability could also provide a greater national service. He was instrumental in creating the Military Assistance to Safety and Traffic (MAST) Program, which provided this service to our nation's towns and rural areas. Neel's innovative and creative ideas led directly to the use of helicopters as a part of the medical health care delivery system.

This book captures the story of DUSTOFF from its conception. It reviews its development and use in both Korea and Vietnam, but focuses on the post–Vietnam years that saw almost constant transformation of unit structure, doctrine and structural command and control, and the development and adaptation of new aircraft and lifesaving equipment. It also chronicles the transfer of the MEDEVAC units from medical to aviation control, a most traumatic event that presented the MEDEVAC community with another set of challenges.

What held steadfast through these times of change was the immutable fact that brave American Warriors on the battlefield executed the nation's wars with the faith that comes from knowing that should they become casualties, the DUSTOFF crews would come. Their heroic efforts were recognized during our nation's military missions in Panama, Desert Storm, Provide Comfort, Bosnia, Afghanistan, and Iraq; the almost continuous support for MAST operations across the nation; and innumerable responses to domestic crises, Hurricane Katrina most prominent among them. Theirs is a stellar legacy, one well recognized and now, well recorded.

Darrel Whitcomb has expertly captured the story of this national treasure—the face of hope in scenes of chaos—the story of the Warriors of compassion. All captured in two quotes – "When I have your wounded" and "I knew you'd come."

Daniel W. Gower, Jr.
Colonel, U.S. Army Retired
Executive Director, DUSTOFF Association

Preface

There is a very interesting togetherness between medicine and aviation with which I have been fascinated over the years.

- Maj. Gen. (ret) Spurgeon Neel, USA[1]

Much has been written about U.S. Army aeromedical evacuation—or MEDE-VAC—as it has come to be known, and deservedly so. Most works have focused on the war in Korea or Vietnam. This project has a larger interest. It will explore the conceptualization of the initial attempts to use aircraft for evacuation, review its development and maturity through those conflicts, and then focus on the history of MEDEVAC post–Vietnam to the transformation of the MEDEVAC units from medical to aviation command in 2003, and the response to Hurricane Katrina in 2005.

By MEDEVAC, I specifically mean the utilization of helicopters to pick up wounded soldiers and rapidly move them to medical facilities in the rear area. I acknowledge that ground vehicles can also perform this function, and those units are also an important part of the story of medical evacuation. The focus in this work will be on the unique use of helicopters to accomplish this mission. It is a fascinating story of the development of a uniquely American innovation, although other nations also conduct it now for their troops.

Some definitions are needed:

MEDEVAC: Medical evacuation is performed by dedicated, standardized medical evacuation platforms, with medical professionals who provide timely, efficient movement and en route care by medical personnel of the wounded, injured, or ill persons from the battlefield and other locations to medical treatment facilities.[2]

Similar and frequently confused with MEDEVAC is:

CASEVAC: A term used by nonmedical units to refer to the movement of casualties aboard nonmedical vehicles or aircraft.[3]

As the definitions show, MEDEVAC is much more than CASEVAC. It is a key component of the overall medical system of the Army that has as its primary mission the conservation of military manpower.

"Necessity," said the Greek philosopher Plato, "is the mother of invention." Military commanders have long recognized the need to move casualties from the field of battle as quickly as possible. Alexander the Great had a medical corps of litter bearers who brought in the wounded and teams of surgeons and medics who practiced the medicine of the day as best they could. The result was fewer deaths and more men returned to duty.

Later armies followed variations of this theme. As the technology of medicine itself advanced, so did the ability to collect the wounded. Armies took advantage of technological progress to facilitate the process. French armies of the 18th century developed special wagons. They called them "Ambulance Volante" or "Flying Wagons," and the lumbering vehicles followed closely behind the battle lines to collect the inevitable result of increasingly lethal warfare.

An evolution of this system was created by United States Army Maj. Jonathan A. Letterman. After witnessing the carnage and lack of good care for Union soldiers in the first year of the Civil War, he was empowered by Maj. Gen. George McClellan, commander of the Army of the Potomac, to establish an evacuation system based on an ambulance corps for the Army of the Potomac to collect the wounded and provide initial care. It would be equipped with ambulances, horses, and necessary supplies and manned by medical technicians who would then deliver the casualties to divisional field hospitals. Specially detailed officers would administer this system, thus allowing the doctors to focus on caring for the wounded. Eventually, they would also use ships and trains to move the wounded to general hospitals in the rear areas. The system worked well and was soon adopted for the entire Army through Army regulations and then an Act of Congress. It established a chain of evacuation that still exists.

As the technology of transportation advanced, so did the implements of medical evacuation. Any new invention was—within a short time—drafted for evacuation duties. Ships, trains, trucks, and automobiles were all adopted, and medical personnel put aboard, thus extending medical capability forward so that casualties could more quickly receive care. When the airplane was developed into something that could carry more than just a pilot, it too was detailed to evacuation duties. It was only natural that the helicopter, with its unique ability to land in nearly any location, would be assigned to MEDEVAC duties. It held the promise of further decreasing the time required to move critically wounded from the point of injury to critical medical care. It seemed to be the perfect device to answer the necessity that spawned the chain of evacuation.

Yet every child has two parents, and while necessity is the mother of MEDEVAC, aviation is its father. He is a stern father with immutable laws of physics that define what those wonderful MEDEVAC helicopters and crews can and *cannot* do. Helicopters do facilitate moving the wounded through the chain of care more quickly than other vehicles, but the physical limits of flight cannot be overridden by medical necessity.

Helicopters can only go so fast and so far, and there are places where helicopters cannot go. These may be defined by weather, terrain, or a vengeful enemy, but those rules are inviolate—no amount of necessity can override them. Any user of helicopters must obey those rules or be prepared to pay a terrible price. This reality has been traced in blood many times over.

These rules apply to any practitioners of the art of aviation. Long ago, aviation pioneers realized that airplanes and their use must be controlled by aviators who understood the reality of flight. Perhaps recognizing this, during the Korean War the Army designated a small number of Medical Service Corps (MSC) officers to attend flight school and become MEDEVAC helicopter pilots. It was—and still is—a good match.

It is evident that in the modern world of aviation and medicine, the MEDEVAC pilots have to serve both masters. They must understand the medical imperative of their task, yet perform it within the limits of physics. They must honor both of their parents to be successful.

In a microcosmic way, the four-person crew of the MEDEVAC helicopter represents this melding of two disparate sciences. In the cockpit, the two pilots, commissioned or warrant officers, understand both specialties. In the back of the aircraft, the crew chief focuses on the operation and care of the aircraft, while his cabin-mate, the flight medic, is the medical technician. His focus is on the application of medical care as necessary to evacuate the casualties to higher levels of medical capability. It is a time-tested system that brings together the best of both specialties.

But which is primary: aviation or medicine? It is a beguiling question. To whom should that crew answer, the medical command that controls the chain of evacuation and medical supplies, or the aviation command that provides the organization and support necessary to facilitate flight?

That appears to be the dilemma, the yin and yang of this story. Is it, in the end, the right question?

One immutable point is crystal clear. That wonderful force of MEDEVAC helicopters and crews is a national treasure that serves our nation in both peace and war.

This story is presented chronologically. Part I looks at the heritage of MEDEVAC from its beginnings in World War II through the bitter battles in Korea, the interwar years, and the long struggle in Vietnam. Part II covers the 1980s, a time of domestic duties and contingency operations. Part III looks at the turbulent 1990s with the end of the cold war, a hot war in the Persian Gulf, dramatic military force reductions, and a call to duty in the Balkans. Part IV stretches into the millennium, covering the terrible events of 9/11, further conflict in Afghanistan and Iraq, the Aviation Transformation Initiative that moved MEDEVAC from medical to aviation control, and the national response to Hurricane Katrina. In general, after Part I, a thematic approach is used, and the chapters are organized with interweaving sections covering doctrine (Service and joint), organization, and operations.

One explanation is necessary. I will mention many specific U.S. Army units in this work. Divisions and larger units will be referred to by their full title, as will medical units down through battalion. Combat battalions will be referred to as per the Combat Arms Regimental System. The MEDEVAC units that are medical companies (Air Ambulance) and medical detachments (Helicopter Ambulance) will be addressed as Med Co (AA) and Med Det (HA), respectively, such as the 57th Med Det (HA) or the 45th Med Co (AA). As the story will explain, in 2005, the MEDEVAC units were reorganized and moved from medical to aviation command and control. At that point, they lost their heritage designations such as the 498th Med Co (AA), and each unit became the Charlie company of a general support aviation battalion like Charlie Company, 2d Battalion, 3d Aviation Regiment, abbreviated as C/2d/3d. These simplifications are in the interest of brevity.

This work has brought me into contact with many wonderful people who have facilitated its creation. I would be remiss not to mention them.

My first research effort took place at the Armed Forces Medical Library in Falls Church, Virginia, where I was well supported by Patrick Walz, Emily Court, and Diane Zehnpfennig. One of the first books that they gave me to read was *DUSTOFF: Army Aeromedical Evacuation in Vietnam,* which was written by Peter Dorland and James Nanney and published in 1982. It is a fine piece of history that effectively tells the evolutional story of MEDEVAC in that conflict, and it helped me set my course to discover the later story.

My next stop was Fort Rucker, Alabama. I attended the 2CF7 Medical Evacuation Doctrine Course at the U.S. Army School of Aviation Medicine (USASAM). I met Lt. Col. Vinny Carnazza, Maj. Ken Koyle, 1st Sgt. Michael Stoddard, and Sfc. Jim Burbach at the USASAM, and conducted interviews with fellow students in the 2CF7 course.

I also spent fruitful time at Fort Rucker with Steve Maxham and Dick Tierney at the U.S. Army Aviation Museum and with Col. Dave MacDonald and his coworkers at the Medical Evacuation Proponency Directorate.

Dr. John Dabrowski, the Army Aviation Branch Historian, gave me a great deal of his time, as did Jill Redington, Jean Southwell, and Janice Haines, who helped me dig through the massive data available in the Aviation Technical Library.

I made several very productive visits to the U.S. Army Center for Military History at Fort McNair in Washington, DC, where I worked with Mr. Stephen Everett and Ms. Patricia Ames. Their help in deciphering Army force structure was invaluable.

The National Archives in College Park, Maryland, are a rich source of information. There, I was well assisted by Rich Boylan and Susan Francis-Haughton who patiently helped me find archival information on units and operations.

I traveled to Fort Bragg, North Carolina. Ms. Donna Barr Tabor, the historian for the XVIII Airborne Corps, helped me recover data on the MEDEVAC units that have served in this unit or at this post. Lt. Col. Scott Putzier of the 56th Medical

Evacuation Battalion helped me find data on that unit. I attended the inactivation ceremony for the 57th Med Co (AA). It was sad to watch as the guidon was cased on this unit that has existed since the Korean War era. Perhaps more than any other unit, it represents the spirit of MEDEVAC.

The medical warriors at Fort Sam Houston, Texas, hosted me for two weeks as I conducted interviews and did primary research on doctrine and force structure in the AMEDD Directorate of Combat and Doctrine Development. Col. Mark Hegerle and his personnel were graciously generous in their support. I must specifically thank Ms. Cecily Price and Mr. Ken Sutton for allowing me to call on their vast historical knowledge of this mission and its doctrine. I also went to Fort Hood, where I visited the 507th Med Co (AA) and the 36th Medical Battalion (Evacuation), two units key to this history.

Several individuals have given me critical "vectors" in this venture. Col. (ret) Dan Gower of the DUSTOFF Association has guided me with invaluable background and historical information, and he has been absolutely selfless in helping me to find and interview key participants in this mission. This project could not have happened without his beyond generous support. His absolute love for and dedication to this mission and community of real heroes is truly humbling.

Col. Randal Schwallie has served as my conduit into the Army Reserve community. The Army Reserve's story of great service as part of the MEDEVAC community has received little recognition.

My work allowed me to visit several more MEDEVAC companies, both active and National Guard. All commanders were wonderful hosts and gave me open access to their histories and troops. Interviewing them was a truly enriching experience. Over the years, there are or have been more than110 units. I could not visit them all or their descendents. But I would like to especially thank 2d Lt. Jasmine Chase of the 112th Med Co (AA), Maine ARNG, who generously shared her unit history with me.

The U.S. Army Military History Institute at Carlisle Barracks, Pennsylvania, is a rich source of information, and I spent two very productive days there under the expert guidance of Mr. Dave Keough.

Capt. Jim Page hosted me for two days at Fort Campbell as I dug into the history of MEDEVAC at that huge post, home to the famous 101st Airborne Division (Air Assault). It is the location for two MEDEVAC units now, the Charlie Companies of the 6th and 7th Battalions of the 101st Aviation Regiment, formed from the remnants of the inactivated 542d and 50th Med Cos (AA), respectively. This visit was critical to understanding MEDEVAC and the key role that "Eagle Dustoff" played in this saga.

I traveled to Germany and visited the pre-transformation 159th Med Co (AA) at Wiesbaden Air Base, the 236th Med Co (AA) at Landstuhl, the 45th Med Co (AA) at Ketterbach, and the MEDEVAC alert facility at Hohenfels. Additionally, Mr. Bruce Siemon, the U.S. Army Europe Historian, hosted me at his office in Heidelberg for a very productive visit to that rich trove of documents.

While visiting Seattle, Washington, I met with Mr. Mark Hough. Mark never served in the military, but has developed a strong and enduring interest in MEDE-VAC. He has published the best single book chronicling the individual histories of MEDEVAC units, *United States Army Air Ambulance*. He generously shared his voluminous files with me and gave me a "tour" of his collection of more than 500 unit patches.

In Atlanta, I spent a day with Lt. Col. Al Koenig, a historian assigned to the First Army. He is leading the effort to capture the U.S. Army response to Hurricane Katrina, and generously shared his extensive files with me. The next day, I visited Lt. Col. Pete Smart at the Redstone Arsenal at Huntsville, Alabama. He works in the Aviation Utility Helicopters Project Office, and he gave me an excellent tutorial on the MEDEVAC fleet of helicopters.

My office mates at the Office of Medical History have been unselfish in their support. Our archivists, Will Edmondson and Lisa Wagner, provided great support in digging out documents from our extensive collections. Tom Gray and Annita Ferencz provided the administrative structure that made the office run. Maj. Lew Barger and Maj. Rich Prior were our active Army counterparts and served as the critical link to our forces operating daily around the world. Drs. Sanders Marble, Jonathan Hood, and Lisa Budreau are all experts in their fields and possess that innate capability to always ask the provoking question. All of this was directed by Dr. John Greenwood, a preeminent historian who, with more than 30 years experience as a prolific historical writer, set the standard for the rest of us. I sincerely thank the team for their support, and Dr. Greenwood for his leadership and guidance. Lastly and perhaps most importantly, I must also thank my dear wife, Chris, for her generous and loving support as my transcriber, editor, and chief taskmaster for this effort. I just could not have done it without her.

This project also gave me the opportunity to become familiar with a very special individual, Maj. Gen. Spurgeon Neel. He—perhaps more than any other single person—created MEDEVAC. As a young major in the late 1940s, he saw the rich potential that helicopters represented as aerial ambulances, and never lost the passion of that vision through the many assignments of his long and distinguished career. Unfortunately, he passed away in 2003. But he was a prolific writer and penned many articles, staff studies, and reports on the subject. Additionally, he granted several recorded and transcribed interviews that are rich in detail, and track so much of the mission as it developed during his career. He is truly the patron saint of MEDEVAC.

I offer a sincere salute to the dozens of soldiers and civilians I interviewed for this project. Their patience is appreciated. There was no way to meet with all of the men and women who have been members of this great community. I do believe that I have interviewed a truly representative slice of them. My interviewees make up four distinct groups: (1) the "old lionhearts" from the Vietnam War; (2) the post–Vietnam transitionals; (3) the post–Desert Storm "zealots," who are the commanders of today; and (4) the young men and women who are the current MEDEVAC force. I have done my utmost to properly record and use their words as accurately as possible, and I hold in confidence those "background" discussions so vital to understanding. To all my interviewees I say, "Your words are the essence, the heart of the story."

Some individuals I asked to interview refused because the memories are too strong. I respect that and accept it. Much of this story is about war. That endeavor touches all who experience it. Some soldiers love it. Some soldiers hate it. All are changed irrevocably by the experience.

And lastly, I offer a dedication.

I dedicate this work to the men and women of MEDEVAC. First of all, it is their story. Most importantly, it is offered for all that they do. Day and night, they are there. Good weather and bad, they are there. Enemy or no enemy, they are there. They give far more than their nation has a right to expect. Their efforts humble us all. They represent the best of our nation, and we must never forget that.

And right now, they are out there at so many locations,
waiting for that call.

Suffused as they are with a focus, a determination, a will that has been
forged in the fire of compassion.

Pray that it should always be so.

Part One

Fulfilling a Need:
From Conception to Combat

Chapter One
An Honorable Heritage

"When I have your wounded."

Maj. Charles Kelly[1]

His name is Andrew Russ. A tall, soft-spoken Californian, he is a brand new 2d Lt. in the U.S. Army. His commission was earned through the Reserve Officers' Training Corps program at San Diego State University, where he graduated in 2005 with a degree in biology.

His initial interest was medicine. But he comes from a family of aviators; his dad was a Navy F-4 fighter pilot and his older brother is already in the Army flying the OH-58D, Kiowa. He could not resist the call to fly as opposed to being a physician.

"It has kind of been a family thing," Russ admitted quietly.

Yet he took his commission in the U.S. Army Medical Service Corps (MSC) because he wanted to fly MEDEVAC as opposed to Navy fighters or Army attack helicopters. Why?

His answer was self-deprecating: "It's a feeling you get when you help someone else. In college, I worked as an emergency medical technician on an ambulance and in an emergency room…. I liked actually being out there to help bring them from where they are to sustained care, because that is really one of the most important parts, getting them there. It's a feeling of satisfaction you get when you take someone from where they got hurt … to where someone else … can fix them."[2]

Russ trained on Black Hawks, graduated as the only MSC officer in a class of 50, and reported to his MEDEVAC Company at Fort Drum, New York. It belongs to the 10th Mountain Division. That unit is heavily involved in the Long War against terror. Russ will see hard duty in places across the globe. He understands the heritage of MEDEVAC and what it will require of him.

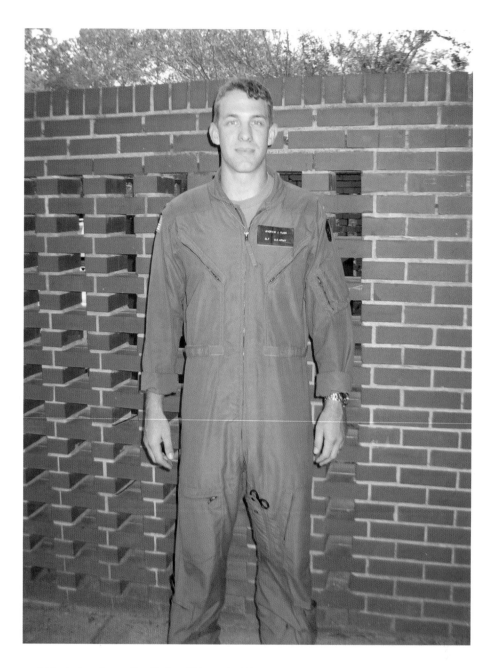

2d Lt. Andrew Russ at Fort Rucker, Alabama, in 2006.
Source: Author.

"Somebody has to do it," Russ said. "Selfless service is one of the seven Army values.... I would like to be part of that heritage."[3]

He and so many other young men and women like him are the future of MEDE-VAC.

Early Efforts

The MEDEVAC heritage to which Russ and his contemporaries aspired to join was slow to develop and had its tribulations and challenges. From the very beginning of modern aviation, the early pioneers questioned the utility of aircraft designed around a rotating wing. Even Orville and Wilbur Wright delved into the concept.

"Like all novices," Wilbur Wright wrote, "we began with the helicopter, but soon saw that it had no future, and dropped it ... If its engine stops, it must fall with deathly violence, for it can neither float like the balloon nor glide like the aeroplane. The helicopter is much easier to design than the aeroplane, but it is worthless when done."[4]

Others were not so despairing. Igor Sikorsky, eventually considered the "gentle genius" of the helicopter community, built his first helicopter in the Ukraine in 1909. He abandoned the project because he could not find an engine that could produce enough power to generate a useful lift capability. This was the fundamental problem, and it would require many years to overcome. Yet he intuitively sensed that when man learned how to hover and take off and land vertically without needing a runway or prepared field, he would truly be able to exploit the third dimension as he and the other aviation pioneers dreamed to do.[5]

Different aviation pioneers saw the utilitarian value of using "fixed" wing aircraft for medical evacuation. In 1910, Capt. George H.R. Gosman, U.S. Army Medical Corps, actually built an aircraft modified to show that casualties could be carried. He submitted a report to the War Department but it was not acted upon. Two years later, the Secretary of War did review another such proposal, but rejected it because he did not feel that aircraft were sufficiently developed for such duty.[6]

During World War I, several countries did experiment with the use of aeroplanes for MEDEVAC. These countries came to the same conclusion as the U.S. Secretary of War: the need was compelling, but the aerocraft were not technologically up to the tasking. The U.S. Army also continued its low-scale developmental efforts. By 1920, four DH-4s were modified to carry two litter patients and a medical attendant. Some were dispatched to duty along the border with Mexico, where U.S. Army troops were keeping a wary eye on developments in Mexico. After several soldiers were so evacuated, an after-action report stated that, "No longer will the luckless recruit ... be jolted for hours in a rough riding automobile over cactus and mesquite, but borne on silvery wings, cushioned by a mile of air, will be conveyed in the twinkling of an eye to the rest and comfort of a modern hospital."[7]

In 1921, the U.S. Army took delivery of a Curtis Eagle airplane that carried four litter and six sitting patients. The aircraft was dispatched to ferry patients from Mitchell Field, New York, to Bolling Field, Washington, DC. Unfortunately, the aircraft was flown too close to a severe electrical storm and crashed, killing all seven on board. This one accident had a chilling effect on any further development of aircraft for aeromedical evacuation before World War II.

However, intellectual efforts continued. One Medical Corps officer, Col. Albert E. Truby, did an inclusive study of airplane ambulance. He predicted that airplane ambulances would be used in the future for the following purposes:

1. Taking doctors to crash sites and bringing the wounded back to hospitals.
2. Transporting patients from isolated stations to large hospitals where they could receive better treatment.
3. Transporting seriously wounded soldiers from the front to hospitals.
4. Transporting medical supplies in emergencies.[8]

Another officer, Lt. Col. G.P. Lawrence, Medical Corps, published an article in the *Military Surgeon* in which he pointed out that any fixed wing aircraft would be limited by the availability of prepared runways. He suggested that the autogiro, a hybrid aircraft with a fuselage-mounted engine for forward thrust but a free rotating or rotor wing for lift, be modified for evacuation duties. It only needed a short runway. They were developed in Europe, and several were imported to the United States in 1928.

Lawrence's article also suggested a tactical plan for incorporating the use of the autogiro in current Army medical regiments. He especially recommended them for medical teams accompanying fast moving tactical formations. Thinking grandly, he also proposed the establishment of an "Ambulance Wing" consisting of 300 officers, 2,300 enlisted troops, and 200 autogiros to directly support a field army. The result would be a vast reduction in evacuation time.

Lawrence wrote, "The patient handled by autogiro would find himself in the general hospital at one jump in approximately half an hour from the time he left the collecting station…" No records indicate that his suggestion was ever acted on or even reviewed.[9]

World War II

When the United States was drawn into World War II, aircraft production was vastly expanded. A variety of aircraft of all sizes was produced and deployed to the far stretches of the globe. Field commanders intuitively used the fixed wing cargo and utility aircraft for medical evacuation. Visionaries, however, had not given up on helicopters. Igor Sikorsky had continued his efforts, as had 300 other companies. All were stimulated by massive increases in military procurement spending and tried to produce a usable helicopter. He led them all when he produced and flew the two-place VS-300, the first successful helicopter to fly in the United States, on 14 September 1939. The United States and Great Britain eventually procured the VS-300, and it served with both of their military forces as the R-4. He considered the unique lifesaving capability of the helicopter as one of its

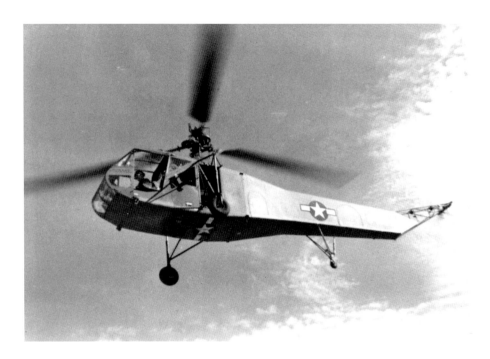

World War II R-4 Helicopter.
Source: Army Medical Department Museum.

most important attributes.[10]

Four of those R-4s deployed with an air commando task force called Project 9 (subsequently renamed the 1st Air Commando Group) to the China–Burma–India Theater in 1943 to support allied forces operating against strong Japanese forces that had attacked into northern Burma. It was co-commanded by Col. John Alison and Col. Philip Cochran. Among their many assigned tasks was the rescue of downed airmen and evacuation of wounded.

Unfortunately, the R-4s did not adapt well to combat. Commanders immediately recognized that they were flimsy and underpowered for the challenges they faced. One was lost en route to the theater when the C-46 carrying it crashed. Another was destroyed when the pilot flew into a power line on a training flight. (This unit ultimately grew into the Air Force Special Operations Command, which now operates worldwide.[11])

As the battles raged in the jungles of Burma, calls for medical evacuation became constant. Fixed wing aircraft from L-1s to C-47s were sent in when airfields could be hacked out of the jungles. They would deliver medical supplies and haul out wounded. This had an immediate and positive effect on troop morale.

"A man could be wounded anywhere in the battle area, and that night, he would be in a hospital in India," wrote Alison in an after-action report. On many occasions, where possible, smaller aircraft would land near the battle lines and bring out the most critical casualties. More than 350 soldiers were saved this way.[12]

On 21 April 1944, one of the Project 9 L-1 light observation aircraft carrying a pilot and three wounded British troops was shot down and crashed in a rice paddy in Burma. The paddy was not adequate for a fixed wing aircraft, but a small, open area was available nearby. The evacuation mission was assigned to 1st Lt. Carter Harmon. "Send the eggbeater…," the alerting message read. Harmon would fly one of the two remaining R-4s to attempt to evacuate those wounded and rescue the pilot. Because of the distances involved, Harmon needed the maintenance personnel to rig an additional fuel barrel onboard so that he would have enough range to get to the downed men and back.

Harmon was concerned that the 175-horsepower engine would not be up to the task. He had to fly over some high terrain. The thinner air at higher altitudes reduced lift capability and occasionally caused the engine to stall in the hover. Too little lift, too little oxygen. He knew that he was pushing his aircraft to its physical limits, but strong Japanese forces were searching for the American pilot and his three British wounded.[13]

To reach the survivors, Harmon leapfrogged through a series of airfields. At one, air commando mechanics removed the fuel barrel and installed a wing tank from a destroyed L-5 observation aircraft. This gave him the capability to overfly his last fuel stop.

While the mechanics were installing the tank, Harmon coordinated a recovery plan with other Project 9 assets. Using a map of the area, they identified a sand bar—which was in a river about 10 miles from the survivors—that was long enough for small L-5 fixed wing aircraft to land and take off. Harmon could only bring out one survivor at a time. He would shuttle all four to the sand bar for transfer, thereby saving a great deal of time.

With the plan set and the new fuel tank installed, Harmon took off. He was led to the crash site by one of the L-5s. As it orbited above, he descended into the landing zone and loaded the first survivor. When all was ready, he pushed the engine to full power and watched the rotor tachometer exceed the "redline." The shuddering aircraft slowly lifted and cleared the trees. Harmon then delivered the wounded soldier to the sandbar and repeated the process a second time. Both survivors were then trans-loaded to L-5s and flown to a main airfield that had a hospital.

When Harmon tried to take off for the third recovery, the engine overheated and had to be shut down. The next morning, the engine was cool enough to start and Harmon recovered the last two persons.[14]

Harmon remained at the forward airstrip for another 11 days and recovered many more soldiers from the jungle. He flew 23 missions before advancing enemy units forced the abandonment of the airfield, and he was ordered to redeploy farther to the rear. The value of the helicopter as a key initial instrument in the evacuation chain had been established. This was tempered with the stark demonstration that the immutable laws of aerodynamic physics defined what helicopters could and could not do.[15]

Other commands heard about Harmon's success. In late June 1945, as U.S. Army forces battled the Japanese Army in the Philippines, helicopters (and fixed-wing aircraft) were used to evacuate wounded soldiers of the 38th Infantry Division, which were engaged in the bitter mountain fighting on Luzon.

The helicopters were a mix of R-4 and newer R-6 aircraft assigned to the 5th and 6th Aviation Repair Units, and they were actually located on U.S. Navy Liberty-Class cargo ships anchored in Manila Bay. After an adequate landing zone was hacked out of the jungle, the helicopters—flown by 1st Lt. James Brown, 1st Lt. Robert Cowgill, 1st Lt. John Noll, 2d Lt. Louis Carle, and 2d Lt. Harold Green—were dispatched and recovered 70 critically wounded personnel, who were then

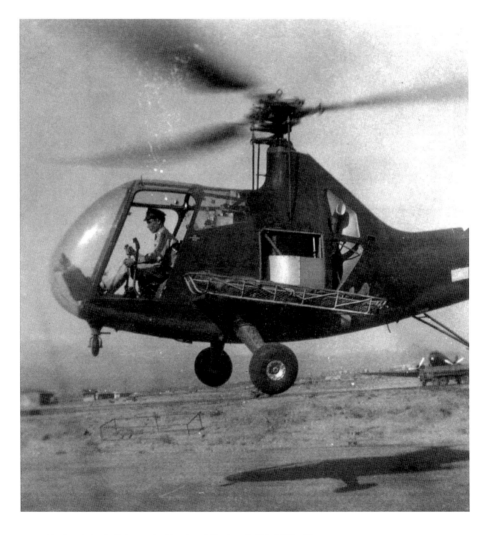

2d Lt. Louis Carle flying an R-6 in the Philippines in World War II.
Source: Dustoff Association.

delivered to hospitals within 30 minutes. Unlike the Harmon recovery, these helicopters encountered sustained enemy resistance, and several were damaged. The effort did demonstrate the efficacy of using helicopters to evacuate larger numbers of wounded troops. The pilots were awarded Air Medals for their efforts.[16]

In his after-action report, the Surgeon from the Air Service Area Command, Maj. E.T. Hauge, recommended that sections of eight helicopters be assigned to each division for aeromedical evacuation. Later, when planning for the possible invasion of Japan, the casualty evacuation plan included the use of helicopters in formed rescue squadrons.[17]

These vignettes were only isolated events. Helicopters were a rarity in this war. Only 385 were produced—mostly in 1944 and 1945—and few made it overseas into the combat zones.[18] Yet their value as critical additions to the evacuation chain was immediately obvious to all who cared to see. Yet the end of the war removed much of the emphasis for their further development and use.

Post–World War II

The Army continued some developmental work with helicopters. However, the major realignment of military forces, which occurred in 1947 and saw the U.S. Air Force created as an independent service, caused great uncertainty about who would perform what tactical missions. The Secretary of Defense, James V. Forrestal, addressed these issues in 1948 at a roles-and-missions meeting held in Key West, Florida. The agreements signed there and implementing instructions called the Joint Army Air Force Adjustment Regulations 5-10-1, which were published in 1949, delineated what tactical missions Army aviation could fly. They were limited to observation, reconnaissance, local messenger and courier service, emergency wire laying, and evacuation. Furthermore, the Air Force also controlled procurement, research and development, and much of the training and maintenance of Army Aviation.[19]

In 1949, a young Maj. Spurgeon Neel, Medical Corps, was serving as the surgeon of the 82d Airborne Division. A few years before, he had seen an old gyrocopter that had been used as a test bed MEDEVAC vehicle. He watched the continued development of the early helicopters and later participated in a test of a Sikorsky H-5 as an evacuation platform.

Afterwards, he stated, "We concluded that it was not only feasible, but it was most desirable that this be pursued." He briefed the results of his test to his division superiors, but nothing was done. However, it generated within him a personal dedication and passion to develop within the Army and perhaps the entire nation a fully developed MEDEVAC capability. He would act on that passion many times throughout his distinguished career. However, Neel's initiative was an isolated event. The real motivator for MEDEVAC would appear in the frozen fields of Korea just a few years hence.[20]

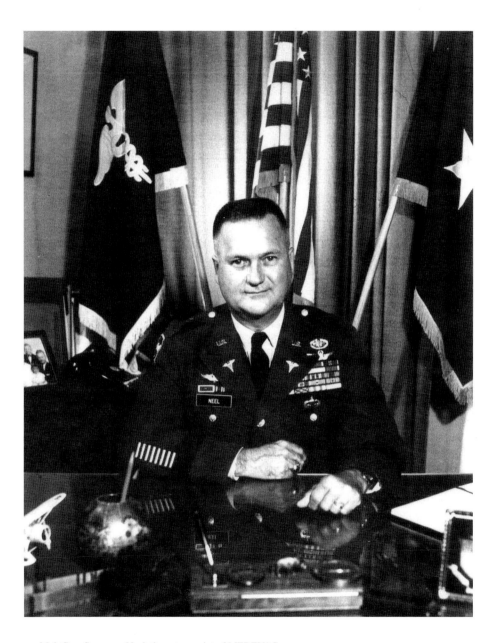

Maj. Gen. Spurgeon Neel, the patron saint of MEDEVAC.
Source: U.S. Army.

The Korean War

On 25 June 1950 the military forces of North Korea attacked South Korea. North Korea was initially opposed by South Korean forces, which could not hold. The South Korean government requested support from the United States and United Nations (UN). The UN responded favorably and requested support from member nations. The United States pledged support, and within days U.S. military units assigned to the U.S. Far East Command, commanded by Gen. Douglas MacArthur, were flowing to the Korean Peninsula. The Army forces were assigned to the Eighth U.S. Army, and U.S. Air Force units were attached to the Far East Air Forces (FEAF).

Almost immediately upon arrival, U.S. forces took casualties. To care for them, the Eighth Army Chief Surgeon, Col. Chauncey E. Dovell, directed the creation and deployment of the 8055th and the 8056th Mobile Army Surgical Hospitals (MASHs) to support the combat units. They quickly deployed from Japan to Korea and were operating by 9 July 1950 behind the 24th Infantry Division and the 1st Cavalry Division.[21]

The terrain of Korea was rugged and forbidding. The primitive road structure had very few prepared surfaces and adequate bridges over the formidable rivers that traversed the country. The combination of these factors made evacuation of the wounded via conventional ground transportation very difficult. The medical doctrine in effect at that time was a holdover from World War II. It defined the basic "chain of evacuation" as "the entire group of successive installations engaged in the collection, transportation, and hospitalization of the sick and wounded."[22]

In response to the North Korean attack, the FEAF deployed several rescue aircraft to the Korean Peninsula on 7 July 1950 including L-5s and C-47s from the 3d Air Rescue Squadron (ARS). They performed search and rescue missions for downed aircrews. By their inherent nature, they could also be used for medical evacuation. However, few usable airfields were available, and after nine days they were flown back to Japan. They were replaced by several Sikorsky H-5 helicopters, which deployed to Taegu airfield, and then moved south to Pusan when U.S. forces were forced back into that enclave. On 5 August 1950 one of the helicopters responded to an emergency call from an Army unit and picked up Pfc. Claude C. Crest, Jr. It was the first recorded MEDEVAC mission of the conflict (actually Casevac since there was no en route medical care).[23]

Dovell was aware of the mission and grateful for the help. He asked the commander of the 3d ARS for a demonstration. An H-5 was flown to Taegu where it landed in a school yard. Dovell's medical technicians examined the aircraft as a medical evacuation vehicle and announced that it was adequate to carry two litters. Dovell had two "patients" loaded in standard litters and climbed aboard. He then had the helicopter take off and land. Impressed with their ability to put it in tight places, he asked for a longer flight. They took off and flew to an evacuation hospital 100 kilometers away. Completely satisfied with the operation, he formally asked the commander of the 5th Air Force, which was subordinate to the

FEAF, for the use of his helicopters for MEDEVAC until the end of 1950.[24]

The Commander of the 8055th MASH, Maj. Isaac Tender, Medical Corps, noted the efficacy of helicopter operations when he wrote the following in the unit history for October 1950: "Helicopters were used to remove patients from the front areas and bring them to the hospital. ... The helicopters proved to be well worth their cost for use in removing patients from the front. ... making a 15 minute air trip which would have been several hours by [ground] ambulance from the front to this hospital."[25]

This expedient was necessary for two reasons: first, the harsh conditions of Korea; second, the Army did not, at that time, have an aviation MEDEVAC (or Casevac) capability, and it would take time to build one. At the beginning of the war, the Army possessed only 56 helicopters, all of which were variants of the H-13 Bell Sioux. None of them was organized into medical units.

Dovell's request for Air Force rescue helicopters to perform MEDEVAC made its way to the Commander of the FEAF, Lt. Gen. George E. Stratemeyer. He endorsed it and sent it to Headquarters, Air Force, in Washington, DC, on 14 August 1950.

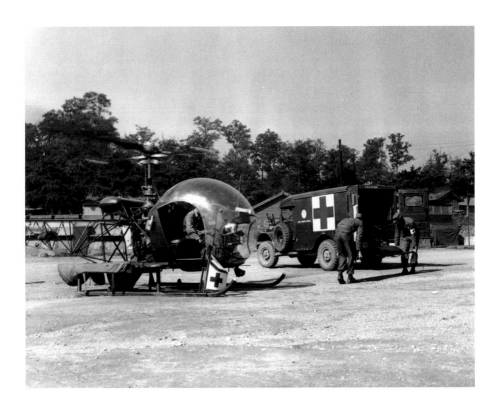

Korea era H-13 Helicopter.
Source: Army Medical Department Museum.

He asked for an "evacuation and utility squadron" of 25 H-5 helicopters and trained medical personnel to perform front line evacuation. This caused some very intense doctrinal discussions on the Air Staff because many analysts thought that the initial evacuation of casualties to front-line aid stations was properly a U.S. Army function. However, the Air Force Surgeon General Maj. Gen. Harry G. Armstrong agreed with the request. He directed to send FEAF 14 more H-5s and to raise the allocation of H-5s for the 3d ARS to 23 helicopters. Yet, the priority mission for the helicopters would remain search and rescue with MEDEVAC a secondary capability, and a specifically designated "evacuation squadron" would not be formed.[26]

Concurrent with this action, Dovell had also forwarded a request through Eighth Army channels for 50 helicopters for MEDEVAC support. MacArthur endorsed it and forwarded it to Army Headquarters in Washington, DC. The request was reviewed and endorsed by the Army Surgeon General, Maj. Gen. Raymond W. Bliss, who had visited Korea and agreed with the need for the MEDEVAC helicopters. Planners began the necessary actions to create several initial helicopter detachments for MEDEVAC duty. The first units and aircraft arrived in Korea in January 1951. Implicit with this action was the understanding that the Army would now have the responsibility for aerial MEDEVAC from front-line aid stations back to the MASHs.[27]

This understanding was formalized in follow-on agreements between the Army and Air Force on 2 October 1951 and 4 November 1952, which made the Army responsible for "battlefield pickup of casualties, their air transport to the initial point of treatment, and any subsequent move to hospital facilities within the combat zone."[28]

However, until the Army detachments arrived, the helicopters from the 3d ARS continued to handle the MEDEVAC calls. To be more responsive, the helicopters and crews sat alert at the MASH locations. Additionally, they carried medical supplies and fresh blood forward when they went for casualties. As of 20 February 1951, Air Force helicopters had MEDEVACed 750 critically wounded soldiers. Dovell estimated that fully half would have died if they had been moved by surface transport. During the conflict, two-thirds of the helicopter missions flown by the U.S. Air Force 3d ARS were for MEDEVAC taskings. U.S. Marine Corps and Navy helicopters also assisted with Casevac, and in one battle in November, retrieved more than 900 wounded from the battle area.[29]

One young Air Force pilot, Capt. Richard Kirkland, documented this service in a personal memoir of his service in Korea with the 3d ARS. Flying the H-5 with a medic onboard, he routinely rotated between duty at one of the MASHs and several forward rescue sites. Kirkland had previously flown fighters in World War II and had watched helplessly as several unit mates had been shot down and not rescued. Initially unhappy with his assignment to helicopters, he realized that the helicopter could serve as a rescue vehicle for airmen. He was surprised, though, at his initial posting to a MASH unit. That changed the next day when he got his first mission and saw the ruggedness of Korea.

"There were roads to most of the battalion aid stations in the combat zone, if you call them roads. But they were extremely rough," Kirkland noted. "And for a critically wounded patient, the rough ride in that vintage of field ambulance was not only agony, but often fatal." He and his fellow rescue pilots also noted, "[We] quickly discovered that enemy gunners used the red crosses on the [vehicles] as targets."[30]

Throughout the autumn of 1950, the Army activated and formed medical helicopter detachments. The 1st and 2d activated on 1 October, followed by the 3d and 4th on 1 November. Each unit was assigned four H-13 helicopters and an equal number of pilots. These pilots were not medical personnel, but were non-branch specific and came from all backgrounds including infantry, armor, transportation, etc. Their assigned mission was to "provide immediate means of evacuating non-transportable and selected critically injured or ill patients needing immediate surgical or medical care not provided by forward medical facilities."[31]

The 2d Helicopter Detachment deployed from Fort Bragg, North Carolina, and arrived at Inchon, Korea, on 22 November 1950. It was attached to the 47th Ordnance Light Aviation Maintenance Company for administration, logistics, and training until 31 December. This "break-in" period allowed the men to adjust to the harsh Korean conditions and train to the mission. It also included a great deal of focused medical training for the pilots provided by medical officers at the MASHs. On 1 January 1951, it was reassigned to the 8085th Army Unit, Eighth Army Flight Detachment, and declared "operational." It became the Army's first aeromedical evacuation unit in combat. It was then attached to the 8055th MASH for missions. Its first call for evacuation came the next day. Two helicopters flown by 1st Lt. Willis Strawn and 1st Lt. Joseph Fowler traveled 120 miles to Wonju, picked up two casualties per aircraft, and brought them to the 8055th.[32]

The next unit to deploy was the 3d Helicopter Detachment. It left Fort Hood, Texas, and arrived in Korea on 2 December 1950. After theater training and orientation, it was attached to the 8076th MASH and assumed alert duties on 25 January 1951. The 4th Helicopter Detachment followed a month later. It formed at Fort Winfield Scott, Presidio of San Francisco, California. After arrival in Korea, it was attached to the 1st MASH, but continuous mechanical problems with its aircraft kept it from operational use. The last unit to deploy was the 1st Helicopter Detachment. It activated at Camp Pickett, Virginia, and arrived in Korea on 21 February 1951. By this point, all units within Eighth Army wanted helicopters, and the 1st Helicopter Detachment's aircraft were stripped away. It never became operational.[33]

The pilots came from all parts of the Army. Capt. Louis Hamner, MSC, was an artillery officer and commanded an aviation detachment with 10 fixed-wing aircraft and 20 officer pilots and observers. Their job was to fly beyond the forward line of troops to collect intelligence and direct artillery. Hamner was surprised when he was notified that he would be reassigned to command the 8193d. It looked like an easy tasking, and the H-13 helicopter seemed like a simple aircraft to fly. Yet he noticed that they lacked radios, internal lights, or even basic instruments for night or weather flying.

Tasking was given to the pilot as a written order or verbally. Hamner's unit remained in the same geographical area, and his pilots became very familiar with its physical features. They hung a situational map in their operations center that was kept up-to-date with both friendly and enemy locations. Settling into the mission, Hamner had only two concerns. First, the troops in the field did not understand the limitations of the helicopter. They always wanted to overload it or expected it to fly at night or in bad weather. They initially did not know how to set up a landing zone both for safety and to expedite the loading and care of casualties. Second, the H-13 was not a very hardy aircraft. It was what they were given, and they made the best of it. With just 11 aircraft flyable at any time on average, they evacuated 1,985 wounded in the first six months of 1951.[34]

On 14 May 1951, by General Order, the Eighth Army changed all of the unit designations. The 1st Helicopter Detachment became the 8190th Army Unit (AU); the 2d became the 8191st AU; the 3d became the 8192d AU; and the 4th became the 8193d AU. The unit designation change was an interim measure. In December 1952, the Army Surgeon General created a Table of Organization and Equipment for a Medical Detachment (Helicopter Ambulance) [Med Det (HA)] that was approved by the Department of the Army. This established these units as medical vice aviation ad hoc units belonging to the Army Medical Service (AMS) and under the administrative and operational control of the Eighth Army Surgeon. Under the new structure, the units were changed:

From	To
8190th AU	37th Med Det (HA)
8191st AU	49th Med Det (HA)
8192d AU	50th Med Det (HA)
8193d AU	52d Med Det (HA)[35]

Two more Med Dets, the 54th and 56th, were activated in Korea in December 1952. Simultaneously, the 53d Med Det (HA) and 57th Med Det (HA) were also activated at Fort Sam Houston, Texas. Instead of Korea, the 53d was slated for Europe, and the 57th remained at Fort Sam Houston. The next September, the 53d deployed to Darmstadt, Germany, where it became operational in February 1954. Also assigned to Europe was the 58th Med Det (HA), which activated at Salzburg, Austria.[36]

In the summer of 1952, now Lt. Col. Spurgeon Neel, a recent graduate of the Army Command and General Staff College at Fort Leavenworth, Kansas, reported for duty as the Chief of the Medical Field Service Branch at the Medical Field Service School located at Brooke Army Medical Center, Fort Sam Houston. He reengaged with his interest in MEDEVAC and did an intense study of MEDEVAC developments in Korea. Based on that review, he developed the basic considerations and doctrine for the helicopter ambulance medical detachment and recommended that they be bunched into companies for better utilization and command and control.

In a prescient article published at the end of that tour, he wrote:

> Speed of evacuation is most important in the severely wounded. Casualties are a 'perishable commodity.' They cannot be stockpiled, but must receive proper treatment as early as possible. A man dies in so many minutes, not over a distance of so many miles. Any measure that will reduce the time lag between wounding and treatment will reduce both the mortality and morbidity of war wounds.[37]

> The precepts established by Neel became the basis for the evolution of MEDEVAC doctrine and the subsequent structure of helicopter ambulance medical detachments and air ambulance medical companies that still exist.[38]

In November 1952, the Office of the Surgeon General in Washington activated an Aviation Section to strengthen medical control over MEDEVAC. It coordinated planning, operations, staffing, and supply of medical helicopter units, and was initially directed by Maj. Leonard Crosby, an MSC officer. He was also directed to develop a plan to train MSC officers as pilots for MEDEVAC duty. Initially, the Army Medical Department considered training medical officers as pilots. The intent was to have a cadre of aviators who understood both medicine and aviation. This was determined to be impractical, and MSC officers were provided the opportunity to volunteer instead. Upon completing pilot training, all were assigned as MEDEVAC pilots. The first seven completed training and earned their pilot wings in April 1953. Initially assigned to the 53d Med Det (HA) at Fort Sam Houston, several were subsequently reassigned to Korea, arriving after the cease-fire. They established the pilot pipeline for MSC pilots to fly MEDEVAC, which still continues.[39]

Throughout the war, the standard Army MEDEVAC helicopter was the H-13. For a short time, the 8192d AU was equipped with Hiller H-23s. They were severely underpowered for the job and replaced with H-13s. Best described as a metallic "grasshopper," with a long, lanky fuselage and large bubble canopy, the H-13 was thrust into MEDEVAC duty for one simple reason: when the need arose, it was the only aircraft available that was capable of doing the mission. Its originally designated mission was observation. Expediency, however, dictated its use for MEDEVAC duties. Yet shortcomings abounded. There was no internal room for patients; they had to be carried on litter rings mounted along each side of the aircraft. This meant that en route medical care could not be provided. Eventually, medics designed a system that allowed for transfusions to be given in-flight. Since the infusion of cold fluids could induce shock, the system was designed so that the tube passed by a hot section of the engine, which then kept the fluids at acceptable temperatures. The troops in the field became experts at practical expediency. The external litters also meant that patients were exposed to the elements. A small metallic forward shield was rigged to protect from the airflow of flight, but it only partly helped. There were a few instances of evacuees freezing to death in flight.[40]

The aircraft were not equipped with any advanced flight instrumentation or gyroscope-based attitude indicators. This limited their capability to fly at night or in weather. Many pilots had to complete missions at night using handheld flashlights to illuminate the instruments. Most pilots developed an intimate knowledge of their assigned areas of operation and used that knowledge to fly "low and slow" below required instrument flight minimums to recover the wounded.

The pilots began to develop a mystique as "intrepid spirits," who—according to the Commander of the 8076th MASH Lt. Col. Kryder Van Buskirk—"saved many lives." One pilot, 1st Lt. William Blake of the 49th Med Det (HA), evacuated 900 casualties in his tour of duty.[41]

After the war, Korea historian, Albert Cowdrey, wrote of them:

> Separated from the crowd, working alone, and pushing their fragile craft ever closer to the enemy, such men came to resemble the pilots of World War I in their singularity and taste for derring-do. Though the helicopter's course still lay from the collecting station to the Mobile Army Surgical Hospital on normal runs, pickups from aid stations became common and some even occurred forward of the battalions. Early on, a marked contrast showed between the rarity and value of the few available machines, which implied great prudence in their use and the spirit of the men who flew them, urged on by the exigencies of war.[42]

The aircraft also did not have any armor protection or self-sealing tanks. Pilots had to be very judicious about where they flew. Almost any enemy ground fire could bring down an aircraft. Perhaps the biggest limitation was the aircraft engine. The 200 horsepower Franklin 0-335-3 piston engine was just not sufficient for the task. It was grossly underpowered for carrying a pilot and up to two casualties across the varied terrain and elevations at which they operated. The engine had a bad habit of shredding fan belts, transmissions, and bearings, as well as fouling spark plugs. Batteries would freeze on cold nights and were brought indoors for protection.[43]

The aircraft had a published maximum speed of 100 mph and a range of 300 miles. Engine fatigue usually limited that to 70 mph and 250 miles. To increase range, some pilots had extra fuel tanks mounted in the cockpit. More common pickup points kept a supply of fuel so that they could refuel more frequently. The aircraft also had limited communications capability. A T-5 series transmitter/receiver was installed, but it only had eight preset frequencies and no in-flight retune capability. As the war progressed, most predesignated casualty pickup points were issued radios and kept them tuned to one of the MEDEVAC identified frequencies. Still, many tactical units in the field who needed MEDEVAC could not tune their radios as necessary for the MEDEVAC aircraft. This forced many pilots to make approaches to locations without final situational updates before landing. In many cases, the pilots were unable to contact aviation command and control or air traffic control agencies that were introduced to better control, coordinate, and de-conflict the movement of aircraft above the battlefield.[44]

However, regardless of the limitations imposed by the aircraft, it was a welcome addition to the medical chain of care for three main reasons. First, it reduced the time necessary to transport a casualty to quality care. Time always runs against critically wounded soldiers, and the helicopter—not constrained by the limitations of ground transport—dramatically reduced that time.

Second, this mode of transport was more comfortable and less traumatic for the patients. One soldier who was grievously wounded in the legs, arms, and stomach was initially moved to the aid station by raincoat, litter, and jeep. It was a miserable travail. He was treated and then picked up by a MEDEVAC helicopter to be transported to a MASH.

His medical report stated that, "The take-off was so gentle he didn't know when it left the ground, and the ride was so soothing he dozed off, and didn't even notice the landing at the [Mobile Army Surgical Hospital]."[45]

Third, the ability of the helicopters to fly in any direction as needed meant that the unit surgeons could direct their most critically wounded to hospitals that had special medical capabilities, facilities, and surgeons.

These positive factors had one major end result. They were a tremendous morale boost to the soldiers doing the fighting because the soldiers knew that if they were wounded, the pilots in the "grasshopper" helicopters would get them and deliver them into a huge medical system that was organized, manned, and equipped to take care of them.[46]

Said one young soldier after he had been MEDEVACed, "When I saw that helicopter land it looked like a mechanical angel coming–it was an answer to a man's prayer."[47]

At the beginning of the conflict, command and control of the MEDEVAC units resided with the Eighth Army Surgeon. With the activation of two corps headquarters (I and IX), he passed that authority to the corps surgeons. All requests for MEDEVAC were forwarded within medical channels through regiment to division to corps. The request had to follow a standard format that included:

- Number of patients and condition;
- Location;
- Landing instructions, to include color of identification smoke;
- Description of site;
- Current tactical situation;
- Number of blankets needed; and
- Amount and type of blood needed in case of in-flight transfusion.

When the corps surgeon approved the request, a mission order was called to the closest helicopter detachment. Because of the limited number of helicopters, the missions were prioritized by the seriousness of the casualties. This task of prioritizing the missions meant that in many cases, the surgeon had to make life-and-death decisions because there were never enough MEDEVAC helicopters to satisfy the demand.

On at least two occasions, divisions asked for their own MEDEVAC helicopters. The 3d Infantry Division sent forward a request that was endorsed by I Corps. Later in the war, the 45th Infantry Division made a similar request, again with Corps endorsement. The Eighth Army Chief Surgeon rejected both requests. He answered that there were not enough helicopters, and the current area support and standby coverage were adequate.[48]

Despite the process being cumbersome, it worked. In one after-action report on MEDEVAC, it "was extremely effective … It was not uncommon for a helicopter to be airborne within eight to ten minutes after a patient reached a medical installation [battalion aid station]. Often, he was on an operating table at a surgical hospital within an hour after he suffered the wound."[49]

In June 1953, all six of the Korea Detachments were again reorganized, this time under the 1st Helicopter Ambulance Company (Provisional). As suggested by Neel, its mission was "to provide adequate tactical, administrative, and logistical support to the helicopter detachment." It was, in turn, assigned to the 30th Medical Group, which was responsible for theater-wide evacuation.

Upon activation, the company commander, Capt. Earl Russell, an artillery officer, conducted a mission analysis. He determined that the detachments were authorized a total of 30 helicopters and 42 pilots. Yet they were assigned only 16 helicopters and 15 pilots. With this level of equipage and manning, he determined that they could perform their primary mission of battlefield evacuation to the surgical hospitals, but not their secondary mission of lateral and rear evacuation. He saw these shortages as acute limitations to mission accomplishment.

Russell also wrote that the policy of assigning combat arms pilots to his helicopter detachments to complete their Korea tours was not working well. Although the intent was to remove them from combat, the pilots realized immediately that picking up wounded from the battlefield was still a continuation of combat. He recommended that only MSC pilots be assigned to the medical detachments.

Russell observed that the H-13—while dependable—was not optimal for medical evacuation. He recommended that the newly produced Sikorsky H-19, with its higher speed, range, and payload be adapted for MEDEVAC duties.[50]

In the last few months of the conflict, the Army shipped two Transportation Companies, the 6th and 13th, each equipped with 20 of the new H-19s, to Korea. These aircraft were much larger than the H-13s; had much improved all-weather flight instrumentation; and, while designed and designated to provide general support such as troop and supply transport, could also perform Casevac, supplementing the MEDEVAC helicopters. On 23 March 1953, several helicopters evacuated an unspecified number of wounded from regimental aid stations and took them directly to a hospital near Seoul.

A month later, H-19s from the 6th recovered 683 sick and wounded UN and Republic of Korea prisoners released by the North Koreans. In July and August, the 13th Transportation Company evacuated a total of 1,547 wounded soldiers as both sides waged local attacks before a cease-fire ended the hostilities.

One after-action report stated, "The greater capacity of the H-19 aircraft make them particularly effective in convoy or mass evacuation."[51]

Just as the cease-fire was taking effect, Neel arrived in Korea to command the 30th Medical Group, the single management headquarters for all nondivisional medical personnel. He had assigned to his group seven surgical hospitals; two evacuation hospitals; several support battalions, companies, and ground evacuation units; and the 1st Helicopter Ambulance Company (Provisional). As the fighting dissipated and casualty flow decreased, he saw the true value of the helicopter as an evacuation tool. He later noted:

I learned that the helicopter is not only a ... good ambulance-type vehicle to move a patient from where he is wounded directly to that hospital which is best situated, equipped, and staffed to take care of his unique condition. But I was most impressed as a manager at the contribution the helicopter makes to the management of overall medical resources: the number of hospitals, the location of the hospitals, the staffing. Instead of trying to put neuropsychiatry in each hospital or neurosurgery, or ophthalmology, or orthopedics, you can have hospital 1 be an orthopedic center, hospital 2 be an eye center, hospital 3 be a chest center. Then you bring the patient to the correct center for whatever his condition is. Now that is predicated on medical control. ... if the surgeon has control of the helicopters, the same guy who has control of the hospitals, then we can use a systems approach.[52]

Two years later, Neel authored a detailed lessons learned for MEDEVAC operations in Korea. In it he made several overarching points:

1. **Organization.** Helicopter evacuation within the combat zone is the responsibility of the AMS. The company-sized unit is superior to small cellular elements. It should remain under the command of the field army or a centralized medical command should one be available. The inherent speed, range, and flexibility of ambulance helicopters dictate against their assignment to subordinate commands.

2. **Control.** Integration of the evacuation and treatment components of the field army's medical service is essential. Helicopter evacuation units should remain assigned to field army or an appropriate central command headquarters. The dispatch of individual helicopter sorties should be the responsibility and function of the corps surgeon who is at a sufficiently high level to determine realistic priorities, yet close enough to the action to keep abreast of the immediate situation. Only AMS agencies should accept evacuation requests. Command surgeons alone know the status of medical treatment facilities, such as surgical lags, location of special treatment teams, and projected displacements of medical installations.

3. **Communication.** No separate communications net is required to control helicopter evacuation. Airborne radio sets should be netted with appropriate Air Force agencies and fire support coordinating centers to provide control of aircraft in flight.

4. **Personnel.** Helicopter pilots, particularly those flying reconnaissance type helicopters engaged in battlefield pickups, should be officers of the MSC. They must possess sufficient medical training and experience to make sudden decisions regarding the destination of patients. MSC pilots should receive greater consideration in the development of career patterns. Greater emphasis should be placed on integrating Medical Service pilots into the overall effort of the AMS.

5. **Aircraft.** Aircraft such as the H-13 allow for recovery from restricted places, and their external mount for casualties provides for quicker loading and unloading. Larger helicopters with internal load capability are also needed. A mix is best. We do not need to provide for enough medical evacuation helicopters to handle all contingencies. When necessary, hospital empty out

for unit movement, mass casualty situations, or supplemental evacuation support can be provided from the Transportation Corps, or another agency. The H-13 needs better flight instrumentation and navigational gear, but not if it will reduce available cargo load capability.[53]

By the end of hostilities on 27 July 1953, the role of the helicopter as a key part of the evacuation chain and continuum of care had been well established. Ill-equipped for the mission, and initially ad hoc in organization, the men and machines of MEDEVAC overcame harsh terrain, primitive conditions, and a brutal enemy to evacuate almost 18,000 casualties. Air Force rescue helicopters also picked up another 8,373 U.S. and UN personnel.[54]

But was it aviation or medicine? As Col. Allen Smith, U.S. Air Force Medical Corps, a medical historian wrote in a postmortem:

> Present military thinking still includes a large segment which considers the sick and wounded as so much impedimenta which must be moved at a certain cost per ton mile to maintain military efficiency. Another quite different kind of thinking, particularly among medical circles, would provide the quickest and best possible medical care. Both viewpoints have validity, but only if both are considered together. The real answer lies not so much in the compromise wherein both viewpoints relinquish certain claims, but in each viewpoint gaining from the other certain additional principles which result from the tremendous advances in transport equipment and techniques and in medical care.[55]

The biggest contribution of the MEDEVAC helicopters was to reduce the time between when a soldier was injured and received care. Maj. Gen. Lawrence Keiser, commander of the 2d Infantry Division, wrote in an after-action report, "The injuries to the majority of these [unit] patients were so severe that it is doubtful if they would have survived evacuation by field ambulances."[56]

Additionally, it is impossible to calculate the number of men saved by the timely delivery of medical supplies or fresh blood delivered by the MEDEVAC helicopters. Overall, the mortality rate for those who died after reaching medical facilities was 2.4%, as opposed to 4.5% in World War II. The MEDEVAC helicopter was undoubtedly a major contributor to that reduction.[57]

Albert Cowdrey, a historian of the war, offered perhaps the best critique of MEDEVAC in Korea when he wrote:

> Costly, experimental, and cranky, the helicopter could be justified only on the grounds that those it carried, almost to a man, would have died without it.... A specialized vehicle of high cost and limited effectiveness, the MEDEVAC chopper won its fame as an evacuation vehicle under conditions that were unique to the Korean War. As a wealthy nation that admired technical innovation and placed a high value on individual life, the United States was well fitted to finance such a pioneering effort. Preexisting medical skills of a high order were necessary to make the trial a success, for only a medical service of great sophistication could have dealt competently with the massive and near fatal injuries that were the helicopter's specialty. The endeavor was not militarily significant, but it boosted morale by demonstrating that, against all purely material considerations, the nation intended to save every possible life. The typically high-cost, low-yield experimental period during the Korean War proved the potential of a vehicle whose future impact on all emergency medicine, both military and civilian, would be great indeed.[58]

The experiences of Korea clearly showed the efficacy of helicopter MEDEVAC and established its place in the chain of evacuation and continuum of care. The spirit of MEDEVAC created in that conflict became the standard. The tactics and techniques established are continuously refined on the battlefields of future conflicts.

Chapter Two

From Korea Through Vietnam

> *"Getting the casualty and the physician together as soon as possible is the keystone of the practice of combat medicine. The helicopter achieved that goal as never before..."*
>
> Col. Spurgeon Neel[1]

A s the United States disengaged from the Korean conflict, the lessons learned from the effort were collected and digested. The Aviation Section in the Surgeon General's office worked tirelessly in the early postwar years to protect the creation of the MEDEVAC force and turn those lessons learned into corrective actions. The need for centralized control of MEDEVAC assets was an accepted fact. Follow-on discussions determined that although the H-13 was unacceptable as a long-term MEDEVAC aircraft, it was not necessary to design and purchase a specific specialized aircraft just for MEDEVAC. The smarter path was to ensure that all future aircraft would be capable of patient transport. Such fleet commonality would lead to reduced training, supply, and maintenance costs, and ultimately an overall better use of resources.[2]

More units were also formed. In early 1954, the 56th Medical Detachment (Helicopter Ambulance) (Med Det [HA]) was moved to Camp Zama, Japan, to transport soldiers evacuated from airfields in Korea to area hospitals. The 274th Med Det (HA) was activated at Fort Sam Houston, Texas, and when trained and equipped was transferred to Vainingen, Germany, later that year. The new 63d Med Det (HA) replaced it at Fort Sam Houston. Additionally, in Germany another unit, the 47th Med Det (HA), was activated at Bremerhaven to serve the large U.S. community in that area.[3]

At about the same time, the Army launched a design competition for a new utility and MEDEVAC helicopter. By now, Lt. Col. Spurgeon Neel had returned from Korea and was assigned to the Army Surgeon General's Office in the Pentagon to establish the aviation medicine branch. When he discovered that a new helicopter was being proposed for MEDEVAC duties, he wrote, "The AMS [Army Medical

Service], which is the only agency in the Army with any real valid experience in air or surface evacuation, should participate in the development of aircraft as well as logistical support policies and procedures." Neel was assigned to lead the assessment team.[4]

Under Neel's leadership, he and several Medical Service Corps (MSC) officers in the Aviation Section became intimately involved in Army efforts to conceptualize, design, and procure a new fleet of helicopters. Working with engineers, transportation specialists, and communicators, they insisted that the aircraft have a cabin with enough space for a medic to provide onboard care, thus making it truly MEDEVAC by today's definition. Post–Korea studies showed that patients who could most benefit from the speed and versatility that helicopters provided also required en route patient care and emergency intervention at the same time. One report stated, "If they needed to go by air, they also needed to be treated en route or else they had little chance of survival."[5]

Neel and his team reviewed 12 proposals from six different manufacturers. In their design plans, all gave first priority to MEDEVAC use. Their efforts were so sustained and persistent that the new helicopter was unofficially called a helicopter ambulance. Later, when the Army had to go before Congress to procure the funds for production of the selected helicopter, Neel was consulted to script briefing papers to explain the medical necessity of the selection as a MEDEVAC vehicle. He liked to remind them that the MEDEVAC helicopter was "…an obstacle crosser, whether it is enemy territory, or traffic in San Antonio, or the Rhine River."[6]

In 1955, several units were pulled out of Korea. The 37th was sent to Fort Benning, Georgia. The 52d was moved to Japan and shared duties with the 56th until that unit was transferred to Fort Bragg, North Carolina, in early 1956. It then converted to H-19 helicopters. The 52d inactivated within a year. The units remaining in Korea still had missions to fly. In February 1957 an Air Force C-124 was forced to ditch at night in the Han River, north of Seoul. Two crews from the 54th Med Det, led by 1st Lt. Charles Heath and 1st Lt. Hugh Beebe, headed up a force, ultimately consisting of 26 Army and Air Force helicopters, which recovered all 137 passengers and crew from the frigid waters of the river.[7]

Again in 1955, another unit, the 82d Med Det (HA), was activated at Fort Sam Houston. It replaced the 63d that was subsequently transferred to Landstuhl, Germany. Located just down the ramp from the 57th, the 82d immediately struck up a strong rivalry with the older unit. At the end of the year, the 58th—still in Austria—was inactivated and its personnel and aircraft dispersed to other units in Europe.[8]

The new helicopter competition was intense, and Neel and his assistants were in the midst of it. The contract ultimately went to the Bell Helicopter Corporation for its XH-40 in February 1955. Designated the HU-1 "Iroquois" in 1957, it garnered the nickname "Huey." It was redesignated the UH-1 (utility helicopter) in 1962, but the nickname remains. By 1962, 158 UH-1As had been built under a general Army contract. All were initially equipped with the Lycoming T53-L-1A turbine engine that produced 800 horsepower. The UH-1's designed useful load lift capability was 2,000 lbs, and it had a predicted range of 115 miles at a cruise speed of 140 mph. It would be the new MEDEVAC helicopter.[9]

During this time, the various units were relatively stable. Most active was the 57th at Fort Sam Houston. Equipped with H-19 helicopters, it supported several Texas communities during heavy flooding. In late 1957 the unit moved to Fort Meade, Maryland.

One year later, the 52d Med Det (HA) reactivated in Germany. The 37th Med Det (HA) moved from Fort Benning to Fort Ord, California, in June 1959. A short while later, it was redesignated as the 47th Medical Platoon (AA) [Air Ambulance], but completely inactivated in 1961.[10]

In 1959 the U.S. Army Reserve (USAR) formed its first MEDEVAC unit when it activated the 317th Medical Company (Med Co) (AA), at Miami, Florida, with its platoons located at Orlando and Tampa, and Atlanta, Georgia. It was equipped with old H-13s. Another active duty unit, the 21st Medical Platoon (AA), was formed with six H-19s at Fort Benning.[11]

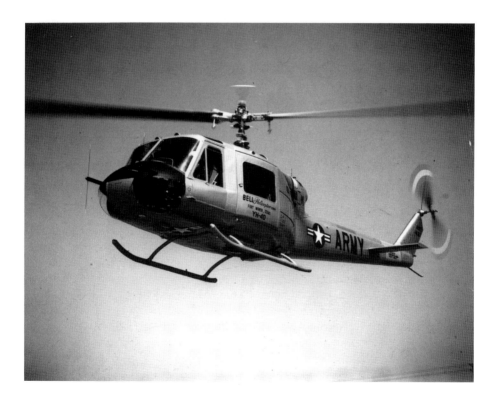

The first YH-40 prototype.
Source: Army Medical Department Museum.

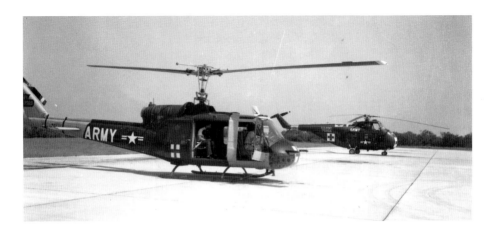

A new UH-1A and old H-19 helicopter in the early 1960s.
Source: Army Medical Department Museum.

This same year, a future MEDEVAC pilot, Doug Moore, graduated from Arkansas State University as a Distinguished Military Graduate of the Reserve Officers' Training Corps and commissioned as a Regular Army 2d Lt. in the MSC. While at Fort Sam Houston for the branch basic course, he requested flight training. However, the tactical units in Germany needed young officers, and he was assigned to the 34th Medical Battalion there. During his tour he commanded the 95th Med Co, which gave him a strong basis of knowledge about Army medicine. Subsequently, he was accepted for flight training and was ordered to report to flight school in 1963.[12]

The 57th Med Det (HA) was reequipped in early 1960 with five new UH-1 helicopters while still maintaining its H-19s. The 56th was also given UH-1s. In May both units were deployed to Chile to provide emergency relief after a series of devastating earthquakes and tsunamis rocked that nation. While the 56th and 57th were in Chile, all medical detachments (HA) were redesignated as platoons (AA). When the two units returned to their home bases, both the 56th and 57th Medical Platoons (AA) were awarded the William J. Kossler Award for 1961 by the American Helicopter Society "for participation in the rescue operations in the earthquake-stricken region of Southern Chile in May and June of 1960." Respective platoon commanders, Capt. Donald Wall and Capt. John Temperilli, accepted the award at the society's annual awards banquet.[13]

A few months later, all medical platoons were again redesignated as medical detachments with a specific identifier (RA) assigned if the unit had been converted to the new UH-1 helicopter. Additionally, when the 56th Medical Platoon (AA) returned from Chile, it was ordered to inactivate. The 45th Med Co (AA) was being formed at Fort Benning and absorbed the 56th personnel and aircraft as well as those of the 21st Medical Platoon (AA).[14]

In 1958 and 1959, the Army Medical Service (AMS) conducted a full review and study of aeromedical evacuation focusing on doctrine, organization, and equipment. Its Combat Development Group was tasked to perform the following:

1. Review and evaluate current doctrine, procedures, and techniques for aeromedical support of joint and service operations.
2. Collect and evaluate experience data relative to current doctrinal, organizational, and operational concepts of aeromedical support.
3. Develop additional or new doctrine, techniques, and procedures for aeromedical support during the time frame 1960–65.
4. Develop future qualitative and quantitative army aeromedical evacuation requirements by type, for the time frame 1960–1965.[15]

Several factors affected the problem:

1. The movement of patients by air to the rear of the combat zone is the primary means of evacuation for all of the military services. Surface transportation is used to supplement aerial movement.
2. Interservice responsibilities for aeromedical evacuation within the army combat zone are prescribed by Department of Defense Directives and include battlefield pickup of casualties, air transport to initial point of treatment, and subsequent moves to hospital facilities within the army combat zone.
3. The feasibility of aeromedical evacuation has been demonstrated clearly during the Korean conflict and confirmed by numerous postwar exercises.
4. To the extent possible, all army aircraft are being developed with the capability of transporting sick and injured as an ancillary mission. (The report noted, as an assumption, that the Bell HU-1A helicopter was scheduled for the medical air ambulance units.)
5. Medical helicopter ambulance detachments are currently organized as per Table of Organization and Equipment (TO&E) 8-500C, dated 30 July 1956, and 2.33 detachments are allocated per corps. They are authorized five helicopters with seven MSC aviators, dually qualified as rotary wing pilots and medical assistants, and 22 enlisted personnel who perform administrative, maintenance, and medical functions. All aircraft are marked with the Geneva Convention Red Crosses and are also used for the emergency resupply of critical medical items such as whole blood.
6. A new TO&E, 8-137D, is being staffed. It will designate a medical AA Company equipped with 25 helicopters and an allocation of one per corps. The company can be divided into platoons. Within a theater, it will be under the operational control of the army surgeon. With this structure, the earlier mentioned detachments could be used for augmentation or to support independent task forces of division size or smaller.[16]

The long and detailed report included 15 conclusions that recognized five main points:

1. Warfare of the future will see the increased use of organic army aviation for emergency and routine aeromedical evacuation.
2. The AMS has the basic technical responsibility for all medical evacuation and timeliness of treatment. The medical service must retain control over all evacuation. This is better than control by nonmedical aviation units that—although it may provide for better aviation economy—places the welfare of the patient secondary to other logistical or administrative considerations; reduces medical control over the movement of the patients; precludes the most effective utilization of critical medical means, doctors, and facilities; and does not provide for the movement and exchange of required and consumable medical supplies and equipment.
3. Medical ambulance aircraft should be special purpose in the sense that they will not be used for any other purpose. They should be manned with medical pilots and crewmembers.
4. The company type organization is superior to the current cellular detachment concept.
5. Medical air evacuation companies should be assigned to a field army or independent corps force. The rotary wing units should be further attached to major medical command headquarters to facilitate decentralized operations and integration with surface evacuation and other medical service support functions.[17]

These points were consolidated into six recommendations:

1. The conclusions should be the basis for the development of army aeromedical evacuation techniques, concepts, procedures, and types of organizations.
2. The AMS should retain the mission and capability of rapid aerial evacuation of severely wounded casualties directly to medical treatment facilities, properly staffed, equipped, and situated for their care.
3. Nonmedical army aviation units should maintain a capability of aeromedical evacuation of routine patients, when required and upon the request of the AMS.
4. The AMS should maintain mission control over all aeromedical evacuation.
5. The AMS should be provided sufficient aircraft for the aerial evacuation of all patients within the combat zone.
6. Organic medical aviation should be reorganized into company type units for the 1960–65 time frame.[18]

On 11 January 1960, The Surgeon General approved the study as the "latest approved organizational and operational concepts of the Surgeon General for the 1960–1965 time frame."[19]

Doctrine

Field Manual 8-55, Army Medical Planning Guide, October 1960

Army doctrine was the basis for all Army operations and organizations. All medical doctrine was encapsulated in Field Manual (FM) 8 series documents. Based on the AMS study, FM 8-55, *Army Medical Service Planning Guide* was rewritten to reflect the increasing use of helicopters. It directed the actual flow of casualties and patients. Efforts would be focused on the movement of those who most needed immediate care, and ground vehicles would be used for those patients considered more transportable. No casualty would be evacuated farther to the rear than necessary to handle his or her medical condition, with the priority being placed on returning those still combat capable to their units as soon as possible. All helicopter MEDEVAC units would be reorganized as necessary, under the new detachment and company TO&Es.[20]

Army National Guard MEDEVAC Units

At about the same time the Department of the Army decided to spread the MEDEVAC mission into the Army National Guard (ARNG). In May 1959 the 123d Med Co (AA), Mississippi ARNG, was formed from a unit that had—at various times—been an armor, aviation, and cavalry unit. Unit lineages belonged to the individual National Guards (there are actually 54 different National Guards), and such combinations were not unusual. The next conversion created the 24th Med Co (AA), Nebraska ARNG, which formed in February 1960. Both units were initially equipped with a mixed fleet of older H-13, H-23, and H-19 helicopters, and small, fixed wing aircraft. Many of the pilots were veterans of service in World War II and Korea. Two months after forming, the 24th flew relief missions under state tasking when spring floods ravaged the eastern portion of the state.[21]

The Berlin Crisis

As 1961 began the MEDEVAC force was still in a state of growth and realignment because of planned relocations and real world events. The 45th Med Co (AA), then commanded by Maj. Rex Medcalf, was moved from Fort Bragg to Germany. Its four platoons were spread out to dispersed locations. Additionally, the 421st Med Co (AA) was also formed in Germany and absorbed the assets and personnel of the 47th, 52d, 53d, and 274th Med Dets. Concurrently, the 15th Med Det (HA) was activated, also in Germany.[22]

In that summer tensions between the United States and its European allies and the Soviet Union and its allies escalated significantly over access to Berlin. East Germany was concerned about the flow of refugees out of its country into the

West. On 13 August 1961, East Germany began to erect a wall along its border and restrict access to Berlin. In response, President John F. Kennedy took strong diplomatic steps supported by firm military measures to protect the right of the Western Allies to freely travel to and from Berlin. He called to active duty almost 150,000 Reservists and Guardsmen—both as members of 113 units and also as individual augmentees—and dispatched reinforcing forces to Europe. The 24th and 123d Med Cos (AA) from the ARNG and the 317th Med Co (AA) from the USAR were activated and reported to their mobilization stations. The 24th reported to Fort Leonard Wood, Missouri, and was equipped with two H-23s and eight H-19s. They performed base support and responded to several local rescue calls as they awaited deployment orders. However, before they or the other mobilized units could be deployed, the crisis was resolved through diplomacy, and all units were released in early 1962.[23]

The Vietnam Era

Europe was not the only area where confrontation was brewing. At the same time, President Kennedy also took the initial steps that led to the U.S.'s lengthy and divisive involvement in the Vietnam War. Long a colony of France, Vietnam had been granted its independence in 1954 after a bloody guerilla war. Two Vietnams were formed. Communist forces controlled North Vietnam, and a western leaning government formed in South Vietnam. However, a residual insurgency in the South turned against the government and attempted to overthrow it. A few American military advisors were dispatched to work with the military forces of the South.

In May 1961, President Kennedy publicly reaffirmed U.S. support for the South Vietnamese government. Over the next few months, the communist guerillas known as the Viet Cong—or VC as they came to be called—launched major attacks against South Vietnamese units. These successes showed that the military forces of South Vietnam were not capable of defending the nation. The President queried his top military advisors who recommended dispatching U.S. combat troops. He was not prepared to do that and instead sent more military advisors to train the Army of the Republic of Vietnam (ARVN) and the South Vietnamese Air Force (VNAF). However, he did send some combat support units to assist the effort.

First MEDEVAC Unit to Vietnam

By December, transport helicopter units and aircraft for the VNAF began to arrive. The next year, the flow of support troops and advisors reached 8,000. They worked directly with the ARVN and VNAF units who sought out the enemy forces. The increased fighting led to an increase in casualties, and Army medical units were designated for deployment. The 8th Field Hospital went first, with several specialty detachments in support. To provide MEDEVAC, the 57th Med Det (HA) would deploy.

Stationed at Fort Meade, the unit was commanded by Capt. John Temperilli, Jr. He and his officers and noncommissioned officers scrambled to prepare their five UH-1 helicopters and unit personnel for the assignment. They deployed in April 1962 and arrived in Nha Trang, a beautiful coastal port town, where they set up next to the 8th Field Hospital. The 57th was assigned to the U.S. Army Support Group, Vietnam (USASGV), which controlled all U.S. Army units in the country and was directly responsible for their administrative and logistical provision. Lacking any support assets, the 57th relied on a collocated aviation unit for its direct logistical support, as well as specialized aviation weather information and flight clearance filing capabilities.[24]

Additionally, planners at the USASGV intended to disperse their aircraft and pilots in single helicopter detachments throughout the country, which was divided into four Corps (I through IV) areas from north to south. Temperilli interceded to prevent this, as well as ensured that the JP-4 fuel that his turbine-powered aircraft burned was available in enough locations for his helicopters to operate. He also asked to have his unit moved to the Saigon area, which was 300 kilometers to the

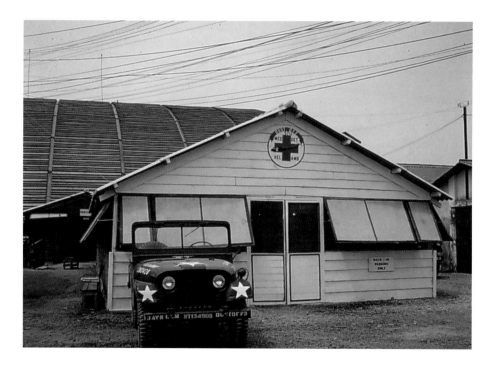

The 57th Med Det (RA) operations building in 1965.
Source: Jim Truscott.

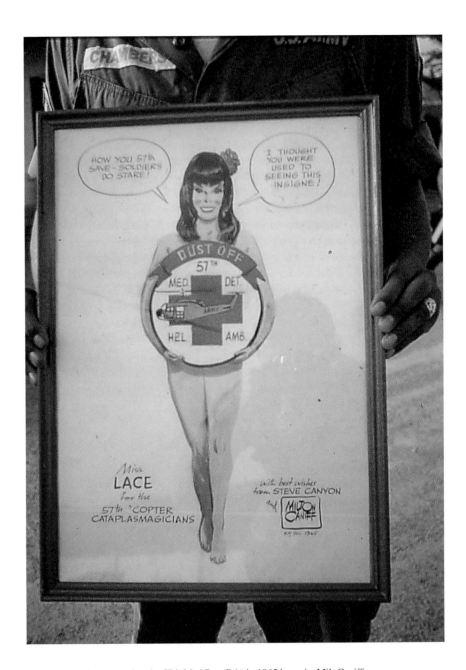

Cartoon portrait presented to the 57th Med Det (RA) in 1965 by artist Milt Caniff.
Source: Jim Truscott.

southwest. Most of the fighting occurred south and west of there, and he wanted to be as responsive as possible. But his request to move was denied. The Saigon area was overrun with units, and there was just no room for the 57th. Temperilli also asked the USASGV staff for a defining mission statement for his detachment. He was promised that one would be developed.[25]

The UH-1s with the 57th were the first of their type in the theater. The aircraft were adorned with the red medical cross on a white background as directed by the Geneva Conventions and U.S. Army directives. Some of the pilots questioned the value of the crosses, citing Intelligence reports that quoted the Viet Cong instructing their fighters that "It is good to fire at ... the red crosses if [a helicopter] is picking up wounded."[26]

The first mission call for the 57th came on 12 May 1962 from Tuy Hoa, another seaside post, about 60 kilometers up the coast, to pick up a Special Forces advisor with a dangerously high fever. He was brought back to the 8th Field Hospital. Soon they were getting regular calls for pickups.[27]

The technical manual for the UH-1 aircraft specified that even though there were positions for two pilots, only one pilot was required to perform the mission, as had been the case with the H-13s in Korea. However, the 57th had more pilots than aircraft and requested a waiver to always fly two pilots. Their request was refused. They believed that the risks of pilot incapacitation by enemy fire outweighed the manual recommendation, and they usually flew with two pilots. Later arriving units would do the same, and eventually the rule changed to allow two pilots aboard at all times. It was overt recognition of the danger of combat MEDEVAC.[28]

Unit Realignments and Activations

While the war in Vietnam was slowly growing, Army MEDEVAC units were being realigned in other areas. In Korea, the personnel and aircraft of the 49th, 50th, and 54th Med Dets (HA) were consolidated into the 377th Med Co (AA) in August 1962. A few months later, the 50th Med Det (RA) was reconstituted at Fort Polk, Louisiana, and the 54th was reconstituted at Fort Benning.[29]

Vietnam Buildup

As the war in Vietnam progressed, the threat only increased. Eventually, the aircraft were upgraded with more armor plating and even body armor to protect the crewmembers.

As U.S. Army Lt. Col. (ret) John Cook later wrote, "The enemy had been quick to learn that the pilots were nothing more than sitting ducks until the patients were loaded. These were lessons that could only be learned in the harsh environment of combat."[30]

The MEDEVAC crew included a crew chief who performed routine maintenance on the aircraft and oversaw the repair of larger discrepancies. He was joined in the back of the aircraft by the medic, a medical technician who actually tended to the casualties. He ensured that essential medical supplies were onboard and provided care for the patients en route back to the hospitals. Most medics also "trained" the crew chief to perform certain basic medical functions, which greatly benefited them when they were carrying more than one casualty or the medic himself was wounded. The medic was the "med" in MEDEVAC.[31]

Noting the necessity of close coordination between the crewmembers, Cook later wrote, "The secret was teamwork. All the good crews had one thing in common – they worked smoothly and efficiently, like four well-oiled parts of a complex machine. The helicopter became an extension of the crews..."[32]

Being the first UH-1 equipped unit in Vietnam also presented unique logistical challenges because the pipeline of replacement parts and supplies was very long. The situation improved somewhat as the U.S. buildup continued, and other UH-1s were shipped in. Then the other units competed with the 57th for the limited parts and supplies available. At one point when a large operation was planned south of Saigon, Temperilli was ordered to ground his aircraft by removing the starter generators and deliver them to other units for the operation. His unit could not fly for a month and only got one of their generators back.

At the same time, the Commander of the USASGV Brig. Gen. Joseph Stilwell considered transferring the 57th from the Medical Service to the Transportation Corps element in Vietnam, which then commanded all Army aviation units in the country. His deputy commander was Col. John Klingenhagen, a career aviator. He managed all aviation units and advised Stilwell that the MEDEVAC helicopters were underutilized as compared to his general service aircraft. Accordingly, he recommended that to spread the utilization rate more evenly the MEDEVAC unit should be combined with the general aviation units. His philosophy was that "aeromedical evacuation is an aviation operation which entails the movement of patients."[33]

This would have violated the hard-learned lessons of Korea, revalidated by the AMS Combat Development Group Study. Temperilli, accompanied by Lt. Col. Carl Fischer, the USASGV Surgeon and commander of the 8th Field Hospital, visited Stilwell and argued that aeromedical evacuation was "a medical operation which entails the use of aircraft." They convinced him to not carry out the reassignment. This was not the last time that this debate would occur.[34]

In January 1963, to better support the increasingly heavy fighting occurring south of Saigon, the 57th was finally moved to Tan Son Nhut Air Base in Saigon. The next month, Temperilli passed command of the 57th to Maj. Lloyd Spencer, and Temperilli and his experienced troops rotated home. As they were leaving, Spencer had his welcoming visit with Stilwell. The unit still had only one aircraft flyable. Stilwell told him that brand new UH-1Bs would arrive soon, and the 57th would get the first five. These aircraft had an upgraded 1,100 horsepower engine that gave it greater lift and climb capability as well as higher speed. It also had a larger cabin and reflected many lessons already learned in this war. By March, the 57th was fully operational again with the new aircraft, and very soon had aircraft on alert in Saigon and upcountry at Qui Nhon and Pleiku.[35]

In August 1963 Headquarters, U.S. Army Vietnam published a mission statement for the 57th Med Det (HA). It expanded on the definition of priority of casualties as urgent, priority, and routine, and had additional rules for personnel based on nationality and civilian–military status. Strict rules dictated the use of MEDEVAC aircraft for nonmedical, administrative, or logistical purposes. It defined a formal format and procedure for a ground commander to request a MEDEVAC. This mission statement was subsequently updated several times throughout the war and applied to subsequent MEDEVAC units as they arrived. However, it was never sufficient to handle the myriad situations that would arise for the MEDEVAC crews.[36]

Sensing an increased need for MEDEVAC capability, the Army created several more units. The 159th Med Det (RA) formed at Fort Riley, Kansas, with five old H-21 helicopters. At Fort Carson, Colorado, the 254th Med Det (RA) formed, and the 283d Med Det (RA) formed at Fort Lewis, Washington.[37]

In Vietnam taskings began to increase. Neither the ARVN nor VNAF had yet developed any MEDEVAC capability. Their MEDEVAC requests were handled by regular aviation units on an "as-available" basis. They began to call the 57th. Spencer sent his crews. On 10 September 1963, they MEDEVACed 197 wounded Vietnamese after VC units destroyed three villages in the Delta region south of Saigon.

Inadvertently, Spencer also established a small but important part of MEDEVAC history. He selected a standard radio call sign for his aircraft—"Dustoff"— after reviewing a list of precoordinated choices. The UH-1 aircraft were known for kicking up quite a bit of dust when they landed or took off, so he grabbed the call sign. It was a natural fit and became the general call sign for their aircraft, although there were some specific exceptions, that is, some aircraft still used the call sign of "MEDEVAC" to honor their heritage from Korea.[38]

In early 1964, Maj. Charles Kelly replaced Spencer. Within days of his arrival, Kelly was ordered to move his aircraft from Qui Nhon and Pleiku back to Saigon and set up a detachment at Soc Trang in the middle of the Delta. Aviation battalions at each location supported the unit. More than 16,000 Americans were involved in the war, and MEDEVAC missions mounted steadily. His crews were increasingly called to fly at night. Based on the lessons learned in Korea, the aircraft were fully capable of doing so.

The USASGV again queried Kelly about removing the red crosses on his aircraft and utilizing the machines for general support missions. He fended off this second attempt to turn his detachment into a utility unit and arranged for the USASGV Surgeon to provide medical supervision to the 57th. He realized that he and his men had to prove the value of aerial MEDEVAC beyond all doubt, and he sent his crews out to look for business. He scheduled single-ship night runs that flew over remote outposts and called them to offer MEDEVAC. The recovery numbers increased, and Stilwell dropped the idea of removing the crosses.[39]

The enemy did not respect the red crosses. Kelly discovered that several times when he listened to the rounds hit the aircraft. Despite the enemy fire, weather, or terrain, if there were casualties to be brought out, he flew. That was his credo. He drilled it into his men and led by example. That dedication cost him his life.

On 1 July 1964, he was on alert duty when an emergency call came in from an ARVN unit near Vinh Long in the Delta region. Kelly and his crew flew to the area. The battle was still raging as Kelly flew low and slow over it to spot the wounded. One advisor called him on the FM radio and told him to leave the area because it was just too dangerous.

"When I have your wounded," Kelly answered firmly. Moments later, a fusillade of rounds hit the aircraft. One of them passed through the side door and struck Kelly cleanly in the heart. "My God," he whispered and then died. The aircraft rolled to the right and crashed.[40]

The rest of the crew survived uninjured and crawled from the wreckage, dragging his body along. They were eventually rescued by another Dustoff. When Stilwell heard of Kelly's death, he wept.

Kelly was awarded the Distinguished Service Cross for his efforts. From that act he received larger recognition. His words and indomitable courage and determination represent the spirit of Dustoff. Capt. Paul Bloomquist assumed command of the 57th.

The Buildup Continued

Back in the United States, the Army published orders to activate another MEDEVAC unit. An entire company, the 498th, formed at Fort Sam Houston that was equipped with 25 UH-1D helicopters and commanded by Lt. Col. Joseph Madrano. Four times larger than a standard medical detachment, it was designed to support an entire corps. Personnel and equipment began arriving in the fall, and by early 1965, the unit was fully formed and ready for any required deployment.[41]

Trouble in the Dominican Republic

While these events occurred in the United States and Vietnam, American attention was diverted for a short period by events closer to home. In the early spring of 1964, long simmering civil unrest in the Dominican Republic, just 500 miles southeast of Miami, Florida, exploded into open warfare between leftist rebels and an interim government installed when a long-term dictator had been assassinated four years earlier. Initially, President Lyndon Johnson ordered U.S. Marines ashore to establish order and protect American citizens and interests. They were joined a few weeks later by a brigade of troops from the 82d Airborne Division. The brigade team was supported with a robust medical task force that included the 54th Med Det (HA).

Security operations were brief and limited, and order was quickly established. As evacuation operations were conducted for all who wanted to leave, the MEDEVAC helicopters supported civic action projects as the medical teams moved out to help the local population.[42]

More Units to Vietnam

Back in Vietnam, the 57th Med Det (HA), later that year, was joined by the 82d Med Det (HA), which deployed from Fort Sam Houston. It was part of increasingly larger numbers of units and men being deployed to the war. Capt. Doug Moore deployed with the 82d. After flight school, he had initially been assigned to the 45th Med Co (AA) at Fort Bragg before coming to the 82d. When he arrived in Vietnam, however, he transferred to the 57th as some of the 57th's experienced personnel helped the 82d quickly come up to speed. Subsequently, he spent his entire tour with the 57th.[43]

1st Lt. Jim Truscott joined Moore in January 1965. Truscott, a 1962 Reserve Officers' Training Corps graduate from Oklahoma State University, received a regular commission and requested the MSC branch and flight school. He was selected into the MSC, but instead of flight school, was assigned to a ground medical unit at Fort Campbell, Kentucky, with the 101st Airborne Division. Two years later, he received his orders for flight school and completed the program at Fort Wolters, Texas. Upon graduation, he was assigned to a MEDEVAC unit in Korea. Most of his classmates received orders for Vietnam. He wanted to go with them and called the Chief of the MSC directly. The Chief asked him if he was volunteering. "Yes sir," Truscott replied. He had his orders within two days.[44]

When the personnel of 82d Med Det (HA) arrived in Saigon, the unit was assigned to the U.S. Army Support Command, Vietnam, which had just replaced the USASGV. They were issued five UH-1B aircraft and dispatched to Binh Thuy, where they replaced the detachment from the 57th, which rejoined its unit at Tan Son Nhut Air Base. Truscott watched the new crews arrive and was not impressed. He started calling his unit "the originals" to differentiate them from the "latecomers." Soon his unit mates joined him, and they even put it on their aircraft. The moniker stuck, and the 57th became known by that title.[45]

In late 1965, though, another type of aeromedical evacuation unit was sent to Vietnam. The 1st Air Cavalry Division (Airmobile) deployed to the Central Highlands region. This unit was unique. Based on studies and tests done before the war, it was created and built around the tactical mobility provided by a fleet of helicopters. This included an air ambulance platoon of 12 new UH-1D MEDEVAC helicopters assigned to the headquarters and support company organic to the 15th Medical Battalion. This platoon did not have an area general support mission. Instead, it was in direct support of the division that also commanded and provided for it.[46]

The platoon also reflected another innovation. Many of the division helicopter pilots were warrant officers. Several were assigned to the air ambulance platoon. Eventually, warrant officer pilots flew in all MEDEVAC units throughout the war, and, as the need for MEDEVAC units increased, they eventually outnumbered the commissioned MSC pilots.[47]

The UH-1D helicopters were a further improvement to the Huey fleet. They had the same engine as the UH-1B model, but longer and larger blades produced more lift that almost doubled the payload. They could carry 4,000 lbs of cargo.[48]

More Med Det (RA) units arrived. On 1 September 1965, the 283d Med Det (RA) deployed from Fort Lewis to Tan Son Nhut Air Base with the 57th, and it provided general support to tactical units in the III Corps area. Two months later, the 254th Med Det (RA) also arrived in Saigon. When its aircraft were delivered, it joined the other two detachments at Tan Son Nhut. It provided direct support to the 173d Airborne Brigade, which also operated in the III Corps area.[49]

More units formed to go to Vietnam. The 498th Med Co (AA) received orders to Vietnam in July 1965. The commander, Lt. Col. Joseph Madrano, flew over early with an advance party and was told that his company would cover all of the III Corps area in general support under the 43d Medical Group. He picked his base locations based on his needs and placed his company at Nha Trang, with platoons at Qui Nhon, Pleiku, and Ban Me Thuot. Such dispersion created logistical challenges, but it provided for the necessary coverage.

The unit had only been in the country a few days when it suffered its first loss. The detachment at Qui Nhon scrambled its alert bird to help a unit in the mountains just to the west. The weather was bad, with low clouds and fog in the valleys. While trying to get into the requesting unit, the crew flew into a mountain. The helicopter was destroyed and burned furiously. The crash killed the crew chief and medic. The two badly injured pilots were recovered the next day. This crash, once again, illustrated that physical limits such as restricted in-flight visibility restrict what helicopters and their crews can do.[50]

While the 498th settled into its mission, the surgeon of the U.S. Army Support Command in Vietnam, Lt. Col. James Blunt, developed a plan to form a new provisional Medical Company that consisted of the 57th, 82d, 254th, and 283d Med Det (RA), all of which operated in the III and IV Corps area. It possessed 22 helicopters and 160 officers and enlisted personnel. Initially named the 436th Med Co (Provisional), it was eventually renamed the 658th. However, the unit never established effective control over the highly individualized medical detachments that had already developed habitual relationships with other aviation and tactical units. It was eventually disbanded and the detachments were spread to other parts of South Vietnam.[51]

As the buildup of American forces in South Vietnam continued, the medical force correspondingly expanded. In January 1966, with 184,000 Americans in the war, the 44th Medical Brigade activated and assumed control of all nondivisional medical units in Vietnam. The brigade commanded subordinate groups, the 67th in I Corps, the 43d and 55th in II Corps, and the 68th in III and IV Corps. Each eventually commanded all of the Med Det (RA) and Med Co (AA) units that served in general support of all of the tactical units in their assigned area.[52]

Back at Fort Sam Houston, another MEDEVAC company formed, the 507th Med Co (AA). Given a collection of older aircraft, it supported training operations all over the United States and became, de facto, a training unit for MEDEVAC crews. The two flight training centers at Fort Wolters and Fort Rucker, Alabama, also expanded pilot output to meet the larger Army needs for pilots in all specialties. All MEDEVAC units experienced the increase in training require-ments as the turnover of personnel assigned to Vietnam steadily increased.

Additionally, the 587th Med Det (RA) formed at Camp Zama, Japan. Many wounded were sent there for care, but the bus rides to the local general hospitals lasted—in some cases—several hours. When Gen. Johnny K. Waters, the Com-mander of the U.S. Army Pacific Command, discovered this problem, he directed the deployment of an air ambulance unit to reduce the transfer time. Moore was a member of the initial cadre. After his tour in Vietnam with the 57th, he had returned to Fort Sam Houston for the MSC nine-month advanced course. To fa-cilitate an earlier return to Japan, he was placed in a shorter reserve component course so that he could join the unit as it formed. When they arrived in Japan, Moore and his compatriots received three UH-1Bs from the 25th Infantry Di-vision, which was deploying from Hawaii to Vietnam. They were subsequently reinforced with five of the newer UH-1Ds direct from the factory.[53]

The flow of wounded soldiers from Vietnam was constant and heavy. Many were evacuated from field hospitals to Japan by strategic airlift. The crews of the 587th would pick up the wounded at the arrival airfields and transport them to the five general hospitals in Japan, similar to the duty performed by the 56th Med Det (RA) in the later stages of the Korean War. The biggest challenge for the pilots was the frequent terrible weather. All had to be excellent instrument pilots by necessity. According to Moore's personal logs, the unit flew 6,450 hours on MEDEVAC missions and carried 62,525 patients during his two-year tour.

Moore recalled, "It was one of those rare assignments where people felt good about themselves nearly every day because we could see the end result of our efforts. Rather than subjecting critically wounded patients to a ride of four to six hours in a bumpy ambulance through horrendous Japanese traffic, we moved them in about 20 minutes, quickly and much more comfortably."[54]

MEDEVAC crews returning from duty in Vietnam enriched units in the United States and Europe. The 421st Med Co (AA), assigned to the 7th Medical Brigade and stationed at Nelligen, Germany, received now Maj. John Temperilli and other veterans. They were the core element in extensive training programs that quali-fied most pilots in mountain operations and instrument flight qualifications. Dur-ing 1965, the unit flew almost 4,600 hours and evacuated 1,021 patients while supporting training operations and the local military communities. The unit also maintained platoons at Illesheim, Grafenwöhr, and Darmstadt.[55]

After a tour with the 57th Med Det in Vietnam, Truscott reported for duty as the commander of the 63d Med Det at Landstuhl, Germany. As a high-time UH-1 pilot, he was very comfortable flying the unit-assigned UH-1Bs. However, the weather was much worse than in Vietnam, especially in the winter when the snow and ice made flying especially challenging. After 18 months, his replacement ar-rived, and he again volunteered for duty in Vietnam. More MEDEVAC pilots were needed there, and his orders arrived expeditiously.[56]

The steady increase of the MEDEVAC fleet in South Vietnam reflected the larger buildup of American forces in the war. In late 1966, the 436th Med Co supported a combined U.S. and Vietnamese force of more than 20,000 troops as they attacked infiltrating enemy forces northwest of Saigon. In the operation, the Dustoff helicopters recovered 3,000 wounded, injured, and sick soldiers. Fourteen of the helicopters were hit by enemy fire, and one was actually shot down. The operation highlighted a problem. Each of the four detachments involved was supporting specific units, and there was no central clearinghouse for the overall control and maximum utilization of assets. So the commander of the 436th developed a command and control net so that all requests for Dustoff flowed through two central dispatch agencies. The centralized control was more effective at coordinating missions and reduced duplication of effort.[57]

The suite of radios aboard the UH-1 consisting of VHF-AM, VHF-FM, UHF, and HF radios facilitated the centralization of control. Using them the pilots or medic onboard could talk to the tactical units in the field making the MEDEVAC request, the control centers, or specific hospitals. This ensured that as soon as the helicopters were airborne with the casualties, they could be routed by a medical regulating officer tied into the overall theater medical system, directly to the specific hospital best equipped to handle the needs of that specific casualty. Additionally, it allowed casualties to be moved directly from the point of injury to those rear area specialized facilities, thus, in many cases, bypassing company or battalion aid stations. It reduced the time necessary to get the casualty to the surgeons, who could now be concentrated in the hospitals.[58]

Additionally, the standard format for requesting MEDEVAC support was further refined. All requests needed to include the following:

1. Location of landing zone;
2. Number and condition of casualties, and types of wounds;
3. Radio frequency of unit involved;
4. Special needs including oxygen and blood;
5. Terrain;
6. Enemy activity at the location; and
7. Weather.[59]

The MEDEVAC crews responded to incoming calls at the command center and tried to be airborne within three minutes of the call.

Another lingering problem was determining when a landing zone was safe enough for MEDEVAC. This was also a subjective call, usually made by the local commander, who—as was to be expected—wanted to get his wounded out of the area. The determinant decided upon—almost ad hoc by the MEDEVAC units—was that if it was "safe enough" for the troops on the ground to be up and moving the wounded, then it was safe enough for the helicopter to land. This put a premium on the helicopter crews establishing radio contact with the requesting unit before arriving.[60]

As ground combat spread throughout the nation, more of it occurred in jungle areas. The natural foliage was thick, and—in many cases—the trees were 200 feet high. Engaged units taking casualties were faced with moving their wounded to open areas while in combat. Such movement rapidly drained a unit of fighting personnel as soldiers left their fighting positions to move the casualties, and it further exposed themselves to enemy fire.

Lt. Col. Hal Moore, at the battle of Ia Drang, noted this when he wrote, "I lost many leaders killed and wounded while recovering casualties. Troops must not get so concerned with casualties that they forget the enemy and their mission. Attempting to carry a man requires up to four men as (litter) bearers, which can devastate a unit at a critical time."[61]

Recognizing the need to bring the MEDEVAC helicopter to units in the jungle, hoists were developed and fitted on the helicopters. They used either a special harness called a "jungle penetrator" or a wire litter if the patient was not ambulatory. However, the hoist created a new dilemma because—to properly use it—the helicopter had to be held in a hover while the litter or penetrator was lowered, the casualty was loaded, and then raised into the aircraft. While doing this, the helicopter was a perfect target for enemy gunners, and several MEDEVAC birds were lost this way. Many crews requested escort attack helicopters for hoist missions. Moore hated hoist missions. He remembered that:

> You are probably hovering 200 feet in the air, dangling a cable down to the ground, trying to get that thing centered where you have no frame of reference… and then once you get somebody hooked up on the ground … the last thing you want to do is lose control and drag him into the trees and kill somebody by catching him in the fork of a tree or else catching the cable and having it break. In the meantime, when you are sitting 150–200 feet in the air, you are clearly visible to everybody for a quarter mile in any direction who has an AK-47.[62]

Interestingly, the U.S. Air Force rescue helicopters, responding to downed aviators all over Southeast Asia, faced a similar problem. They developed the same solution, that is, they dispatched the rescue helicopters as part of a task force that included A-1 attack aircraft or other fighters to provide the necessary close-in support. Then, the recovery helicopter was held in the hover and the hoist lowered to the survivor on the ground.

As 1967 began, American forces continued to increase in South Vietnam to 450,000. An analysis of overall theater needs indicated that for predicted casualty expectations, the Army in Vietnam needed 120 MEDEVAC helicopters. Yet the fleet consisted of only 64 aircraft. The Commander Gen. William Westmoreland addressed his needs to his higher commanders. At the same time, within theater, his subordinate commanders used non-MEDEVAC helicopters with medics onboard as a stop-gap measure.

Another MEDEVAC unit, the 571st Med Det (HA), activated at Fort Meade and subsequently moved to Nha Trang, Vietnam. Almost concurrently, the 45th Med Co (AA) at Fort Bragg was ordered to Vietnam. It had been equipped with old H-19 helicopters, remaining from Korea. These were replaced with 25 UH-1H helicopters, the newest variant of the Huey, direct from the factory. These aircraft had more powerful engines and were fully equipped with instrumentation for night flight. Additionally, all were also eventually equipped with a hoist for jungle recoveries. After receiving their aircraft, the 45th was based at Long Binh, just north of Saigon.

One of the first pilots to join it was Capt. Jim Truscott. When he arrived, he was asked what call sign he wanted to use. The unit pilots used "Dustoff" with a numerical suffix. Jim stated that he wanted to be "Dustoff 13."

The operations officer was taken aback. "That is an unlucky number," he responded. Truscott explained his logic. "Wait a minute, I volunteered to come back for my second tour. Every mission we go on we get shot at. Most of our missions are at night in bad weather, and a call sign is going to be bad luck? Give me a break!" He flew as "Dustoff 13" throughout another full tour and logged about twice as many hours as he had on his earlier tour with the 57th. He then returned in early 1969 to Fort Sam Houston for the MSC Advanced Course as a new major.[63]

Almost simultaneously, several more medical detachments also deployed. The 159th Med Det (RA) went to Cu Chi in III Corps in a general support role. The 50th Med Det (RA) arrived at Phu Hiep in southern II Corps. It provided general support for the 173d Airborne Brigade and Republic of Korea units in the area.[64]

The 54th Med Det (RA) deployed to Chu Lai on the northern coast in the southern portion of I Corps and provided direct support for the 23d (American) Division. The unit included 1st Lt. Jerome (Jerry) Foust. Foust entered the Army in 1966 when he received his draft notice. As a college graduate, he opted instead for a direct commission into the MSC. His first assignment was to a medical holding company at Fort Sam Houston. After being detailed to manually pay 770 soldiers, he volunteered for flight school. He graduated in June 1967 and reported to the 54th at Fort Benning, which was commanded by Capt. Bob McWilliam. Two months later, the unit—newly equipped with six UH-1H helicopters—departed for Vietnam, and flew missions by the end of August.

The 54th's operations officer was Capt. Pat Brady, who returned to the war for a second tour. He pushed his crews hard and wanted them off of the ground within two minutes of receiving a MEDEVAC request. On 29 September 1967, the unit had all six aircraft and another borrowed from a sister unit shot down while supporting ARVN units sweeping an enemy-controlled area. To compensate for the losses, the unit was assigned older UH-1C and Ds until new aircraft were available. Foust flew with the 54th until March 1968 when he switched over to the 45th Med Co (AA) to complete his tour.[65]

Additionally, all MEDEVAC units converted to the newer more powerful UH-1H helicopters.

Helicopter Comparison

Through 1968, all MEDEVAC units converted to the UH-1H. It was a definite improvement over the earlier models. During the War, the U.S. Army used four variations of the UH-1 for MEDEVAC duties:

Model	Engine/Horsepower (hp)	Seats/Litters	Range (nautical miles)
UH-1A	T53/860 hp	6/2 + medic	230
UH-1B	T53L5/960 hp	7/3 + medic	260
	T53L11/1100hp		
UH-1D	T53L11/1100hp	12/6 + medic	230
UH-1H	T53L13/1400hp	14/6 + medic	276[66]

Second Combat Tours

As the war continued, more of the men who earlier served in the war began to return for second tours. Moore returned to serve with and command the 159th, still stationed at Cu Chi. He was promoted to Major and moved over to the 45th Med Co (AA), serving as the unit operations officer. Chief of the Medical Service Corps Brig. Gen. William Hamrick visited Moore's unit and advised him to get a master's degree. Moore then applied for and was accepted to Baylor University upon his homecoming.[67]

More MEDEVAC units were also activated. The 68th Med Det (RA) formed at Fort Bragg as did the 236th Med Det (RA) at Fort Polk, Louisiana, the 237th at Fort Meade, and the 247th at Fort Riley.[68]

Reserve Component Units

As the overall MEDEVAC fleet expanded, the Department of the Army also provided helicopters to several states so that they could form more MEDEVAC units within their National Guards. By the summer of 1968, the following units activated, although equipped mostly with older H-23 helicopters and a few small fixed wing aircraft:

Alabama	133d Med Co (AA)
Arizona	997th Med Co (AA)
Maine	112th Med Co (AA)
Mississippi	123d Med Co (AA)
Nebraska	24th Med Co (AA)
New York	249th Med Co (AA)
Oklahoma	245th Med Co (AA)
South Dakota	1085th Med Det (HA)
West Virginia	146th Med Det (HA)[69]

However, some units began to receive newer equipment. That summer, the 24th Med Co (AA) received 25 UH-1D helicopters, making it the largest MEDEVAC unit in the ARNG. Additionally, under a U.S. Department of Transportation test project called Operation SKY-AID, the unit signed letters of agreement with several local hospitals to provide neo/natal transfer flights and on-call MEDEVAC for the recovery and transport of highway crash victims to the emergency rooms at those hospitals.[70]

Through 1970, the Department of the Army continued the buildup of MEDE-VAC units in the ARNG. The following units were added, again with a mixture of older H-23 and H-19 helicopters and small, fixed-wing aircraft:

Hawaii	2929th Med Det (HA)
Kentucky	441st Med Det (HA)
New Hampshire	397th Med Det (HA)

In addition, the USAR continued to recruit soldiers for the 317th Med Co (AA), at Miami, Florida, with its platoons located at Orlando and Tampa, and Atlanta, Georgia. It was still equipped with old H-13s, but received replacement H-34s within the year.[71]

A Medal of Honor

On 6 January 1968, Maj. Patrick Brady of the 54th Med Det (RA) flew a mission to rescue wounded U.S. and ARVN soldiers in the mountains west of Chu Lai. On a previous MEDEVAC tour, he flew with Maj. Charles Kelly and was impressed with his professionalism and desire to accomplish the mission regardless of weather, terrain, or enemy. Flying through thick fog, he made several trips to several different locations and, despite heavy enemy ground fire, recovered all of the wounded. When his aircraft was damaged, he procured another and flew to a different site to recover soldiers trapped in a minefield. When that aircraft was damaged by a mine detonation, he launched in a third helicopter and recovered 51 seriously wounded men, many of whom would have perished without prompt medical treatment. For his actions, he was awarded the Medal of Honor.[72]

Last MEDEVAC Deployments

In early 1969, the last iteration of MEDEVAC units deployed to South Vietnam. The 68th, 236th, 237th, and 247th Med Det (RA) all joined those units operating in the theater, and the fully matured MEDEVAC fleet reached its peak in late early 1969, as did the overall U.S. force in Vietnam by March, when 540,000 Americans were fighting in that country. Fifteen MEDEVAC units—two companies, two divisional platoons, and 11 detachments—were deployed to and operating in South Vietnam.

At this time, the overarching medical command in Vietnam was the 44th Medical Brigade. It commanded four medical groups: the 43d, 55th, 67th, and 68th. They subsequently controlled a plethora of medical units that consisted of numerous specialty detachments, support battalions, and 23 field, surgical, and evacuation hospitals. The groups controlled all air ambulance detachments and companies, except for the air ambulance platoon of the 15th Medical Battalion, 1st Cavalry Division. However, the actual command and control structure was in constant flux as units came to and then departed from the theater during the war.[73]

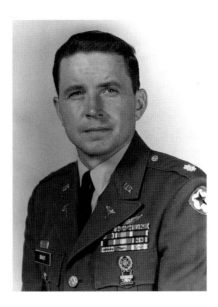

Maj. Patrick Brady, Medal of Honor.
Source: Office of the Chief, MSC

This left only one active duty unit—the 507th Med Co (AA) at Fort Sam Houston—that effectively acted as a training site for MEDEVAC. To address the shortage, another unit, the 212th Med Det (RA), activated at Fort Meade. Assigned six UH-1D aircraft, the unit was rapidly filled with Vietnam veterans and assigned to provide general support to Army hospitals and units in the central Atlantic seaboard area.[74]

Other Theaters

While the ongoing operations in Vietnam filled the headlines, MEDEVAC operations were being conducted in other areas of the world. On 15 March 1969, a MEDEVAC helicopter from the 377th Med Co (AA) in Korea crashed near the DMZ between South and North Korea at night after recovering three wounded soldiers. The four crewmembers were killed, but another Army helicopter recovered the patients. Unfortunately, that helicopter then crashed, killing those soldiers. The MEDEVAC personnel killed in the double loss were Maj. J.C. Rothwell, Capt. Benjamin Park, S.Sgt. Carrol Zanchi, and Sp4c. Edwin Stoller of the 377th.[75]

In Europe, the various MEDEVAC units were consolidated as the 15th Med Det (HA) and 63d Med Det (HA) were placed under the control of the 421st Med Co (AA). Additionally, the units were full of Vietnam veterans like Foust who served as the 421st operations officer. He enjoyed his time in Europe and became a fully qualified instrument pilot. He also shared his experiences with the younger pilots. That year, the units also received improved UH-1D aircraft to replace their UH-1Bs and ancient CH-34s. They flew a regular regimen of intra-theater transfers, field casualty pickups, and blood supply runs through some very demanding weather.[76]

Vietnam High Point

From 1969 on, the MEDEVAC units in Vietnam constantly redeployed all over the country to support operations as necessary. In another reorganization, the 50th Med Det (RA) inactivated, but reconstituted as the Air Ambulance Platoon of the 326th Medical Battalion, 101st Airborne Division (Airmobile), and relocated to the division main base at Camp Eagle, near Hue. The commander of the 326th, Lt. Col. Bernard Mittemeyer, became Lt. Gen. and served as the Army Surgeon General from 1981 to 1985. The platoon quickly picked up the moniker of "Eagle Dustoff" and worked in direct support of that division similar to the air ambulance platoon assigned to the 15th Medical Battalion, 1st Cavalry Division.[77]

The buildup of MEDEVAC units in Vietnam mirrored the larger growth of aviation forces in general. To provide them with necessary air traffic control and coordination, an extensive system of air traffic navigational aids and control centers was established throughout the country. It allowed for extensive traffic control under instrument conditions when the weather dictated it and for procedural control at other times, which provided for positive flight monitoring. This system also advised aircrews of dangerous and restricted areas. The MEDEVAC commanders had to ensure that their crews received the daily updates and were trained and prepared to utilize the traffic control system controlled and operated by the 125th Aviation Company.[78]

Vietnam Drawdown

The drawdown of U.S. forces in Vietnam began in 1969, and the long process that saw the growth and maturity of the MEDEVAC force shifted into reverse. Slowly at first, the various combat and medical commands were inactivated or sent home, and unit consolidations were commonplace. In general, as the major field forces left, the MEDEVAC units followed, although at a somewhat slower pace since they still had to cover the remaining forces. Yet, there was still much hard fighting to do in South Vietnam, Cambodia, and even Laos. Wherever the fighting was, MEDEVAC was there.

As the forces were being drawn down, another innovative reorganization was attempted. To provide better command and control for the disparate detachments, a proposal was sculpted for a medical evacuation battalion. Such a unit commanded several MEDEVAC units in an integrated and coherent fashion. In February 1970, the 44th Medical Brigade redesignated the 61st Medical Battalion as an evacuation unit. It lost its ability to treat patients and took control of all nondivisional ambulances in the northern half of South Vietnam. That included six helicopter ambulance detachments, one bus ambulance detachment, two ground ambulance detachments, and one air ambulance company. Its defined mission was to command and control air and ground transport to move not only patients, but also medical personnel, supplies, equipment, and whole blood as a coherent system.

The reorganization proved successful as aircraft availability rates rose 20%, and all units passed all command inspections. In May 1970, the 58th Medical Battalion was similarly converted to an evacuation unit with a like assignment of companies and detachments and designated responsibility for the southern half of the country. The two units subsequently performed their designated functions until June 1971, when both were inactivated and the 67th and 68th Medical Groups assumed their responsibilities. The concept was short-lived, but a seed had been planted that would return full bloom in the future.[79]

A Second Medal of Honor

On 2 October 1969, Chief Warrant Officer Michael Novosel from the 82d Med Det (RA) flew a mission to Kien Tuong Province in response to a request for MEDEVAC. He arrived in the midst of an ongoing battle. Disregarding frequently intense enemy fire, which damaged the aircraft and eventually wounded Novosel, he made 15 extractions and saved the lives of 29 allied soldiers. For his actions, he received the Medal of Honor.[80]

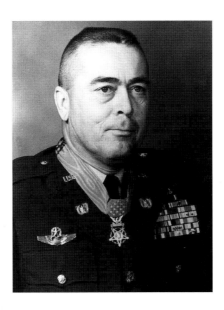

CW3 Michael Novosel, Medal of Honor.
Source: Office of the Chief, MSC

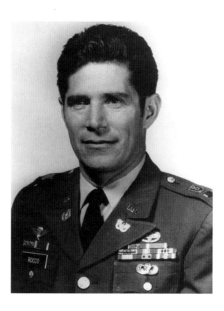

S.Sgt. Louis Rocco, Medal of Honor.
Source: U.S. Army

A Third Medal of Honor

On 24 May 1970, a MEDEVAC helicopter from the Air Ambulance Platoon of the 1st Cavalry Division responded to an emergency call from an ARVN airborne unit operating a few miles inside Cambodia. Sfc. Louis Rocco served as a medic advisor with the ARVN unit and volunteered to go as an additional medic. Enemy fire shot down the helicopter as it approached the pickup zone. Rocco survived the crash, but sustained a fractured wrist and hip. Seeing that the other four crewmembers were all more severely injured and in some cases unconscious, he repeatedly returned to the burning aircraft to recover them, even though he was severely burned. He carried them to the safety of an ARVN fighting position and cared for them until all could be rescued. His actions saved the lives of three countrymen and earned him the Medal of Honor.[81]

Stateside

After graduating from the MSC Advanced Course, new Maj. Jim Truscott was assigned to the 18th Medical Brigade at Fort Meade as the S-1 (personnel officer). Still on flight status, he flew with the 212th Med Det (RA), also stationed at Fort Meade, to maintain his currency. The unit regularly flew missions moving patients from Andrews Air Force Base to the Walter Reed Medical Facility in Washington, DC, or to other regional hospitals. On occasion, he flew the Army Surgeon General to locations outside Washington. A year later, he was transferred to the Surgeon General's staff and worked on avionics and navigational equipment upgrades for the MEDEVAC helicopters. He further enhanced his career when he was selected to attend the Army Command and General Staff College at Fort Leavenworth, Kansas. He remained in Kansas for another year to complete a master's degree at the University of Kansas. He was being prepared for bigger and better things.[82]

Doctrine

FM 8-10, Medical Support Theater of Operations, April 1970

Based on its experiences in Vietnam, the Army Medical Department updated its doctrinal manuals. The FM that defined and directed support for an army in the field was FM 8-10, which was out of date and revised in April 1970. The manual described concepts of operation in broad terms. From it would cascade more specific guidance to lower echelon units, primarily in the form of tactics, techniques, and procedures, for specific equipment or the accomplishment of specific missions. It defined aeromedical evacuation as "...the movement of patients to and between medical treatment facilities by aerial vehicles that are specially crewed and equipped to accommodate patients and to provide required in-flight medical care."[83]

It also detailed eight principles for care and treatment including the following:

1. Health services must be continuous for best chance of survival.
2. Higher echelon commands will evacuate patients from the lower echelon units.
3. No soldier will be evacuated farther to the rear than his physical condition warrants or the military situation dictates.
4. Control of medical support resources must rest with the medical staff officer or commander having responsibility for providing health services within the command.
5. The medical means must be as close to the casualties as time/distance factors and the tactical situation permits. Early collection, sorting, and treatment of patients must be provided.
6. Medical support must be flexible and adaptive to changes in tactical plans or operations that may require redistribution of medical resources.
7. Medical units must have mobility comparable to that of the units they support.
8. Medical support must conform to the tactical plan and should be provided adequately at the right place and right time.[84]

This manual indicated that in a theater of operations, a medical brigade would be assigned to the field army support command. The brigade would command, control, plan for, and operate the field army medical support system. It could command and control as many medical groups as necessary to provide needed medical support. Normally, the 25-ship air ambulance medical companies would be assigned to the various groups. Helicopter ambulance medical detachments would be assigned at the brigade, group, or subordinate battalion level as necessary to provide necessary evacuation support. The air ambulance companies and detachments would be responsible for evacuating all categories of patients to designated medical facilities and would be on an "on-call" basis, with priority given to those most seriously wounded. Aeromedical evacuation was the preferred means of evacuation, as part of an overall integrated evacuation system that was designed quickly to move the wounded to needed medical care.[85]

FM 8-35, *Transportation of the Sick and Wounded*, which was published in 1970, further amplified the guidance in FM 8-10. This FM, which focused on patient movement, was a "how to" manual that provided specific and detailed tactics, techniques, and procedures for the manual carrying of patients and their transport using rotary-wing and other vehicles.[86]

Based on the updated doctrinal guidance, over the next year, the AMS also developed updated TO&Es for the various MEDEVAC companies and detachments. The detachments could be equipped with up to six aircraft and generally be assigned to a field army medical brigade, theater army medical command, or an independent corps, division, task force, or special action force. Their specific mission was to perform medical evacuation functions where units of less than company-size were needed, or to increase the evacuation capabilities of fixed-strength units where increments of less than company-size were needed. Generally, one detachment was allocated for each division or equivalent force supported and two for each corps or equivalent force supported. They were designed for highly mobile operations, but required a great deal of logistical support from supported units.[87]

The companies were assigned up to 25 aircraft and could be subdivided into as many as four platoons, each similar to a detachment. The companies generally were assigned to a field army medical brigade or a major medical command of an independent corps or task force on a one-per-one basis. The companies were robust units and could maintain 24-hour operations as well as perform their own organizational maintenance on all equipment except medical items and aircraft avionic equipment. They also relied on higher echelon units for more general support.

Their specified tasks for both the detachments and companies were to provide the following:

1. Aeromedical evacuation of selected patients;
2. Emergency movement of medical personnel and accompanying equipment and supplies; and
3. Uninterrupted delivery of whole blood, biologicals, and medical supplies.[88]

All companies and detachments were organized under these two TO&Es. Again, there was one organizational exception. Units like the 101st Airborne Division (Airmobile) that were designed around the air mobility inherent in helicopters, would maintain—within its medical battalion—its air ambulance platoon of 12 aircraft that were organic to the unit and integrated into the medical structure. The platoon was usually located near the battalion headquarters for quick response, but could be forward-located with maneuver units. The platoon also had an aircraft maintenance section for organizational maintenance. Division aviation mainte-nance units provided higher level maintenance to the air ambulance platoon.[89]

More New Units and Redeployments

In 1971, several MEDEVAC units were formed. The 32d Med Det (RA) acti-vated at Fort Ord under the command of Capt. Merle Snyder; the 78th Med Det (RA) activated at Fort Carson; and the 151st Med Det (RA) activated at Fort Bragg. Additionally, units started returning from Vietnam. The 498th Med Co (AA) redeployed to Fort Stewart, Georgia. Throughout the year, the flow of units coming back to the United States was continuous. Many of the units inactivated or consolidated with others.[90]

Foust left his assignment with the 421st Med Co (AA) in Germany and reported to Vietnam in June 1970 for a second tour. Initially, he served as a safety officer with a medical battalion. In April 1971, he was assigned as the commander of the 237th Med Det (RA). The unit was based near the ancient city of Hue, not far below the Demilitarized Zone. Initially, his crews supported units throughout Mil-itary Region One. When other units departed for home, the 237th was given four more aircraft and crews and functioned as a company minus. His unit supported the Vietnamese incursion into Laos called Lamson 719, and had one aircraft shot down and many shot up. Foust logged more than 2,000 hours of combat flying and returned home after 18 months when his unit was subsequently redeployed to the United States. He reported again for duty at Fort Sam Houston.

After attending the MSC Advanced Course, he joined the 507th Med Co (AA) for an 18-month tour as the operations officer and became an instructor in the Academy of Health Sciences. He used his combat experiences to instruct, mentor, and mold another generation of both rising Medical Corps and MSC officers.[91]

As 1972 began the 236th Med Det (RA) redeployed from Vietnam to Fort Sam Houston. 1st Lt. Art Hapner, who had been drafted into the Army in June 1969 just as he graduated from college, joined the 236th. While training to become a pre-ventive medicine specialist, he had a chance encounter with Capt. Ray Salmon, a Vietnam MEDEVAC pilot veteran, who asked him if he had a college degree and wanted to become a MEDEVAC pilot. Hapner answered in the affirmative and within six months he was a brand new MSC 2d Lt. Then he attended flight school at Fort Wolters and Fort Rucker and returned to Fort Sam Houston as a pilot with the small flight detachment at the Brooke Army Medical Center. He met and flew with several Vietnam veteran pilots like Capt. Hank Tuell, who took him out on several missions and taught him the finer points of flying. Tuell and those senior highly ex-perienced warrant officers also taught him the value and importance of mentoring.[92]

By February 1972, only five detachments—the 57th, 159th, 237th, 247th, and the 571st—remained in Vietnam to provide general support to the rapidly decreasing combat and support units. The air ambulance platoons left with their divisions. The 101st Airborne Division realigned as an air assault unit and retained the air ambulance platoon assigned to its 326th Medical Battalion. The 1st Cavalry Division restructured as an armored division, and its 15th Medical Battalion lost its air ambulance platoon.[93]

The remaining detachments continued to fly combat, especially when the North Vietnamese Army invaded South Vietnam in March. The enemy brought with them the very deadly SA-7 heat-seeking missile that directly threatened low flying aircraft such as the UH-1. This missile dictated a change in tactics. No longer could MEDEVAC helicopters hold a hover for any time for jungle recoveries. They had to stay in motion at very low altitude until landing. Until countermeasures could be developed for the aircraft, this was their only defense.

Europe

In May, disaster struck the MEDEVAC community in Europe. A series of terrorist bombs exploded in front of the officer's club at the headquarters of the V Corps in Frankfurt, Germany. Thirteen people were wounded in the blast that also killed Lt. Col. Paul Bloomquist, veteran of two MEDEVAC combat tours in Vietnam and a former commander of the 57th Med Det (RA). He had been honored as the Army Aviator of the Year in 1965 and selected by the U.S. Chamber of Commerce as an outstanding young American. A few years later, the medical headquarters in Ziegenberg, Germany, was named for him.[94]

Last Units Out of Vietnam

Later that year the 159th Med Det (RA) redeployed back to the United States. In February 1973, the 237th, 247th, and 571st ceased operations. Three weeks later, the 57th flew the last American MEDEVAC mission of the war when it picked up a patient with a severe appendicitis. The 57th—known forever as the "Originals"—was there from first to last.

In tribute to the contribution of the MEDEVAC units in the conflict, Gen. Creighton Abrams, then the commander of U.S. forces in Vietnam, said of them:

> Courage above and beyond the call of duty was sort of routine for them. It was a daily thing, part of the way they lived, and it meant so much to every last man who served there. Whether he ever got hurt or not, he knew 'Dustoff' was there.[95]

Before Vietnam, Lt. Col. Spurgeon Neel had written recommendations for MEDEVAC employment based on experiences in Korea. Vietnam validated some and discredited others. He had recommended company-sized organizations as opposed to cellular detachments. The first two MEDEVAC units that went to Vietnam were the 57th and 82d, both cellular detachments, which depended on collocated aviation units for sustenance, logistics, and some maintenance. Eventually, two independent companies were deployed. However, they were broken into dispersed platoons and suffered some of the same problems. Two air ambulance platoons were created within the medical battalions assigned to the 101st Airborne and the 1st Cavalry Divisions. They called on the resources of those larger units for necessary logistical support. Overall, it seemed that the arrangements for support for the MEDEVAC detachments were ad hoc and depended on whatever arrangements the commanders could orchestrate at their assigned location.[96]

Neel had also written that there was no real requirement for a separate communications net for the control of MEDEVAC. Events in Vietnam contradicted this. It was clear that the radio suite provided to the UH-1 gave the crews and medical regulating officers the ability to speak with whoever was necessary to facilitate the movement of the wounded or sick soldier directly from point of injury to the facility best able to provide for him.[97]

Additionally, Neel wrote, "…helicopter evacuation within the combat zone is the responsibility of the [AMS]." In Vietnam, initially, the first two units were assigned to the U.S. Army Service Group, Vietnam. Both were collocated with aviation units that provided their support. During this period, proposals were made at least twice to use them as general purpose units. It was not until 1966 that the 44th Medical Brigade activated and assumed control of all Army medical units in the country. It operated until all units were finally withdrawn in 1973. The two air ambulance platoons assigned to divisions were under division control. The officers within these platoons were MSC officers and knew how to plug their units into the medical system within the country. No patients were delivered to a hospital without talking to a 44th Brigade medical regulating officer.[98]

Results

How did MEDEVAC do in Vietnam? The numbers are staggering and suggest that the system worked beyond all expectations.

- From May 1962 to March 1973:
  - 496,573 Dustoff missions were flown,[99] and
  - 900,000 casualties/patients were airlifted.[100]
- The Medical Department lost 199 helicopters in Vietnam from all causes. The loss rate of MEDEVAC versus non-MEDEVAC helicopters was 1.5 times higher. Hoist missions were the most dangerous with one of 10 hits reported on MEDEVAC helicopters occurred on hoist missions. Four hundred seventy pilots were killed or injured by enemy action or crashes. Of the crew chiefs and flight medics, 121 were killed and 545 were wounded.[101]
- Two officers, one warrant officer, and two enlisted soldiers are still listed as missing-in-action.[102]
- Two MEDEVAC pilots and one medic were awarded the Medal of Honor for their heroic actions:
  - Maj. Patrick H. Brady, for actions near Chu Lai, Republic of Vietnam on 6 January 1968.

- ○ CW4 Michael J. Novosel, for actions in Kien Tuong Province, Republic of Vietnam, on 2 October 1969.
  - ○ Both pilots were on their second MEDEVAC tours.
  - ○ Sfc. Louis R. Rocco, for actions near Katum, Republic of Vietnam, on 24 May 1970.
- Three MEDEVAC officers, three warrant officers, and three enlisted soldiers were awarded Distinguished Service Crosses.
- One MEDEVAC officer was awarded the Navy Cross.

Perhaps the best single analysis of MEDEVAC in Vietnam was written— again—by now Maj. Gen. Spurgeon Neel, who noted toward the end of the conflict in 1972:

> Getting the casualty and the physician together as soon as possible is the keystone of the practice of combat medicine. The helicopter achieved that goal as never before.… The technical development of the helicopter ambulance…the growth of a solid body of doctrine and air evacuation procedures, and the skill, ingenuity, and courage of the aircraft crewmen and medical aidmen who put theory into practice in a hostile and dangerous environment made possible the hospitalization and evacuation system that evolved in Vietnam.[103]

To those who had argued that "Aeromedical evacuation is an **aviation mission** which entails **the movement of patients**," the actions of men like Charles Kelly, Patrick Brady, Mike Novosel, Louis Rocco, and so many others counterargued and proved through their actions that no, aeromedical evacuation was really "a **medical operation** which entails the **use of aircraft**."[104]

These accumulated experiences brought to fruition the vision of Neel. They established MEDEVAC as a military medical mission that needed its own doctrine and units of detachment and company size, and all under medical control—very possibly in the form of a medical evacuation battalion structured to treat MEDEVAC as a system designed to bring forth the best of the combination of medicine and aviation. They showed that the ever improving helicopter could be a key element in the evacuation process that brought wounded soldiers into the hands of those medical specialists and physicians who could properly treat his wounds. They showed that a cadre of officers and soldiers who were well founded in the intricacies of both elements of that system was needed to forge that "togetherness between medical and aviation" advocated by Neel.

*   *   *   *

It was a proud heritage, one that would carry the MEDEVAC community into the future with confidence and pride, as rising young officers like Doug Moore, Jerry Foust, Jim Truscott, Pat Brady, and so many others mentored the newer troops and made MEDEVAC and the Army even better. It was the kind of heritage that could attract young soldiers into selfless service.

But the MEDEVAC community as well as the Army at large needed time to recover from the strain of the long Vietnam War before addressing new challenges that would arise.

Part Two

Domestic Duties
&
Contingency Operations

Chapter Three
Quiet Years, 1973–1980

"MAST has saved several lives in Texas and has rendered invaluable aid in a large number of cases. I hope that the project will be maintained as a regular program and indeed expanded to every extent possible."
Sen. John Tower[1]

Return to Garrison

Societal Change

With the final withdrawal of Army units from Vietnam in 1973, the MEDEVAC force was either returned to the United States or dispersed to Korea and Europe. Personnel rosters showed that there were 359 Medical Service Corps (MSC) aviators, most of whom with vast combat experience. For them, the remainder of the decade brought few changes to organization, some updating of doctrine, a steady but not overly burdensome operations tempo, and the addition of a new mission, one focused on domestic needs.

The garrison Army to which they returned was very different from the one that had dispatched them to war a decade earlier. Like the nation in general, it had dramatically changed. Vietnam took a toll on American society. The growing antipathy to the war that developed in the late 1960s and early 1970s was in many cases transferred to the soldiers. In numerous documented cases, young soldiers were scorned when they returned home. "Baby killer" was an epithet shouted at many, and soldiers were not welcome on most college campuses. Racial tension was common on the bases because of the social revolution of the 1960s. Many soldiers returned from the war with drug addictions and behavioral and psychological issues. The Army returned home rife with low morale, poor discipline, and reduced military effectiveness. Career officers and noncommissioned officers (NCOs) were severely challenged by these difficult problems.[2]

One young MEDEVAC officer witnessed these developments. 1st Lt. Frank Novier entered the Army in May 1971. He was commissioned into the MSC and posted to a ground job with the 82d Airborne Division at Fort Bragg, North Carolina. A few months later, he was reassigned back to the Army Medical Department Center & School at Fort Sam Houston, Texas, in casual status awaiting a slot in flight training. He received orders to join the 421st Med Co (AA) in Germany after graduating in November 1974. Arriving in early 1975, he did his share of staff duty officer tours while getting mission-qualified. One evening, he handled a major discipline problem when some soldiers were throwing wall lockers out of a barracks. He also noticed that there were places on the post where it was unsafe to walk at night. At the time, he recalled, "Germany was not a real fun place."[3]

He also noticed that most of the pilots were excellent flyers, but highly individualized in their procedures. Many were downright sloppy in their dress, and he did not enjoy flying with them. However, they did teach him a passion for the mission. What was missing was unit pride and cohesion.

Novier said, "They were a reflection of the Army of the 1970s. It was not a very strong Army; it was beaten down from Vietnam. These guys were individual heroes, you didn't have this cohesive feeling of being a unit." He also noticed that the unit did not do any field training. Occasionally, a crew or two would fly out to be near a field exercise. They would land on a hill and monitor their radio for calls. Yet, he sensed that it was all done half-heartedly.[4]

With the end of the military draft on 30 June 1973, the Army had to compete for young men and women in the labor market instead of being infused each year with a new cohort of young soldiers as it had been since World War II. Many wondered if an organization as hidebound as the Army could openly compete or if the nation was prepared to pay a competitive price for young men and women who had other choices. A Presidential Commission was formed in 1969 to study the problem and make recommendations. One commission member, the renowned economist Milton Friedman, argued that it was the only way that a democracy with an open market economy could maintain a standing military. He made his case in a testy exchange with Gen. William Westmoreland, Army Chief of Staff, and former theater commander in Vietnam.

Westmoreland told the commission that he did not want to command an army of mercenaries. Friedman asked, "General, would you rather command an army of slaves?" Westmoreland responded, "I don't like to hear our draftee soldiers referred to as slaves."

Friedman retorted, "I don't like to hear our patriotic volunteers referred to as mercenaries. If they are mercenaries, then I, sir, am a mercenary professor, and you, sir, are a mercenary general; we are served by mercenary physicians, we use a mercenary lawyer, and we get our meat from a mercenary butcher." Friedman's argument carried the day, the military draft was eliminated, and the Army became all volunteer.[5]

To attract qualified young men and now women in the numbers needed to sustain the force structure, the Army initiated a recruiting program. The Army adopted the slogan "Be all that you can be" to attract new troops.[6]

Recruited into the Reserve Officers' Training Corps (ROTC) earlier, Bill Thresher raised his right hand and recited the oath of commission on 21 December 1973, as he became a 2d Lt. in the MSC. Thresher was a recent graduate of Henderson State University, Arkadelphia, Arkansas. He initially intended to take his commission in the armor branch, but he changed his mind when he learned that his chances of flying were better in the MSC. When he reported for active duty, he was ordered to Fort Bragg for duty with the 5th Combat Support Hospital as a medical logistics officer. It lasted a little more than a year as he awaited orders to flight school. However, it was an eventful tour. Thresher was impressed with the sense of mission that permeated all of the units assigned to the XVIII Airborne Corps.

He remembered: "Everything there was about urgency. You have got to be ready to go, constantly under the gun for emergency deployment readiness exercises." He also saw the key part that the MSC officers played as the facilitators for the clinicians. It gave him a keen appreciation for the role they played serving both the profession of medicine and the profession of arms. It also gave him a strong fundamental knowledge of Army medicine that benefited him later. After 14 months at Fort Bragg, he was assigned to Fort Rucker, Alabama, for his flight training.[7]

Operations

Garrison Duty

After graduating from flight school in February 1976, 2d Lt. Thresher was posted back to Fort Bragg to serve with the 57th Med Det (RA), led by a tough commander, Major Bob Rose. Rose was a Vietnam veteran and a rigorous leader. Thresher found that same sense of urgency he had experienced on his earlier assignment and saw that it made perfect sense for a MEDEVAC unit. Another Vietnam veteran, Capt. Bill Kruse, who was the consummate pilot and held nearly every qualification possible, also mentored him. Thresher wanted to fly a lot, and Kruse taught him all manner of tactics and techniques in the cockpit that were hard learned in Vietnam. It was invaluable mentoring and the key way that flight experience was passed to new pilots. No fully standardized flight procedures existed then, and published flight manuals offered only the barest explanations of tactics and techniques.

Thresher's very first operational mission was to recover a soldier from the Sicily drop zone who was killed when both of his parachutes failed. Loading that soldier and another with a broken leg sustained in the jump onto his aircraft delivered to the young lieutenant the reality of his chosen career field. Thresher learned the basics quickly, and with barely 50 hours in the UH-1, he was upgraded to aircraft commander. As he steadily logged missions and hours, he grew to enjoy the mission and flying, and developed a deep appreciation for what it was giving him.

He said:

> It was a great grooming ground for responsibility because when you are the pilot in command of your aircraft with a kid in the back who has deviated his spine on Holland Drop Zone … and your copilot has got less time than you do, you learn responsibility pretty quick. …and this soldier in the back is depending on you. His mother and father are depending on you; his kids are depending on you. It's an obligation and you can't let him down. …The reason he is alive today, theoretically, is that you were able to get there within seven, eight minutes and get him to a hospital within twelve minutes so somebody then could do their job. … The medic on the ground who treats the guy when he is first hurt and the doctor who saves his life at the hospital—they are both critical but you are the glue between the two of them. That's what the 57th meant to me.[8]

In general, the MEDEVAC units did not suffer the same type of discipline problems rife throughout the Army then. In part, this resulted from the fact that all medical personnel were volunteer specialists of some sort who had to score higher on their entrance exams and then complete difficult training to get their jobs. In December 1977, now Capt. Bill Thresher was abruptly removed from flying duties and assigned to command the 429th Med Co, a ground ambulance unit. He inherited a poorly performing unit with a number of discipline problems that required him to issue several nonjudicial punishments or even discharges. Initially, he feared that his strong actions would alienate his other troops. However, he found that by taking firm actions against the recalcitrant ones, the good troops rallied to him. He instilled in them the sense of urgency he had learned in his previous units and turned the 429th into a very sharp unit.[9]

But Thresher's experiences were somewhat the exception. The Army also had to take internal steps to change the way it fundamentally did business. It had to get soldiers back to the basics of soldiering by hiring civilians to perform the mundane chores such as KP, grass cutting, and guard duty.

Training had to be refocused to provide more exciting and meaningful endeavors. It also had to be redesigned to encourage the development of initiative, self-reliance, moral and physical courage, and mutual confidence. Soldiers had to be encouraged to take advantage of educational opportunities—both on and off base—and develop a logical learning progression that would last throughout their career. The Army reenergized its programs to develop professional leadership for both officers and NCOs. It had to establish an NCO educational system for the development of sergeants at all levels. It also had to realign the officer assignment system to allow for stabilized tours for commanders, something that had been badly broken by the personnel turbulence caused by the rapid buildup and just as rapid inactivation of units for the Vietnam War.

Perhaps most important, it had to improve the quality of life for the soldiers. The barracks needed to be upgraded to allow for privacy. Better housing had to be built for Army families. Facilities on base such as the post exchanges, personnel offices, and gymnasiums needed to be improved. Health care had to be expanded, with longer clinic duty hours more convenient for the troops. Soldier pay needed to be improved to make it competitive with what an enlistee could earn on the outside. All of these items required increased funding, and Congress supported them with increased appropriations starting in fiscal year 1973.[10]

In the mid-1970s, Lt. Col. Pat Brady was given command of the 326th Medical Battalion, 101st Airborne Division, at Fort Campbell, Kentucky. He had not served directly with troops for a while, and was shocked at what he found. Much of his time was taken up with disciplinary problems and drug use.

Brady remembered the following: "There was a permissiveness coming out of society that overflowed into the Army. I think probably the best way to describe it was the slogan of the time… 'Today's Army wants to join you.'" He believed that many of the troops that were entering the Army then were inferior to the soldiers with whom he had served in Vietnam and other earlier assignments. He further believed that too many of recruits brought with them "disciplinary problems that detracted from training."[11]

Maj. Doug Moore watched these developments from his position as the deputy commander for administration at the U.S. Army Medical Department Activity at Hunter Army Airfield, Georgia. In the summer of 1973, as a new Lt. Col., he reported to Fort Leavenworth, Kansas, to attend the Army Command and General Staff College. While there as a "token medic," he wrote a paper about the future uses of air ambulance units. His unpublished paper, titled "Air Ambulance Support for the Combat Division," was a forward-looking analysis of necessary air ambulance unit structure based on projected threats and missions. He proposed increasing the number of air ambulances necessary directly to support a division from six to 10. He also raised questions about the proper way to command and control them, provide for aircraft maintenance, and deal with the increasing sophistication of communications, navigation, and airspace control. He also suggested that MEDEVAC doctrine needed to be updated with these changes—all prescient thoughts as future events would show.[12]

Recruitment

Initial results for the new recruitment program were disappointing. During the fiscal year ending June 1972, only 68.5% of the needed quota of new enlistees was met. However, by Christmas, recruiting began to bottom out. By the end of fiscal year 1973, the enlistment rates exceeded 100%. Two reasons were cited for the turnaround: (1) The Army was smaller than it had been since well before the Vietnam buildup; and (2) Congress also helped by providing recruiting bonuses for 32 critical skills and incentive bonuses for recruiters.[13]

At the same time, a reduction-in-force for officers was enforced. The buildup of forces in Vietnam had created a huge bulge in the officer corps in year groups 1967 to 1970. Before Vietnam, officer strength had comprised about 11.6% of the total Army manpower. By 1972, it swelled to 14.9%. For long-term stability, it had to be reduced to 13.7%. In 1972 and 1973, reduction-in-force boards were held, and 4,900 officers were released.[14]

Another paradigm shift was the active recruitment of women. Since 1948, the Army had limited the number of women to no more than 2% of total end strength.

They were restricted almost exclusively to the clerical and supply fields. Married women could not join, and women who became pregnant were discharged.

These restrictions were slowly lifted. In 1973, 10,900 women joined the Army. Capt. Jerry Foust, serving as an instructor at the Academy of Health Sciences at Fort Sam Houston, saw some of the first to come into the medical branches. He was impressed. "The first women who went through the school did just fine," he said, "They were smart." The numbers steadily increased, and by 1978, there were more than 53,000 women in the service. Female recruits were a key factor in the Army achieving its recruitment needs.[15]

As numbers increased, restrictions on assignments for women were relaxed, and they spread into almost all elements of the Army. In 1976, women were allowed into the U.S. Military Academy at West Point, and 119 entered the class of 1980. In the Reserve Components, female membership also steadily rose. By 1982, more than 38,000 women were serving in the U.S. Army Reserve (USAR). Women were also strongly encouraged to enter the ROTC program, and their numbers exceeded 5,000 active participants by the end of the decade. The integration of women into the Army was so successful and complete that the Women's Army Corps, in existence since 1942, was disestablished in 1978, and women were assigned to branches just like the men.[16]

The introduction of women into what had traditionally been an all-male environment led to a rapid increase in incidents of sexual harassment and fraternization. The Army soon realized that it needed to establish new rules and procedures to regulate soldier behavior. Firm guidelines were established that defined improper fraternization, especially between superiors and subordinates. The problems were never completely solved, but the trends turned positive as women began to firmly establish themselves in their chosen fields as professionals fully capable of doing their jobs and fully deserving of the respect due to them as professionals. The Army was truly no longer "your father's Army."[17]

Moore witnessed those changes. After staff college he attended airborne qualification training at Fort Benning, Georgia, and then reported to Fort Bragg, to command the 307th Medical Battalion, 82d Airborne Division. It was an intense two-year assignment because the division always had to have a brigade-sized force ready to deploy, and that included a company from his battalion. At the end of that assignment, he was directed to attend the Army War College at Carlisle Barracks, Pennsylvania, and was one of only six MSC officers selected.

He mixed with a broad swath of Army and other service officers, plus rising leaders from other governmental agencies and even other nations. It was a time of learning as they collectively struggled with the issues roiling the Army and nation. They discussed the efforts to rebuild and restructure the military. This experience was a good foundation to his next assignment with the Inspector General of the Army.[18]

In 1977, the MSC of the Army made a concerted effort to increase the number of females serving in that branch. At the MSC's request, the Recruiting Command conducted surveys among women already serving. Most indicated satisfaction with the progress of their careers, although many complained of sexual bias. More than two-thirds preferred the MSC to other branches. The MSC made some positive changes to its recruiting effort, and the results were very positive. From a low of just 7 female officers in 1968, the MSC had 544 serving by 1987, most joining after 1977. Some joined to fly as MEDEVAC pilots.[19]

In February 1979, in response to the increased recruiting efforts to bring more women into the MSC, 1st Lt. Karen Anderson graduated from flight training at Fort Rucker and became the first female MEDEVAC pilot. She joined the 247th Med Det (RA) at Fort Meade, Maryland, as a medical evacuation pilot.[20]

Organization

Units

In September 1973, the active Army MEDEVAC units were located at the following places:

United States

498th Med Co (AA)	Fort Benning, Georgia
507th Med Co (AA)	Fort Sam Houston, Texas
54th Med Det (RA)	Fort Lewis, Washington
57th Med Det (RA)	Fort Bragg, North Carolina
	(replaced the 151st Med Det that inactivated)
68th Med Det (RA)	Schofield Barracks, Hawaii
237th Med Det (RA)	Fort Ord, California
	(replaced the 32d Med Det that inactivated)
247th Med Det (RA)	Fort Meade, Maryland
283d Med Det (RA)	Fort Bliss, Texas
571st Med Det (RA)	Fort Carson, Colorado
AA Platoon, 326th Med Battalion, 101st ABN Div	Fort Campbell, Kentucky

Germany

421st Med Co (AA)	Stuttgart – with platoons also at Schweinfurt and Darmstadt
15th Med Det (RA)	Grafenwöhr
63d Med Det (RA)	Landstuhl
159th Med Det (RA)	Bremerhaven
236th Med Det (RA)	Augsburg

Korea

377th Med Co (AA)	Yongsan, Korea[21]

Throughout the decade, units would be reassigned and moved. In 1975, two more units, the 36th Med Det (RA) at Fort Polk, Louisiana, and the 431st Med Det (RA) at Fort Knox, Kentucky, were activated. In October 1979, the 283d Med Det (RA) moved from Fort Bliss to Fort Wainwright, Alaska. The next year, the 247th Med Det (RA) was moved from Fort Meade to Fort Irwin, California.[22]

Personnel Movements

Like the units, the personnel of MEDEVAC were also periodically reassigned as they progressed steadily through their careers. After graduating from the Army Command and General Staff College in June 1973, Maj. Jim Truscott went to Headquarters, European Command, located near Stuttgart, Germany, as an operations officer, an assignment that gave him a unique opportunity as a relatively junior officer to participate in joint and combined operations. A year later, he was reassigned back to the 63d Med Det (RA), now at Landstuhl, the same unit that he had commanded six years prior, but now equipped with six UH-1H helicopters and a full complement of pilots, medics, and support personnel. Their mission was to provide evacuation of sick and injured essentially from locations along the Rhine River to hospital locations. They were under the operational control of the 421st Med Co (AA). The unit received its logistical support from aviation maintenance and logistical units in the area. Truscott rapidly developed the skills necessary to work with both the medical and aviation communities to perform his mission.[23]

One hundred and eighty miles to the southeast, 1st Lt. Art Hapner and the 236th Med Det (RA) had settled into their facilities just northwest of Augsburg. Their six UH-1Hs had all flown in Vietnam and were completely refurbished. The pilots were a mixed lot, with one-half also Vietnam veterans. Many were not fully trained to fly in instrument conditions, and the unit had to set up an internal program to do so. The unit primarily supported field units, but also had occasional taskings to support the local communities. The pilots occasionally flew to Garmisch to pick up patients. Pilots in the unit became very adept at instrument and international flying. Hapner served with the 236th until 1976, when he was sent back to Fort Sam Houston for the MSC advanced course.[24]

Reserve Component Units in the Total Force

Another fundamental change was afoot within the Army. The active component was always supported by a large Reserve Component that had two subcomponents: (1) the USAR, and (2) the 54 Army National Guards (ARNGs) of the individual states, Washington, DC, Puerto Rico, Guam, and the Virgin Islands. In times of war, the units from both subcomponents were activated for federal service and fought alongside their active duty fellow soldiers. However, during the Vietnam War, for political reasons, there were only minor activations of Reserve Component forces. As the nation withdrew from the conflict, Secretary of

Defense Melvin Laird announced in 1970 a "Total Force" concept that would reintegrate the active and Reserve Components so that in future wars, both would be relied on to serve the nation. In 1973, this concept became official policy, and more force structure was moved into the two Reserve Components.

Traditionally, the ARNG units had been composed primarily of combat type units while the USAR consisted mostly of combat support and combat service support formations, especially medical units. But the break was not clean. Congressional pressure and constant intervention resulted in each component having units of all types. During the Vietnam War, Secretary of Defense Robert McNamara tried to combine the ARNG and USAR. He was decisively blocked by congressional action and while the traditional split was maintained in theory, in reality, both components received authorizations for combat, combat support, and combat service support units protected by yearly appropriations laws that were subject to constant congressional involvement.[25]

To make these forces more capable of rapidly activating and operating with the active duty Army units, they received newer equipment and authorizations for more full-time personnel to ensure continuity of training and administrative matters. Additionally, the current Army Chief of Staff Gen. Creighton Abrams believed that the nation had made a terrible mistake in the Vietnam War by not calling on the ARNG and USAR to participate in the conflict. He saw the early and committed use of the Reserve Components as vitally necessary for sustaining the national will in time of war. Thus, he directed the Army to take specific steps to structure its combat forces so that it could not be committed to anything more than short duration contingency operations without calling on its Reserve Components. By the end of 1973, two-thirds of the combat support and combat service support units needed to sustain the Army in the field were in the Reserve Components. Although Reserve Component manning initially dipped during the 1970s, the units received new equipment and grew in later years.[26]

This restructuring affected the MEDEVAC force. More units were authorized for both components. The USAR activated new detachments. In most cases, the various states converted already existing ARNG units into MEDEVAC companies and detachments. In the mid 1970s, the following units were active in reserve status in the two components:

Army Reserve (USAR)

145th Med Det (RA)	Marietta, Georgia
273d Med Det (RA)	Tomball, Texas
321st Med Det (RA)	Salt Lake City, Utah
343d Med Det (RA)	Hamilton AFB, California
347th Med Det (RA)	Miami, Florida
348th Med Det (RA)	Orlando, Florida
412th Med Det (RA)	Louisville, Kentucky
872d Med Det (RA)	Lafayette, Louisiana[27]

Army National Guard (ARNG)

24th Med Co (AA)	Nebraska
112th Med Co (AA)	Maine
123d Med Co (AA)	Mississippi
126th Med Co (AA)	California
1187th Med Co (AA)	Iowa
142d Med Det (RA)	North Dakota
146th Med Det (RA)	West Virginia
397th Med Det (RA)	New Hampshire
400th Med Det (RA)	Washington, DC
441st Med Det (RA)	Kentucky
470th Med Det (RA)	Kentucky
670th Med Det (RA)	Tennessee
717th Med Det (RA)	New Mexico
812th Med Det (RA)	Louisiana
813th Med Det (RA)	Louisiana
841st Med Det (RA)	Washington
867th Med Det (RA)	Missouri
868th Med Det (RA)	Missouri
920th Med Det (RA)	Kansas
986th Med Det (RA)	Virginia
1022d Med Det (RA)	Wyoming
1059th Med Det (RA)	Massachusetts
1085th Med Det (RA)	South Dakota
1134th Med Det (RA)	Alabama
1136th Med Det (RA)	Texas
1150th Med Det (RA)	Nevada[28]

A New National Mission for MEDEVAC

Operations

Military Assistance to Safety and Traffic

Concept. As the active duty Army struggled with the difficult challenges of the post–Vietnam era, several of the stateside MEDEVAC units received taskings under a new program called Military Assistance to Safety and Traffic (MAST). Many individuals participated in its development including Spurgeon Neel, a key contributor, who throughout the 1960s constantly wrote and spoke about the use of helicopters in medical care. His efforts drew the attention of civilian medical leaders who asked for a civilian version of MEDEVAC.

In February 1969, Dr. Charles Atkinson, a physician from Florida wrote to then Col. Neel, serving as the Director of Plans, Supply, and Operations on the Office of The Surgeon General staff. Atkinson read one of Neel's articles and was interested in possibly procuring Army MEDEVAC support for his community.

Neel replied:

> The concept of using air ambulances in the highway safety program appears to be a very valid approach to the problem of getting the patient to professional care as soon as possible....The helicopter air ambulance is solving our major evacuation problems and I believe will solve yours also.[29]

Two months later Neel wrote an article for the *Journal of the American Medical Association* in which he stated: "The experiences that the Army Medical Service has gained in the utilization of helicopter ambulances can and, I believe, must be translated into comparable civilian emergency health programs." He also pointed out that Army MEDEVAC elements at Fort Rucker and Fort Sam Houston had performed local rescues of highway accidents on an ad-hoc basis since 1966.[30]

Others within the Army also pushed the concept. Lt. Col. Robert Sears, a career aviator, proposed an "Air Medical Evacuation System" in his master's thesis while attending the School of Engineering at Arizona State University in 1968. His paper proposed a "concept of utilizing helicopters as a means to transport the seriously injured to a medical facility capable of treating the specific injuries, with complete independence from road and traffic conditions ..." He specifically noted that, "The U.S. Army has pioneered the field of helicopter evacuation and has proved the effectiveness of the concept."[31]

After graduating from Arizona State University, Sears served in the office of the Assistant Vice Chief of Staff of the Army, Gen. William E. DePuy. He briefed DePuy on the program and concept. DePuy gained approval for Sears to develop the idea and initially send it out for staff coordination on feasibility. The responses were generally favorable with questions raised about financing, legal authorities, etc. The ARNG was especially supportive, seeing its units as key participants, but noting that they would have to be reequipped with newer helicopters.[32]

Concurrently, the Departments of Transportation and Health, Education, and Welfare also considered similar proposals. Operation SKY-AID, the test program run by the 24th Med Co (AA), Nebraska ARNG in 1968 and 1969, had shown the efficacy of domestic MEDEVAC and portended great promise. After the Secretary of the Army, Stanley Resor, was briefed on the Air Medical Evacuation System proposal, he sent a memorandum to Melvin Laird, Secretary of Defense, stating that he believed that the project held great promise. For several months, Laird discussed this very idea with the Secretary of Transportation. In response, Laird appointed Resor and the Army to serve as the executive agent for the Department of Defense (DOD) on the matter, making him (Resor) the decision authority for all Air Medical Evacuation System matters involving the DOD and directing him to initiate an interagency study group to determine the best course of action.[33]

Test. The interagency study group formed and worked through the fall and winter. The Department of Transportation actually chaired the study group because it had already funded several test projects under the Highway Safety Act.

In April 1970, the study group visited Fort Sam Houston to observe the 507th Med Co (AA). The group also considered Army Reserve Component units for the program and visited the 24th Med Co (AA) at Lincoln, Nebraska, to hear about its success with Operation SKY-AID. In May, they presented a development plan for a test of the now renamed MAST program. The 507th Med Co (AA) was directed to be ready by June to provide coverage over San Antonio and the adjoining 10 counties. The test began 1 July and ran until the end of the year. Each governmental department would fund its own incurred costs.[34]

Subsequent discussions between DOD and the Department of Transportation determined that the initial test would be expanded to five locations, none of which would initially include a Guard or Reserve unit. The sites were selected based on the location of military units, a state government's expression of interest and support, a rural environment contiguous to adequate medical facilities, and different climate and terrain conditions.

First Mission. The operation at Fort Sam Houston started 15 July 1970. The first call came two days later. A young man had been run over by a tractor in Dilley, Texas, 84 miles away, sustaining a broken leg and shoulder and internal injuries. Two minutes after the call was received, a 507th MEDEVAC helicopter under the command of Capt. Sam McLamb lifted off and sped to the scene. The subsequent return flight to the hospital took 30 minutes, well short of the 90 minutes required by a ground ambulance. The value of MAST was immediately clear. Later, McLamb stated that, "It was the closest thing to a Vietnam Dustoff mission one could imagine. It included the same tension and speed … everything but the hostile fire."[35]

Additional Army operations were started on 6 August with the 78th Med Det (RA) at Fort Carson and the 54th Med Det (RA) at Fort Lewis. The U.S. Air Force also participated and opened MAST operations with detachments of the 42d Aerospace Rescue and Recovery Squadron at Luke Air Force Base, Arizona, and Mountain Home Air Force Base, Idaho, on 1 September 1970. At each location, the operation was crafted with the support of local authorities. It was clearly understood that military usage would not replace or compete with local services. The helicopters would not be used in areas where ground ambulances could better respond. Requests for helicopter assistance were based on the judgment of medical or emergency personnel at the scene who believed that the medical situation was life-threatening and required expeditious helicopter transport to a facility capable of providing the necessary care.[36]

Secretary Laird made a trip to San Antonio to observe the program. Watching a 507th helicopter deliver a patient injured in an automobile accident, he pointed out that highway accidents were the greatest killer of young men in America. He added, "When I saw the rapid evacuation and treatment of casualties in Vietnam, I thought this was one lesson we could apply at home."[37]

The test ran through December. The 507th logged 114 missions and recovered 138 patients. All other units were dramatically lower, with the Mountain Home and Luke units only logging four and five missions, respectively, because they

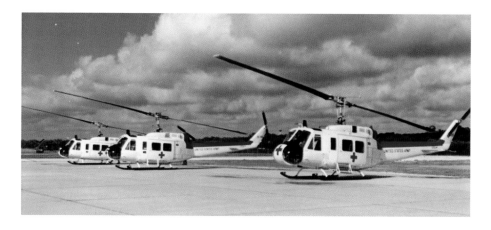

White UH-1s from the 507th Med Co, Fort Sam Houston, Texas, performing MAST duty in the 1970s. Source: Army Medical Department Museum.

only made crews and aircraft available for a limited period each day. The 54th at Fort Lewis flew 34 missions and carried 41 patients. Unfortunately, one of its crews suffered a fatal crash, and subsequently, the local authorities were reluctant to call them out, fearing another accident.

Limitations in communications gear were noted, and localized procedures had to be resolved. Overall, the program was successful. Some local resistance occurred because a few local ambulance companies perceived the use of the military assets as unfair competition. From a military perspective, the report noted that:

> It proved desirable from the standpoint of training and motivation for the medical unit in particular. Aeromedical evacuation procedures developed for combat situations are readily transferable to civilian applications. Public acceptance of the concept was clearly established and reflected most favorably upon the military. ... MAST operations were a 'natural' for the medical company ... [38]

The Interagency Group completed the test phase with several conclusions:

1. Even though the short test was based on limited operational experience, the concept appears to be sound from a military and civilian perspective.
2. The military possesses significant capability for providing assistance that does not necessarily exist within civilian companies due to financial considerations.
3. Army MEDEVAC units are particularly well suited for the missions that provide realistic training and motivation for assigned personnel.
4. Tactical aviation units can provide the support, but it diverts them from their primary mission.
5. Air Force rescue units have limited manning and equipment and require augmentation to provide 24/7 coverage.

6. The test indicates that participating units suffered no degradation of unit integrity, effectiveness, training, or ability to do their primary mission.
7. Availability of military assets does not mean that the local communities will necessarily use it.
8. Less than full-time availability of assets restricts community requests for the services.
9. The local community emergency medical system must be capable of integrating with the military unit for proper and timely notification, coordination, and communication.
10. The general public and medical and law enforcement officials show a high degree of acceptance of the program.
11. Military units supporting MAST operations do not require any additional money, personnel, or aircraft.[39]

At Fort Rucker, the home of Army Aviation, Commander Maj. Gen. William J. Maddox, Jr. watched the process very closely and was pleased with what he saw:

> I examined the interim test report… and decided that MAST was well within the capability of Army units to handle… I concluded that the MAST program was in line with the readiness objectives we have for Army units because it provides a method of giving our people an opportunity to have a life saving and operational mission as opposed to a routine training mission.[40]

Continued Operations. Even though the MAST test was concluded, the operations did not stop. As word of the program's success spread, more units wanted to participate, and discussions began about utilizing Guard and Reserve units. Many received newer equipment, and their close relationships with their communities ensured early acceptance of the new capability. The governors of Nebraska and Idaho asked to participate. The Governor of Arizona was especially interested. He was aware of Sears' work at Arizona State University and requested that the 997th Medical Company (AA) of the Arizona ARNG be included in the program. However, ARNG participation needed legal determination before it could occur.

Enabling Legislation. Political support for the program began to develop. Congressmen J.J. Pickle and Abraham Kazan of Texas both submitted statements of support for the program into the *Congressional Record*. Senator John Tower, also from Texas, wrote a strong letter to the Secretary of Defense in which he stated, "MAST has saved several lives in Texas and has rendered invaluable aid in a large number of cases. I hope that the project will be maintained as a regular program and indeed expanded to every extent possible." Numerous city mayors from across the nation, like Franklin Keller of Lacoste, Texas, copied his efforts. Keller wrote, "Please do all you can to have the lifesaving service of MAST continued and expanded throughout our area. I feel this is a very worthwhile service and should by all means be continued."[41]

In 1971, President Nixon called for increased medical support for rural areas as national policy. Political support continued to grow for MAST as congressional and executive branch offices received letters of endorsement and city council resolutions of support. The next year Congress passed and the President signed Public Law 93-155, authorizing (but not requiring) the use of DOD helicopter resources in a continuing medical emergency transport role in the civilian community. The law also specified some limitations:

1. Assistance could only be provided in areas where military units able to provide assistance were regularly assigned, and military units could not be transferred from one area to another for providing such assistance.
2. Assistance could be provided only to the extent that it did not interfere with the performance of the military mission.
3. The provision of assistance would not cause any increase in funds required for the operation of the DOD.[42]

In addition to these limitations, the Secretary of Defense set several more restrictive policies for the program:

1. Military units would not compete for emergency medical evacuation missions in areas where civilian operators could provide comparable support.
2. Military support would be accomplished only as a by-product of and within the Military Department's annual training program and without adverse impact on the primary military mission. MAST sites would be established adjacent to installations only where air ambulance or rescue units were regularly assigned and aeromedical personnel and equipment were available.
3. MAST operations could be discontinued with little or no advance notice because of DOD priorities.[43]

By January 1974, the five original MAST designated units had flown 2,456 missions and carried 2,773 patients.[44]

Within the next several months, several more units received MAST taskings. The 57th Med Det (RA) at Fort Bragg, the Air Ambulance Platoon of the 326th Medical Battalion at Fort Campbell, the 68th Med Det (RA) at Schofield Barracks, the 82d Med Det (RA) at Fort Riley, Kansas, the 237th Med Det (RA) at Fort Ord, and the 498th Med Co (AA) at Fort Benning with platoons at other locations all assumed MAST duties to the great delight of their local communities. Two years later, the 273d Med Det (RA), an Army Reserve unit at Tomball, Texas, became the first Reserve Component unit to also assume MAST tasking. There were many more within the next year, as MAST became a major consumer of the services of the Army's active and Reserve Component MEDEVAC community.[45]

At Fort Sam Houston, Capt. Jerry Foust became a self-described "talking dog" for MAST. He was sent to cities and towns across Texas, Louisiana, New Mexico, and the midwest to relay the positive things that MAST could do for their communities. He loved the assignment.[46]

At one point, Foust encountered a young lieutenant named Dan Gower, who had graduated from Texas A&M University in 1970 and commissioned into the infantry. He asked for and received orders for flight school. While at Fort Rucker, he and his wife were injured by a tornado. Consequently, he had to request a humanitarian assignment back to Fort Sam Houston after graduation.

There he was assigned to the 507th. Foust liked Gower and convinced him to branch transfer to MSC. Gower transferred and flew his fair share of MAST missions.[47]

In addition to his flying obligations, his first position in the unit was to serve as the administrative officer that thrust him into the myriad social issues prevalent then. He had troops in trouble for drugs and alcohol abuse, and several had to be discharged. He dealt with racial tensions. In general, Gower noticed that the soldiers who came to MEDEVAC were a bit more mature and stable than troops in other units. They understood the importance of MEDEVAC and accepted the necessary training and focus necessary to accomplish the mission.

During his time with the unit, the 507th received some of the first women to enter the MEDEVAC mission area. Their first female medic was Spc. Donarita Czerwinski. Her first real mission after qualification was a MAST scramble to recover a farmer who fell into a combine that chopped his legs off just below his groin. She handled the difficult mission because the "old head" Vietnam veterans had trained her. Gower was proud of her and his other soldiers. He served with the 507th until 1977 when he attended the MSC advanced course and transferred to the 68th Med Det (RA) in Hawaii.[48]

MAST Continues to Grow. The next unit to join the MAST program was the 431st Med Det (RA) at Fort Knox, Kentucky. Activated in the spring of 1975, it began participating in MAST almost immediately. By September 1976, more than 8,200 MAST missions had recovered 8,613 patients. Helicopters from Army and Air Force units—both active and Reserve—were on call at 22 locations across the United States. Missions came in all varieties. A crew from the 571st Med Det (RA) at Fort Carson was launched to pick up a young soldier's wife who was going into labor four weeks early. They picked her up for transport to the Fitzsimons Army Medical Center in Denver. However, en route at 8,000 feet she gave birth to a four-pound daughter who was delivered by the flight medics, Sp5 Tom Haverkorn and Pfc. Debra Kleinfelter.[49]

In another incident, a backpacker fell on Mount Rainer and slid down 1,500 feet, receiving severe internal injuries, fractured ribs, etc. He suffered from exposure to the harsh elements. Park rangers were notified late at night and determined that it would take several hours to rescue him with a ground team. They called the 54th Med Det (RA) at Fort Lewis for help. At first light they launched a UH-1 MEDEVAC helicopter. The backpacker was on a glacier with jagged ice at 9,500 feet elevation. The pilot held the helicopter on one skid as the crew recovered the man. They evacuated him to a hospital in Takoma.

The Air Ambulance Platoon of the 326th Medical Battalion at Fort Campbell also became very busy with MAST calls. In two days in June 1976, both aircraft and

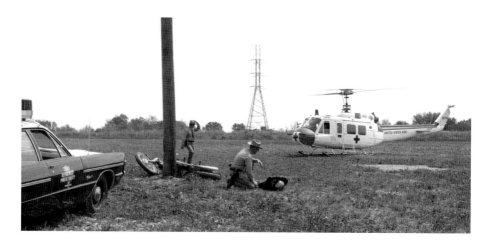

A 507th Med Co crew responding to a MAST call.
Source: Army Medical Department Museum.

crews on call were dispatched six times to answer various calls to do the following:

1. Respond to an aircraft accident;
2. Transport a burn victim;
3. Carry emergency blood supplies (twice);
4. Transport a patient with a brain tumor; and
5. Transport a day old baby with birth defects.

These flights provided needed services to the communities involved and excellent training for the crews involved.

In California, a bad storm capsized a small boat off of Santa Cruz in the Monterey Bay. A patrol boat tried to save the occupants, but was itself swamped, and its crew of two had to swim to shore. A UH-1 from the 237th Med Det (RA) at Fort Ord was dispatched and rescued the crew of three in 15 minutes.

In still another illustrative incident in 1976, a butane truck exploded in Eagle Pass, Texas. Ten people were killed and 40 were injured. The 507th Med Co (AA) at Fort Sam Houston was called for help. The unit launched six helicopters that stopped at local hospitals to transport needed on-site medical personnel. Then the helicopters made seven trips back to several San Antonio hospitals to deliver 22 injured people. Representative Abraham Kazan was deeply appreciative and wrote a thank-you letter to the unit. "Be assured of my continued support of the MAST program and my deep appreciation for your aid to people in need...."

A witness to the entire incident, Texas Highway Patrolman Ken Phillips, also wrote to the unit. "I hope the MAST program will be expanded to include other areas in Texas that are remote from expert medical care." The dedication, courage, and skill of the men and women of the MAST units proved its worth in saving lives, obtaining prompt medical attention for the seriously injured, and reducing suffering. MAST brought the military and local communities together while also providing excellent training for the crews. The program showed success beyond its expectations, and the Eagle Pass mission was recorded as one of the most memorable. By March 1977, the 507th and its two separate platoons had recorded the recovery of 2,000 patients.[50]

Crash Rescue

The MEDEVAC units were also considered for other missions. One was crash rescue. A small number of UH-1s was outfitted with fire suppression kits for use in recovering aircrews from burning aircraft. The helicopters were modified with an extendable boom that could spray 50 gallons of water forward of the aircraft. Theoretically, the spray could suppress flames long enough so that the medic and the crew chief—who was specifically trained in firefighting—could dismount, enter the wreckage, and pull out the trapped survivors.

Three units, the 132d Med Det (RC) at Fort Bragg, commanded by Capt. Glen Flint, the 214th Med Det (RC) at Fort Belvoir, Virginia, and the 218th Med Det (RC) at Fort Hood, Texas, were activated in 1971. Each unit had two aircraft, five pilots, three medics, and three crew chiefs, plus a small maintenance team. All were fully operational within a year. However, there was little need for their services. By 1975, all three units were inactivated. Their personnel and equipment returned to conventional MEDEVAC units that were then assigned crash and rescue duties as a secondary mission, but without the fire suppression kits.[51]

Refocusing on the Future

Organization

Europe

At mid-decade, the MEDEVAC units in Europe focused primarily around the field Army units located in central and southern Germany. The 421st Med Co (AA) located at Nellingen with its 1st and 3d Platoons owned or controlled 49 aircraft. Its 2d Platoon was located at Schweinfurt, and its 4th was at Darmstadt. The 421st also had several individual detachments assigned to it. The 15th Med Det (RA) was at the Grafenwöhr training complex where large combat units routinely rotated through for weapons training. The 63d Med Det (RA) was at Landstuhl and primarily performed intra-theater transfers. The 159th Med Det (RA) at Nürnberg and the 236th Med Det (RA) at Augsburg provided general support to large Army units in their area. All could be called upon to support Army dependents who were sick or somehow injured. Commanders also developed local relationships similar to the MAST program in the United States, which allowed the MEDEVAC units to respond to requests from the local German governments for medical help.[52]

Commanders wrestled with the unique issues facing MEDEVAC flying in Europe. The single biggest challenge was the weather. Europe experienced four distinct seasons, and the flying there, especially in southern Germany, could be very challenging. The units required all pilots to become proficient at all-weather flying.

There were other challenges. The improving capabilities of the Soviet and Warsaw Pact forces to the east could not be ignored. MEDEVAC pilots had to be proficient at low-level or nap-of-the-earth flying to avoid improved enemy air defense weapons. One company commander, Maj. William Wood, wrote: "A pressing need exists for an Army-wide reassessment of air evacuation employment on the European battlefield… In many areas MEDEVAC doctrine remains to be developed." Those were prescient words, shared by others in other arenas. But change sometimes comes slowly.[53]

In 1976, Maj. Jim Truscott took command of the 421st. Although organized as a company command, it actually functioned as a battalion, and he found the challenges daunting. With his units scattered all over Germany, he constantly coordinated

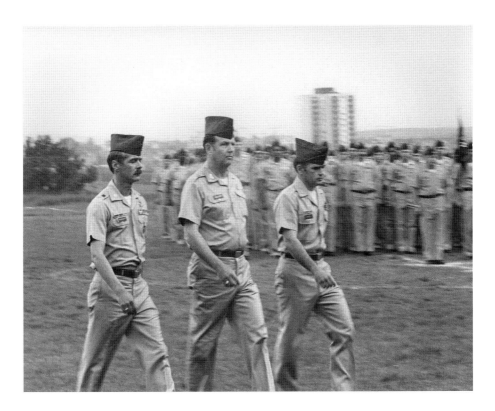

Lt. Col. Jim Truscott (left), with Col. Jim Walker, commander of the 30th Med Group, as Truscott passes command of the 421st Med Co to Maj. Tom Scofield (right) then located at Stuttgart, Germany, in June 1978.
Source: Jim Truscott.

with and answered to several widely dispersed commands. His unit provided on-call service for local German governments, similar to MAST in the United States. Theoretically, they were only supposed to fly when German assets were not available. However, the Germans only flew in the daytime, which meant that the 421st received frequent calls at night. Truscott realized the value of such missions. Almost all were flown single-ship, which meant that all pilots learned rapidly how to make tough operational decisions. Additionally, he pushed them to develop their instrument flight skills to deal with the challenging weather, and he instituted an internal instrument course for some pilots who had weak skills. He removed several pilots from flight status because they either could not or would not improve their flight skills to handle the challenging European weather. When the weather was fine, he encouraged them to fly nap-of-the-earth and develop their tactical skills. His pilots rose to the challenge and enjoyed the flying. He also stressed strict risk management techniques. During his two-year command of the unit, they had no accidents. Truscott's talent and potential were both recognized, and he was promoted to Lt. Col.[54]

Doctrine

Field Manual (FM) 100-5, Operations, July 1976

Moving away from the searing experiences of Vietnam, the Army began an intensive effort to look forward and, as necessary, redefine its warfighting and supporting doctrine for the threats of the future. There existed cause for concern. Although the nation had been exhaustively engaged in that conflict, the Soviet Union and its client Warsaw Pact countries had steadily built up their forces arrayed across the central plains of Europe, both in terms of quantity and quality. New tanks, artillery, and air defense weapons indicated that perhaps the eastern forces were preparing— at some point—to move against the North Atlantic Treaty Organization alliance nations in a bid to establish hegemony over the entire region. The power of Soviet doctrine and technology was validated in 1973 when Arab nations allied with the Soviet Union dealt a devastating blow against Israel, a nation that had designed its defense force around western doctrine and equipment. American soldiers who later toured the battlefields of that conflict saw firsthand the lethality of current Soviet tanks, artillery, antitank weapons, and antiaircraft missile systems, and knew that they presaged a new and vastly more dangerous future for conventional war.[55]

Leading this reexamination of basic doctrine was Gen. William E. DePuy, now the commander of the newly formed U.S. Army Training and Doctrine Command. He had served as an infantry officer in World War II and commanded the 1st Infantry Division in Vietnam. He was personally and professionally well versed in the sting of battle. After reviewing several deep historical analyses, he determined that the future threat suggested war more along the lines of that experienced by the Army in World War II. He personally led the effort to rewrite FM 100-5, *Operations,* the Army's key operational doctrine manual of the time. Given the threats of the day and their geographical location, it focused on the primacy of the defense as opposed to offense and began moving the Army away from its modus of operation during the Vietnam War. Over time, this doctrine would be further redefined into what would become the doctrine of "AirLand Battle." DePuy further dictated that these rediscovered concepts should be taught at the U.S. Army Command and General Staff College in Fort Leavenworth. There the doctrine was buttressed with historical examples and used to train a new generation of rising officers.

The concept called for new technologically superior equipment that could over-come the massive forces of the Warsaw Pact. Although design efforts for this equipment had been ongoing, developments in speed, survivability, rapid com-munications, night vision capability, target acquisition, and fire control fit well into the new doctrine, and they led to the development and acquisition of five new weapons systems:

1. The M1 Abrams main battle tank;
2. The M2 Bradley infantry fighting vehicle;
3. The AH-64 Apache attack helicopter;
4. The Patriot air defense missile; and
5. The UH-60A Black Hawk utility helicopter.

The UH-60A was designed to replace the fleet of UH-1s and was a very high priority with the infantry branch. Its speed and range would fit well with the fast-er armor formations and could be procured for air assault, utility support, and MEDEVAC.[56]

AirLand Battle focused on fighting battles in three areas: (1) close, (2) deep, and (3) rear. It called for the primacy of armor as the pivotal element, supported by the other arms, and closely integrated with tactical airpower. With its fleet of attack helicopters the Army would provide much of that airpower. As the forces received the projected new equipment, they would be reorganized under a program called "Division 86," which optimized that level of command with structured forces to take advantage of the evolving technology being fielded. The entire concept called for new arrangements of support functions to support fast-moving opera-tions. Assignment of MEDEVAC detachments to divisions was considered and then discarded. (The 101st Airborne Division was not reorganized under "Divi-sion 86" and retained its AA platoon with helicopters.) The combat service sup-port operations were required to reorganize and refine their subordinate doctrine to support these concepts. Specifically, the traditional division medical battalion was inactivated and its companies reorganized with a main support company to remain with the new division support command and three forward support medi-cal companies to deploy with brigade-level forward support battalions.[57]

Field Manual 8-35, Evacuation of the Sick and Wounded, January 1977

The Army began to update its FMs from its Vietnam era versions. The first was a rewrite of FM 8-35. It replaced the 1970 version and was vastly more expansive in definition. No longer just focusing on casualty loading tactics, techniques, and procedures, it specified that:

> Medical evacuation is the process of moving any person who is wounded, injured, or ill to and or between treatment facilities. The medical evacuation and treatment of the sick and wounded begin at the place of injury/onset of illness and continue as far rearward as the medical condition of the patient requires. The military services accomplish these functions as rapidly, as orderly, and as effectively as possible, keeping the welfare of the patient as the primary concern.[58]

It included a section on the advantages of evacuation by air, indicating that the speed, range, and flexibility of helicopter ambulances shortened the time needed to move the sick and wounded to that medical facility best manned and equipped to deal with the specific needs of the patient. This made for much more efficient use of highly specialized personnel and equipment that existed only in limited numbers. The helicopter ambulances were not as constrained by terrain as ground vehicles and provided a smoother and comfortable ride for the patients.

The change also discussed some problems with air evacuation. Medical doctrine specified keeping wounded soldiers as far forward as possible so that they could be returned to duty if their wounds allowed. Helicopters, with their speed and responsiveness, made it too easy to very rapidly move patients to the rear, thus over-flying intermediate facilities that could handle their needs. The new FM emphasized that the flow of patients must be monitored and controlled within the medical chain of control to prevent this movement. It reiterated the command and control arrangements laid out in the April 1970 version of FM 8-10, and reemphasized the differing roles for the 25-ship companies and 6-ship detachments, repeated their basic missions, and added an on-call capability for air crash rescue for selected units.[59]

The document also recognized that aviation was inherently dangerous. Although the newer generation of helicopters was equipped with advanced avionics and flight instruments that made them fully capable of flying at night or in inclement weather, Army units in the field did not necessarily have navigational aids that the air ambulances could use in instrument conditions.

The new FM 8-35 also included a section on the dangers of mountain flying, especially at night, or instrument conditions. Varied or heavily treed terrain could force the use of hoists. Although most air ambulance helicopters were equipped with hoists, their use was challenging and required specific training for the crewmembers.

Lastly, the evolving serious threats to MEDEVAC aircraft were addressed. Advances in enemy antiaircraft weapons, especially massed guns, new missiles, and enemy aircraft, were highlighted. As a countermeasure, low-level or nap-of-the-earth flying was taught to all pilots. For the Vietnam era pilots, it was just a return to the ways that they flew in that conflict. The FM also included discussion of the threat posed by advancing friendly weapons systems, thus highlighting the need for procedures to properly coordinate the movement of MEDEVAC helicopters across the modern battlefield in a safe and expeditious manner.[60]

FM 8-10, Health Service in a Theater of Operations, October 1978

In support of this doctrinal shift outlined in FM 100-5, the Army also reviewed and revised its medical doctrine. The key document, again, was FM 8-10. It stated:

Health service support is a single integrated system for providing, in the shortest possible time, the sick, injured and wounded soldiers in the theater of operations with the required care and treatment. This support… includes all health services utilized in the theater of operations… patient evacuation and medical regulating. The objective of military medicine *to conserve trained manpower* dictates that patients are examined, treated, and returned to duty as far forward … as possible and that health service support resources are employed to provide the utmost benefit to maximum personnel in support of the mission.[61]

Within any theater, the Army theater commander was responsible for the medical care of his soldiers and was assigned a medical command (MEDCOM). The MED-COM commander also usually served as the Army Surgeon. The MEDCOM could be of various sizes based on the size of the forces assigned to that theater. Usually, it was a medical brigade, with necessary subordinate units task organized for the mission assigned. Air ambulance units, either companies or detachments, were assigned to the brigade on a basis of two detachments per division supported, one per independent combat brigade, or as necessary to hospital centers to meet the aeromedical evacuation needs of the theater. They were commanded and controlled by the brigade, or as necessary, subordinated to medical groups or even medical battalions.[62]

The new FM also laid out the responsibilities for evacuation. It clearly stated, "To the maximum extent feasible, air ambulances will be used in the combat zone for the evacuation of all patients with any category of precedence…" Tactical combat units were responsible for initial care and evacuation from the point of injury to an initial unit aid station. Division assets, either ground ambulance or air ambulance detachments, evacuated from there to division-level medical facilities. Corps ambulance units, again, either ground or air, then evacuated them to higher levels of care to prepare them for evacuation from theater, if necessary. At any point, any level of care could be bypassed if the condition of the patient required it and the means of evacuation was available.[63]

The Quiet Years Continue

Operations

MAST

As the MAST program continued to expand, it was only natural that Army National Guard MEDEVAC units were considered for the mission. It was something that could very naturally be incorporated into their role as state or federal assets. However, when the MAST program was established, guidance available at that time did not clearly determine that those units could participate. Before federal activation, Guard units were under the control of their state (also, Washington, DC, Puerto Rico, the Virgin Islands, and Guam). Legal opinions had to be developed before a decision could be made. That process was finally completed in May 1978, when the Under Secretary of the Army, Walter B. LaBerge, signed a memorandum authorizing National Guard units to participate in MAST.[64]

As expected, the various Army Reserve Component units received oversight from their Army gaining commands. Many rising MSC officers performed this duty. After completing his series of assignments at Fort Sam Houston in early 1977, Maj. Jerry Foust was assigned as a reserve advisor with the 89th Army Reserve Command in Wichita, Kansas. More than half of all MEDEVAC units were in the Reserve Components, and this afforded him an excellent opportunity to become acquainted with that community of citizen soldiers. Before leaving the assignment in 1979 to attend the Army Command and General Staff College, he visited every MEDEVAC unit in his area and actually flew with most of them, watching very closely for lapses in professionalism and safety. This was very critical because MAST flying itself could be very dangerous, a point sadly reinforced early in 1978 when the Air Ambulance Platoon of the 326th Medical Battalion at Fort Campbell suffered a tragic loss of a MAST crew responding to an automobile accident in the Great Smoky Mountains. That crash killed Captains John Dunnavant and Terrance Woolever, and Sgt. Floyd Smith.[65]

Foust observed many of the Guard units, such as the 24th Med Co (AA) from the Nebraska ARNG, and the 717th Med Co (AA) from New Mexico, as they deployed for summer training or exercises and flew MAST missions. In general, he was impressed with their professionalism, enthusiasm for the missions, and vast experience. Most pilots were older than their contemporaries in the active duty units and were mostly airline pilots in their civilian careers. However, he could also clearly see that their unit tactics still reflected the experiences of their predominantly Vietnam era crews and needed upgrading.[66]

Lt. Col. Pat Brady spent a great deal of time with ARNG and USAR units. Working as the medical coordinator at Sixth Army headquarters in San Francisco, he regularly visited their MEDEVAC units. He found that most of the crewmembers were Vietnam vets and had—on average—1,600 hours of flight time on mission, which was about double the hours flown by "experienced" active duty MEDEVAC crewmembers. The Guardsmen and reservists all chose to remain with MEDEVAC and possessed a wealth of experience that they put to good use.[67]

In 1978, after a very successful series of assignments in Germany, Lt. Truscott was transferred back to Fort Sam Houston to serve as the aviation staff officer at the Health Services Command Headquarters. He traveled worldwide as part of a survey team that visited units to review procedures and operations. This afforded him the opportunity to visit almost all MEDEVAC units. Although he saw a veritable panoply of problems and challenges, one issue kept appearing. He noticed that many units had enthusiastically embraced their MAST taskings. They realized that it provided good training, led to excellent community relations, and was great publicity for the Army. However, many of the units had also lost their tactical edge. Truscott had many intense conversations with local garrison commanders who kept their MEDEVAC units focused on MAST and would not release them for field exercises or training. He reminded them that the MEDEVAC units were go-to-war units and had to be ready. Yet, this was a time of relative peace and in many cases his message was not enthusiastically received.

After two years with the Health Services Command Headquarters, Truscott went to the Army Medical Department Center and School and became Chief of the General Subjects Branch and then the Chief of the Command and Staff Branch, both under the Military Science Division. He worked directly with the Officer Basic and Officer Advanced Courses and the Non-Commissioned Officer Courses. He had a direct and personal opportunity to mentor rising young officers and NCOs.[68]

Serving at Fort Sam Houston as the commander of the Health Services Command, Maj. Gen. Spurgeon Neel maintained his interest in MEDEVAC and watched the development of MAST. He applauded the increased involvement of the units in their local communities, but also recognized that it was affecting their purely military prowess. He commented that, "It is going to take some doing to get them out on a maneuver or get them back into a war."

However, he saw the clear value of the training, especially for the medics. "We feel that the best way to train our medical technicians is to let them take care of actual patients under actual conditions. It is the only way. You can't simulate patients. There is a certain urgency about someone bleeding or not breathing."[69]

Concerning the training provided to the pilots, he was less sanguine. He later said, "To be perfectly candid, this is not the best training for our pilots because there is no war, this is a peacetime situation and we always follow the FAA [Federal Aviation Administration] regulations and we fly fairly high. So the pilots, after accomplishing their MAST mission, still have the requirement over and above that to maintain their proficiency in tree-top flying, nap-of-the-earth flying, night flying, and all of that."[70]

Capt. Bill Thresher also developed a strong opinion of MAST. In April 1979, he moved to Fort Sill, Oklahoma, to command a platoon of the 507th Med Co (AA). What he found when he arrived concerned him. The unit was heavily committed to MAST and basic base and range support, but was undermanned with crews which meant that each had to fly more missions each month. He could see the chronic fatigue in his personnel. More importantly, however, the unit had not had any field training in several years and had lost its tactical edge. To Thresher, the inherent complacency and lethargy in his soldiers' actions were blatantly obvious indicators that the unit and his soldiers needed some redirection.

Thresher was in a quandary. He could clearly see the value of MAST both in terms of what it provided to the local community and the training it provided for his medics. The flying trained the pilots to be very good at instrument procedures since they almost always flew with flight plans under Federal Aviation Administration air traffic control. However, the unit was a designated "go-to-war" unit, and intuition told him that it was just not ready to meet its designed tasking. Thresher addressed the problems forthrightly. He requested and received more aircrew-members to spread out the mission requirements. He also received the unit's full issue of field equipment and began taking his troops to the field for training exercises. Soon his troops were out "soldiering" again, and morale and performance began to improve.

On one of these excursions, Lt. Col. Eldon Ideus, who recently replaced Truscott as the aviation officer at the Health Services Command, under Neel, visited the unit. Ideus had been to many of the MEDEVAC units and shared Thresher's concerns. He was pleased at what he saw at Fort Sill and shared with Thresher a large project that he was working on to develop training manuals designed to standardize flight procedures across the Army. His effort was drawing heavily on the experiences of the disappearing Vietnam era mass of pilots who were beginning to either retire or otherwise leave flying. Thresher enthusiastically supported the work, feeling that it was necessary to stanch a recent increase in flight accidents.[71]

New Personnel

Other Vietnam MEDEVAC veterans touched the new troops in similar ways. In the summer of 1978, Scott Heintz graduated from the ROTC program at Morehead State University in Kentucky. During his summer camps, he was exposed to the combat branches but did not hear much about the support and service support organizations. Fortunately, a friend was going to volunteer for the MSC and told him about its mission. It appealed to him, so he made it his first selection, and as a distinguished graduate of ROTC, he received his choice. Attending the MSC basic course that summer, he was subsequently assigned to be a ground ambulance platoon leader with Charlie Company, 15th Medical Battalion, 1st Cavalry Division at Fort Hood.

The 15th had commanded an air ambulance platoon with the 1st Cavalry Division in Vietnam. Its current commander, Lt. Col. Ernie Sylvester, had flown with great distinction as a MEDEVAC pilot in the war. He and the Charlie Company commander, Maj. Gerry Nolan, a Vietnam era MEDEVAC pilot, took young 2d Lt. Heintz under their wings and regaled him with stories about the mission. They took him to the Fort Hood airfield where a platoon of the 507th Med Co (AA) was located. They pushed him to take the Flight Aptitude Skills Test. He passed it with exceptional scores and was accepted for flight training.

Heintz was also fortunate to have assigned to him an excellent platoon sergeant, S.Sgt. Otis Smith, who guided him on "how to do things right." Heintz later recalled, "The late 1970s, drugs were still an issue. We had some knuckleheads. It was a little bit of a challenge." Smith gave him the training and structure that he needed to handle and learn from those experiences. In December 1980, Heintz reported to Fort Rucker for flight school.[72]

Organization

New Aircraft

Starting in early 1979, the Army began to take delivery of production models of the UH-60 Black Hawk. The first aircraft went to the aviation battalions and companies, with the expectation that some would be assigned to MEDEVAC units to replace their aging UH-1s. The MEDEVAC variant of the UH-60 was designed to carry four litter patients on a rotating carousel, which eased loading, or up to 14 ambulatory patients. It had a projected cruise speed of 160 knots at sea level with a sprint capability of 180 knots, and an un-refueled range of 300 miles. It was equipped with a powerful hoist so that it could work above deep forest, and deicing gear, so necessary in Europe and Alaska. Its assignment to MEDEVAC duties ensured that the medical community was equipped with the most up-to-date aircraft so that it could support the combat units being reorganized and equipped to bring reality to AirLand Battle doctrine. In December 1980, plans were announced for the entire MEDEVAC fleet to be converted to UH-60s by 1990.[73]

Monitoring this development from afar since he had retired from the Army in 1977 with more than 43 years of service, Maj. Gen. (ret) Spurgeon Neel had mixed feelings about the Black Hawk. He saw the value of having a common aircraft across the Army fleet and appreciated its strong engines and upgraded avionics. However, he felt that the new machine was too big and made an inviting target. He remembered that many times, soldiers were wounded in "ones and twos." With bigger, more expensive helicopters, the temptation would exist to hold the patients forward until more were wounded so that a larger helicopter could carry several at once, thereby being more efficient from a transportation perspective. He counseled that, "We don't want to become efficient to [the point] where we let [a casualty] die while we are waiting for 16 more."[74]

New Personnel

In May 1980, Pauline Lockard graduated from Rutgers University in New Jersey. She was the top Army ROTC graduate in her class and took great delight in serving as the first female battalion commander at a school that had originally been all male. Lockard had entered ROTC three years earlier when her brother returned from a tour with the Army in Germany and recommended that she do so. She discovered that the Army was especially keen to recruit capable young women, so she signed up.

After receiving her commission, Lockard reported to her first duty assignment as a platoon leader with the 36th Medical Clearing Company at Fort Bragg. While going through her initial unit training and still awaiting a slot in the MSC basic course at Fort Sam Houston, she met some of the MEDEVAC pilots from the 57th Med Det (RA). It only took a short conversation with them to convince her that she wanted to fly. In checking with her assignment officer, she was informed that she would have to serve a two-year tour with the 36th before she could go to flight school.

While attending the basic course, she submitted a request package for flight school, which required a letter of recommendation. After a course lecture one day, she had a chance encounter with the school commander, Brig. Gen. Quinn H. Becker. The next day, she went to his office and asked him directly for a letter of recommendation. His staff was dumbfounded. Having commanded the 15th Medical Battalion in Vietnam in 1970–71, he knew a bit about MEDEVAC and just looked at her and smiled. "Anybody that has the nerve and audacity to do what you just did deserves a letter to flight school," he said, as his staff drafted the letter. The letter worked and she was accepted, but with the proviso that she serve out her assignment at Fort Bragg first.[75]

Pete Smart, a 26-year-old college graduate and school teacher, wanted to be an Army pilot, but could not afford to fly on a teacher's salary. He spotted an Army recruiting poster that said that aspiring enlistees could be an Army pilot in 40 weeks by becoming a warrant officer. That sounded just perfect. When he approached an Army recruiter, the sergeant wanted him to take a commission. Smart was interested, but then discovered that he would have to pick a branch like armor, infantry, or artillery. That would have required an initial assignment other than flying and would not necessarily allow him to get into flight school. Smart told them that he wanted to be a warrant officer so that he could fly, and they signed him up.

Reporting to the Warrant Officer Candidate Course at Fort Rucker, he found it surprisingly easy for someone who had grown up both physically and mentally fit and was four years older than anybody else in the class. After graduating as a new warrant officer, he remained at Fort Rucker and entered flight school, intent on becoming a MEDEVAC pilot. He was challenged by the formalized and rigid course, but enjoyed the camaraderie of his fellow students, many of whom would become lifelong friends.

As graduation approached, Smart hoped for an assignment to a MEDEVAC unit. Unfortunately, the only MEDEVAC slot for his class went to another student. WO1 Smart ended up with an assignment to the Charlie Company of the 501st Combat Aviation Battalion, 1st Armored Division, as an OH-58 pilot in Illesheim, Germany. He reported to the unit in August 1981. His plans for MEDE-VAC would have to wait.[76]

Operations

Disaster Relief for the Eruption of Mount Saint Helens

The MEDEVAC community received another challenge from a completely unexpected quarter when the nation's attention was dramatically focused on events in the state of Washington in May 1980. On 18 May, the top of Mount Saint Helens, located 100 miles south of Seattle, was blown into the clear northwest sky in the single most devastating volcanic eruption in the United States.

Doug Moore had survived his "learning experience" with the Army Inspector General and was promoted. He escaped the Pentagon and served at Fort Lewis as the commander of the 62d Medical Group, which had a MEDEVAC flying unit, the 54th Med Det (RA) with 6 UH-1H helicopters assigned to it, and also had operational control of a medium-lift helicopter company with CH-47 Chinook aircraft.

When Moore assumed group command, he discovered that the 54th had become so deeply enmeshed in its MAST taskings that it no longer functioned as a

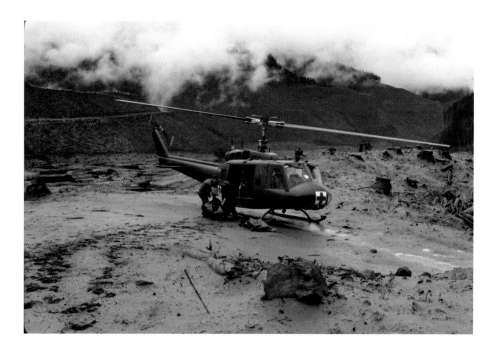

UH-1V from the 54th Med Det (HA) responding to the Mt. St. Helens disaster.
Source: Col. (ret) Doug Moore.

tactical unit. He took some very direct actions, including personnel replacements and unit realignments to return the unit to its primary mission. That was painful, but part of being a commander.[77]

Now, a mountain had blown up in his backyard, and his unit became directly involved in the response and recovery efforts.

Seismic activity near the mount had been detected several months earlier indicating volcanic activity, and as early as March some state level planning efforts had started. Moore's direct participation started early in May when the commander of the 9th Infantry Division, also at Fort Lewis, called him into his office and informed him of the worrisome seismic reports that indicated that a cataclysmic event might be looming. Moore immediately began working with the Washington ARNG and other state and local agencies to develop a coordinated response as necessary.[78]

The mountain exploded on a bright Sunday morning. Moore was at home when his assistant operations officer called him with the news. He looked outside and saw the ugly boiling mass of black and gray debris laden clouds building to the south. The 54th Med Det had aircraft on alert for MAST tasking, and Moore immediately directed them to launch their first aircraft to the area. Other units began to initiate response plans as Fort Lewis went on full alert. The overall state coordinating center was aware of the explosion and had diverted state assets into the area. It asked the Fort Lewis forces to hold and stand by.

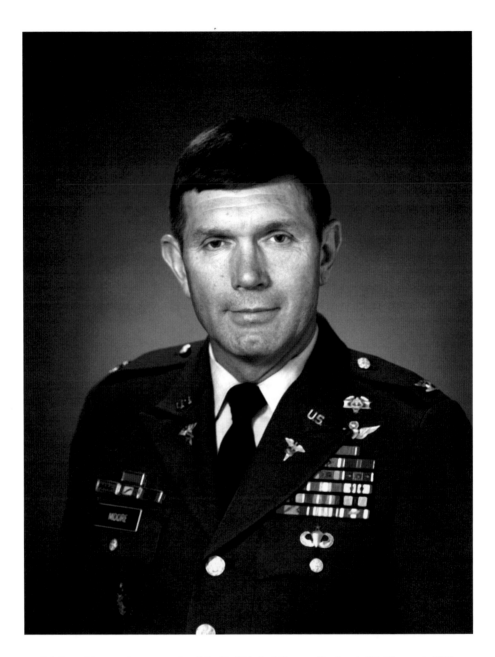

Col. Doug Moore as the commander of the 62nd Medical Group at Fort Lewis, Washington, in 1980.
Source: Col. (ret) Doug Moore.

Secondary eruptions continued into the next day as rain clouds moved in and blanketed the area with a steady rain. People drove with their headlights on and snowplows cleared the roads of debris and mud.

On 19 May, Moore was informed that the state was having problems mounting a coordinated rescue operation. President Jimmy Carter had visited the area that day and in a meeting with the Governor of Washington, Dixy Lee Ray, promised any necessary federal aid. One of his first requests was rescue support, and Moore was directed to lead the effort. He departed Fort Lewis at 0300 in a large convoy of support equipment for the airport at Toledo. Arriving at sunrise, he found a chaotic mess of intermixed agencies, personnel, and equipment. Observing it all was a crush of press personnel there to record the effort.

His troops immediately set up a rudimentary command center and by noon had established a modicum of control over events. Then he had a series of meetings with local police and sheriff commanders to establish an overall rescue and recovery program. Several of these individuals had to be flown to the Toledo airfield in 54th Med Det helicopters because the roads were blocked. Once these jurisdictional issues were resolved, Moore turned his attention to the coordination of aircraft from the Army, Coast Guard, several state National Guards, and many more federal, state, and private organizations.

While doing this, Moore always had to remember that he and his units were in a supporting role. The governor of Washington was in charge of the recovery effort, and Moore ensured that he had a proper chain of command to maintain that relationship. He discovered that his best course of action was to work through the local county sheriffs, and began direct coordination with their designated leader, Sheriff Bill Wiester of Lewis County.

Moore immediately asked Wiester to use his deputies to organize the airfield for continued operations to include an expanded search and rescue flight operations center, a collection point for concerned families and visitors, a gathering area for the ever expanding press teams, and a mortuary.

With those issues addressed, Moore then expanded the search and rescue operations. Pilots from the 54th and other flying units developed a communications plan with the sheriffs and other ground agencies. They agreed on map protocols and the identification of common points so that air and ground search could be coordinated. However, the eruption had so transformed the shape of the mountain that in the most devastated areas, the maps were of only minimal use. Before the eruption, there had been a beautiful lake on the north side of the mountain. The blast and subsequent magma flow literally moved the lake three-quarters of a mile to the northwest and raised it 200 feet. The lake was covered with a layer of dead trees and ash. It took some very skillful flying by some 54th pilots to determine its location and danger to anybody who tried to cross that apparent open area on foot. When the weather finally improved enough to allow steady flight operations, the aircraft started intensive search and rescue flights. However, they still contended with intermittent low clouds, rain, falling ash, and even snow. The magma that spewed forth from the eruption was still warm, and its heat combined with the humid air to generate thick morning fog in the valleys. The Federal Aviation Administration established a special restricted zone around the mountain. Unauthorized aircraft still entered the area and caused several near misses.

Moore was onboard one of the first helicopters to fly over the mountain. They determined that as much as 1,300 feet of the mountain had blown away. A press team picked up their report, and his words were quoted in the papers the next day.

The crews from the 54th and support units flew up and down the valleys daily looking for and recovering survivors, remaining aware of the threat of fog banks full of rock outcroppings, towers, shattered trees, and power lines.

When the weather cleared for several days, another problem arose. The ash and dust that blanketed the area was easily disturbed. Any helicopter takeoff or landing generated clouds of dust. Fortunately, most of the military helicopter pilots were Vietnam vets and handled the challenge well. The thick ash was also very abrasive on the aircraft, and maintenance procedures had to be modified.

The crews picked up more than 200 survivors, including one media team that had disregarded all restrictions, entered the restricted zone, and came close to being killed by the harsh conditions. The crews also recovered 57 bodies, people caught in the horror of the eruption and subsequent fallout. Many of the bodies were horribly mangled, and reminded Moore and the other Vietnam vets of scenes they had seen in that conflict.

The crews from the 54th and other attached units operated out of Toledo until 29 May when the operation was terminated. While there, they were equipped to provide for themselves. Within a few days of their arrival, folks from the local communities brought hot meals to them. Day and night, the informal "chow hall" was open with fresh hot food and endless coffee for "our boys," as the locals called them. For men organized and trained for and experienced in war, the recovery missions flown to help their fellow citizens of southwest Washington devastated by the horrific eruption of Mount Saint Helens were some of the most satisfying missions of their entire careers.[79]

Tactical Training

As the decade ended the Army activated the National Training Center at Fort Irwin in the eastern deserts of southern California. This 1,000-square-mile complex was designed and built as a realistic training area structured to allow brigade-sized forces to practice the evolving doctrine contained in FM 100-5. Ten brigades a year, each with up to 3,500 soldiers, rotated through so the troops could "train as they would fight" in the expanses of the dry canyons. A large cadre of observers and controllers was emplaced to direct and train them.

The units maneuvered on a live-fire range with pop-up moving enemy targets and then through a fully instrumented battle arena against a well-trained opposing force, and actively learned and practiced the tenets of the AirLand Battle doctrine. The National Training Center was eventually joined by the Combat Maneuver Training Center, at Hohenfels, Germany, and the Joint Readiness Training Center, at Fort Chaffee, Arkansas, later moved to Fort Polk.[80]

In October 1980, the 247th Med Det (RA) moved from Fort Meade to Fort Irwin to support the National Training Center. They directly supported the brigades in their training and provided base medical support. In the following decade, this facility provided the Army with an opportunity to develop the ability to fight and defeat the massed forces of the Soviet Union and Warsaw Pact, should they ever attack any of the nations of the North Atlantic Treaty Organization.[81]

MAST Continues to Expand

In November 1980, the 412th Med Det (RA), an Army Reserve unit based in Louisville, Kentucky, signed a memorandum of agreement with the 431st Med Det (RA) at Fort Knox, to augment and on occasion replace it to provide MAST support to Fort Knox and the surrounding area.[82]

As the decade ended, the MAST program noted its 10th anniversary since its conceptual beginning. Missions were being flown from 29 different base locations and involved both Air Force and Army units to include units from their Reserve Components. Records showed more than 18,500 missions had flown consuming more than 43,000 flight hours. The following was in one historical report:

> MAST is an outstanding and durable example of military and civilian community cooperation. The civilians benefit from the life-saving service, and the supporting military unit receives the opportunity to maintain mission proficiency under conditions which cannot be duplicated in a training environment. The reason for the success of the MAST program ... is the personnel assigned to the helicopter ambulance and rescue units. They cared about saving the life of an injured backpacker in a remote area of the Colorado Rockies and a critically ill premature infant in a small community hospital in southwest Texas – and they'll care about the people who will need them in future decades.[83]

* * * *

The 1970s had been a relatively docile period. With the return of American forces from Vietnam, the nation enjoyed a quiet respite and had generally turned inward. The Army was given a chance to reform, rebuild, and refocus. That also benefited the MEDEVAC community as it reconstituted itself, updated and revised its doctrine in line with larger doctrinal and operational changes, entertained thoughts of a new aircraft, and actually picked up a new mission—the MAST tasking—which forced it to integrate with local governments across the nation.

However, ominous events were occurring overseas. Iran experienced a bloody religious revolution and its new anti-U.S. government seized 52 American hostages. They were held for 444 days before diplomatic efforts brought them home. A military rescue effort was mounted but failed. MEDEVAC forces were not involved. That event was perhaps a harbinger of increased American involvement in that region of the world.

Worrisome events also occurred closer to home. In 1979, a communist cabal overthrew a pro-U.S. government in Nicaragua. That led to a leftist insurrection in El Salvador and potential instability in other nations of the region. Central

America had long been considered a quiet backwater. These events began to draw the attention of the nation to that region and portended possible increased involvement there.[84]

On a lighter note, in February 1980 veterans of MEDEVAC units from Vietnam and Korea came together and formed the *Dustoff Association*. Their objectives were to capture their history, recognize their outstanding performers through a Hall of Fame, and link with the current generation of MEDEVAC personnel to perpetuate their heritage. These veterans, like old soldiers from all conflicts, realized that the bonds that they had forged in the sting of battle were not ephemeral but enduring and enriching.[85]

Chapter Four
New Challenges: Near and Afar, 1981–1990

> *"I am satisfied that the recommendation of the [Surgeon General] is in the best interests of the Army and will best ensure continued satisfaction of the aeromedical mission."*
>
> Maj. Gen. Norman Schwarzkopf,
> Acting Deputy Chief of Staff for
> Personnel[1]

Rumblings in Central America and Elsewhere

As the 1980s began, memories of Vietnam were still fresh on the minds of most Americans. However, a few national leaders were concerned about the communist takeover of Nicaragua and the potential for a similar revolution in nearby El Salvador.

El Salvador was a lot like Vietnam, with its rugged terrain, deep jungle, and hot climate, but America was still inwardly focused. As the situation to the south deteriorated, the American people had no interest in getting involved in another counterinsurgency effort. Instead, leaders in the U.S. government decided on a combination of economic sanctions, political initiatives, and limited military support to the friendly nations in the region. The Army had roles to play that were limited in both scope and size, and MEDEVAC units were required only in proportion to any deployment of conventional combat units. America and the Army were still at peace, and as the decade passed, that tranquility changed in response to these developments in Central America and other developing threats, and a renewed national willingness to use military force emerged. These forces affected the organization and doctrine of MEDEVAC units and directed their participation in operations at home and abroad—sometimes in parallel fashion, but always in interrelated ways.[2]

Operations

Europe

After attending the Medical Service Corps (MSC) advanced course in 1976, Capt. Art Hapner was posted with his family back to Landstuhl, where he served as the property book officer for the 2d General Hospital. It was a nonflying position, but he made friends with the troops of the 63d Med Det (RA) stationed at the Landstuhl airfield. When his assignment ended in 1980, he became the operations officer for the 63d, then under Maj. Tom Reed's command. Reed returned to the United States the next year, and newly promoted Maj. Hapner took command of the 63d.[3]

Primarily, the 63d was involved with patient transfer. Many of its passengers were personnel being moved to the 2d General Hospital at Landstuhl from other locations in Germany. Occasionally, the unit moved patients to hospitals all over Germany and even into France and Belgium. The pilots all became well versed in both instrument and international flight procedures, and they also supported calls for medical assistance from the local German communities. Similar to the Military Assistance to Safety and Traffic (MAST) program, but not as formally established, Hapner's crews remained alert 24/7 and responded to calls from throughout the area. Most of their taskings came from a joint operations center at nearby Ramstein Air Force Base, just a few miles northeast.

Some of the missions were very challenging, but Hapner trained his crews well and trusted them. As much as possible, he devolved launch authority to them. He explained:

> We had a daily briefing for the crew coming on board, an operational briefing. We left it with the pilot in command—that was one of the responsibilities they were given... And the pilot in command had control of the mission and responsibility for the aircraft... If the weather was marginal, then the operations officer or the commander, whoever was on that call for that night, would then be called in or at least called and consulted. 'This is what the situation is. The weather is at this point in time.' We would then talk through the scenario and then give the okay or turn the mission down.[4]

Hapner spent a lot of time developing and mentoring his younger troops. He constantly stressed the importance of teamwork, emphasizing that each member of the crew made a valuable and critical contribution to the mission's overall accomplishment. He always admonished his troops to remember that, "Our best day is somebody else's worst day."

Hapner also witnessed the results of the Army's efforts to recruit more female soldiers. While he commanded the unit, he received two female pilots, one officer and one warrant officer, a crew chief, a medic, and an operations specialist. All fit in well. He commanded the unit until June 1982 when he was reassigned to Fort Bragg, North Carolina.[5]

Organization

Eagle Dustoff

The soldiers of the air ambulance platoon of the 326th Medical Battalion, 101st Airborne Division at Fort Campbell in Clarksville, Tennessee, considered themselves proud members of the division and "Eagle Dustoff" was their moniker. In September 1981, they received three new UH-60s for evaluation as MEDEVAC aircraft. Carousels were inserted into the cabins for ease of patient care. These aircraft were initially assigned to the division's lift units. However, the division commander, Maj. Gen. Jack V. Mackmull, wanted his MEDEVAC unit to have the same mobility as the rest of the division and diverted them. Other MEDEVAC units were not programmed to get them for several more years.

Capt. Frank Novier commanded the platoon at the time. He received a visit from Lt. Col. Tom Scofield, who was an action officer and the aviation consultant on the staff of the Office of The Surgeon General. Scofield was an "old MEDEVAC hand." He graduated from Troy State University in Alabama, with a double major in chemistry and mathematics, and joined the Army in 1964 after receiving his draft notice. Accepted for a commission, he branched into the MSC and then went to flight school at Fort Wolters in Texas. Subsequently, he served multiple tours in Vietnam with the 498th Med Co (AA), the 68th Med Det (RA), and the air ambulance platoon of the 15th Medical Battalion, 1st Cavalry Division. After the war, he worked in Army flight test programs with the Medical Research and Development Command and played a small role in the initial development of the UH-60. After attending the U.S. Army Command and General Staff College and completing a tour in Europe with first the 7th Medical Command and then as the commander of the 421st Med Co (AA), he took his vast and detailed knowledge of MEDEVAC to the Office of The Surgeon General in Virginia. He was one of those old Vietnam era "lionhearts" who provided key leadership to the MEDEVAC community in the postwar years.[6]

Scofield was at Fort Campbell to observe the test. He had recommended the UH-60 as a fine MEDEVAC vehicle to the Surgeon General. It was an ongoing battle, though, because other officers on the Army staff opposed its selection. Instead, they pushed to keep MEDEVAC in the UH-1 or even reequip the units with smaller helicopters designed to carry only one or two patients at a time, and without a medic onboard. Scofield worked diligently against such pressure and needed this test to go well. Perhaps to emphasize its importance, he put his arm around Novier's shoulder and said, "Frank, you know, we need to test this and your unit is going to do this." The test was successful, and the carousels made patient loading and unloading much easier, reinforcing Scofield's case for the MEDEVAC UH-60. Shortly after the test concluded, the platoon was upgraded to Delta Company of the 326th Medical Battalion, with the expectation that several more UH-60s would replace its Vietnam era UH-1 aircraft.[7]

Returning to his office in Washington, Scofield perfunctorily reviewed the stack of pilot application packages. He knew that the Army was working hard to create opportunities for women and was pleased to see the application from 2d Lt. Pauline Lockard. However, he was taken aback by her letter of recommendation from Brig. Gen. Becker, so he called her, and she confirmed the encounter. He subsequently worked with her assignment officer and got Lockard released from her posting to the 36th Medical Clearing Company so that she could start flight training at Fort Rucker, Alabama, in October 1981, as one of three female aviators in her class.[8]

Back at Fort Campbell, Novier was pleased that his unit was being upgraded to a company. He also liked having the unit directly assigned to the 101st, believing that it helped his troops to develop a strong kinship with the other soldiers who "wear the same patch." Even though his company belonged to the medical battalion, he had individual teams that developed habitual relationships with the brigades, continually working, training, and deploying with them as part of their support element. It was part of plan and practice, enshrined in "the Gold Book," the division's standard operating procedure.[9]

Even though his duties as the commander kept him busy, Novier sought to mentor and lead by example so he stayed on the duty roster, regularly flew missions, maintained combat ready status, and earned his senior and master Army Aviator badges. He loved the assignment, but left the unit in 1982 for an assignment in Saudi Arabia with the United States Military Training Mission.[10]

In August 1983, Delta Company, 326th Medical Battalion, gained some operational experience with its new Black Hawks when a detachment of six aircraft, crews, and support personnel deployed to Palmerola Air Base, Honduras, as part of a medical task force from the 41st Combat Support Hospital, which was home-based at Fort Sam Houston, Texas. They supported Operation AHUAS TARA II, which ran until February 1984. Delta Company, 326th Medical Battalion, then commanded by Maj. Morris Jackson, flew 843 sorties and carried 7,571 patients, including one soldier wounded by hostile fire. The unit also supported 135 medical civic action program missions and carried medical personnel and supplies to numerous remote locations. With improved speed, range, and communications capabilities, the aircraft proved its value as a MEDEVAC aircraft, especially in the recovery of patients from remote sites in hilly country. The only real challenge for the unit was the procurement of accurate maps, which were critical for navigation in the mountainous region.[11]

A few weeks after Delta Company deployed, Lt. Col. Jerry Foust arrived at Fort Campbell to assume command of the 326th Medical Battalion. He held a series of meetings with the aviation commanders to ensure that Delta Company was properly integrated into the overall division aviation plan. He also ensured that the battalion was integrated into the overall communications plan.

Foust's position allowed him to fly and he quickly qualified in the new UH-60. He pushed his pilots to develop and maintain proficiency in the latest generation of night vision goggles (NVGs) because he realized there was a tactical advantage to flying and operating at night.

Foust also put increased emphasis on the training of his medics. He acquired extra funds for medics to acquire advanced cardiac life support and advanced trauma life support. Some medics became emergency medical technicians, making them some of the best medics in the Army and foreshadowing later changes to the overall Army medic program.

The battalion also gave the crew chiefs rudimentary medical training. Foust's logic on this was simple: "It's a second pair of hands and eyes. You get a patient who turns sour on you, you need help."[12]

While Foust commanded the battalion, Delta Company had a continuing commitment for MAST tasking. He gave launch authority to the company commander or his operations officer. When a mission was assigned, the pilot in command of the crew prepared to fly and then briefed the commander or operations officer on whether the mission was a go or not as per established risk criteria. Foust pushed for that system to be streamlined as much as possible and wanted his helicopters airborne in five minutes. That same requirement existed in combat, and he constantly urged his MEDEVAC commanders to integrate fully with the aviators so that it could happen. Foust commanded the 326th until July 1986, when he left to attend the Army War College at Carlisle Barracks, Pennsylvania. It was, he remembered, a "very successful tour."[13]

While at Fort Campbell, Foust also actively mentored his young officers and troops. One of those was a young lieutenant named Dave MacDonald, who graduated from James Madison University in Virginia in May 1983, and was commissioned into the MSC. After his basic course he was assigned as a medical platoon leader with the 2d Battalion, 5th Cavalry Regiment, 1st Cavalry Division, at Fort Hood, Texas. MacDonald wanted to fly, but had failed his flight physical when he indicated that he suffered from allergies. After 18 months at Fort Hood, he requested and was assigned to the 101st Division at Fort Campbell where he was placed in command of the clearing platoon of the 326th. He excelled in the assignment and impressed Foust, who subsequently assigned him to be the executive officer of Charlie Company of the battalion. He also asked MacDonald if he had any interest in flying. MacDonald told him about the failed physical. Foust asked him how he knew he had allergies. MacDonald replied that in the summer, he sneezed frequently and just marked on his physical form that he had allergies, but had no medical diagnosis to substantiate it. Foust urged him to retake the physical and not indicate allergies in his medical history. He did as instructed, passed the physical, and then reapplied for flight school. The request went in with Foust's strong endorsement, and in 1985 MacDonald traveled to Fort Rucker to become an Army pilot.[14]

Doctrine

Field Manual (FM) 100-5, Operations, August 1982

During the early 1980s, the Army continued its intellectual debate and modified its AirLand Battle concept laid out in FM 100-5 to emphasize that the Army had to be prepared to fight outnumbered and win the first battle of the next war. This implied that the Army had to ensure that it had a trained and ready peacetime force. The Army rewrote the manual to focus on battle between massed armor forces as the heart of modern warfare, with the tank as the most important weapon in the army arsenal. Four basic tenets were presented: (1) initiative, (2) depth, (3) agility, and (4) synchronization, and would take part in three forms: (1) the deep battle, where U.S. forces would attack enemy elements before they attacked U.S. main force units; (2) the close battle, where those forces would openly engage; and (3) the rear battle, where the enemy would attempt to attack U.S. support elements, logistical units, and C2 centers.

To be successful the armor-centric forces had to be properly supported by the combat, combat support, and combat service support elements. Commanders were taught to seize the initiative, act faster than the enemy, conduct operations extending through the depth of the battlefield over extended time, keep the enemy off balance, and synchronize both ground and air power at the decisive point of battle.

This change also acknowledged advances in technology. AirLand Battle was redesigned and refocused to take advantage of those advances to allow U.S. forces to fight and win against enemies such as the Soviet Union and Warsaw Pact, with its large array of heavy divisions.[15]

FM 8-35, *Evacuation of the Sick and Wounded, December 1983*

In late 1983, the Army published an updated version of FM 8-35, but it was mostly a repeat of the 1977 version, with an almost total emphasis on patient movement tactics, techniques, and procedures. However, it did include a section on the proper loading procedures for the new UH-60A MEDEVAC aircraft.[16]

FM 8-55, *Planning for Health Service Support, February 1985*

Two years passed before the refocusing on AirLand Battle appeared in medical doctrine. The first changes, which were noticed in the rewrite of FM 8-55, embraced the new warfighting concept, but noted that, "The opposing forces on that battlefield will rarely fight across orderly, distinct lines. There may be little distinction between rear and forward areas." It also recognized that to maintain the initiative, subordinate commanders had to act independently based on a clear knowledge of the commander's intent. The importance of synchronization was highlighted as critical to providing maximum combat power through unity of effort.

The new version also reinforced the point that health service support (HSS) overall played a key role in maintaining combat power. However, the extended battlefield stretched HSS capability. This was especially true of MEDEVAC units because the distances that they flew were longer and potentially over enemy-controlled terrain.

The FM also slightly changed the planning factors for MEDEVAC units. The basis of allowance became one company per four divisions or per task force as required. Detachments became allotted as two per division, one per separate brigade task force sized element, or one per hospital center.[17]

Operations

Domestic Disaster Response

In January 1982, an Air Florida Boeing 737 crashed on takeoff in a heavy snowstorm at National Airport, just south of Washington, DC. It slammed into a major bridge over the Potomac River, killing 78 persons and causing a huge traffic jam. Civilian and military units from throughout the region responded with emergency help. The 400th Med Det (HA), an Army National Guard unit from Washington, DC, joined the recovery force. Crews launched in three of their UH-1s to provide on-scene support, search for survivors in the frigid river, and evacuate survivors to local hospitals.[18]

Duty in the Sinai

In early 1982, an 11-nation task force designated the Multinational Force and Observers (MFO) was created and deployed to the Sinai Peninsula to enforce the ceasefire between Egypt and Israel negotiated by President Jimmy Carter at the Camp David Peace Accords in 1979. The MFO included a U.S. Army infantry battalion, and a support organization, the 1st U.S. Army Support Battalion (1SB), which included an aviation company. Each parent division supplying the infantry battalion was expected to provide the aviation assets for the 1SB on six-month rotational tours.

By 1987, planners realized that the operational environment was too demanding for rotational pilots, and the Aviation Company was converted to a permanent TDA (table of distribution and allowances—literally, units permanently assigned to a specific location) unit, equipped with 10 UH-1 helicopters, and assigned 100 personnel, including medical specialists. Crews were assigned for one-year tours.

The UH-1s were adorned with a white and orange paint scheme for easy international recognition, and the pilots used the call sign "Nomad." One of their assigned missions was MEDEVAC, and the unit had flight medics attached to it for that mission. Given the genesis of its creation, the activities of the "Nomads" were very politically sensitive. Yet they provided support to all of the various national task forces assigned to the MFO.

The aviation company was split between the two main camps: (1) North Camp at El Gorah, Egypt, just a few miles west of Gaza; and (2) South Camp, located at the far southern tip of the Sinai near the city of Sharm El Sheik.

Most missions were routine. The MFO teams were spread out over the entire expanse of the Sinai, and aviation support was critical to the mission. The Nomads had one of the highest operational tempos of any aviation unit in the Army, with some of the 1969 vintage aircraft logging on average, 2,100 hours of flight time a year.[19]

Aviation, a New Branch for the Army

Organization

Determining the Need

On 12 April 1983, John O. Marsh Jr., Secretary of the Army, signed the necessary documents approving Army aviation as a separate branch of the service. This event was the end result of tireless efforts on the part of numerous individuals, multiple studies, and the lessons of war. The long conflict in Vietnam conclusively showed the value and importance of tactical aviation. Army aviation grew almost exponentially during that conflict, and the community of aviators to fly all of those aircraft tripled. Aviation showed that on its own, it was a major combat power that no longer needed to be inextricably tied to the ground units.[20]

During that conflict, all officers who wanted to fly had to first serve in their assigned branch, such as infantry, artillery, etc. Many of those officers had advanced in rank and were having difficulty maintaining aviation skills while serving in branch-directed but nonaviation assignments. Additionally, in 1974, Congress passed stringent requirements concerning aviators drawing aviation incentive pay. To address these challenges, many of the Army's senior aviators discussed the idea of a separate branch for aviation. Additionally, they believed that aviation was unique enough that it needed its own branch to manage the aviators and provide them a structured environment in which they could pursue a full Army career. This discussion made its way to the Army Chief of Staff, Gen. Bernard Rogers, who was personally aware of the problem because his son was an Army aviator and infantry captain. Rogers directed a study, but—more importantly—queried all of his other four-star generals. Although the generals acknowledged the problems faced by the aviators, they were opposed to a separate branch. Rogers chose not to act, but sent a field message addressing "Commissioned Aviator Career Management." The message said that providing a viable career pattern for commissioned Army aviators required changes to the Officer's Personnel Management System. Specialty Code (SC) 15 became an entry specialty. New officers were accessed directly into that SC or SC 71, aviation materiel management, SC 15M, military intelligence, or SC 67J MSC. Officers were still required to enter a specific branch. Those desiring the SC 15 were required to select either Infantry, Armor, Field Artillery, or Air Defense Branches. Those selecting SC 71 had to select the Transportation Corps. Those selecting SC 15M were required to select Military Intelligence. Those selecting SC 67J went into the MSC.[21]

In the summer of 1979, Rogers went to Europe to serve as the Supreme Allied Commander of the North Atlantic Treaty Organization and Commander in Chief, U.S. European Command. Gen. Edward Meyer became the Army Chief of Staff. He was also aware of the issue but was unable to address it until 1981. While at Fort Rucker for a conference, he directed Maj. Gen. James H. Merryman, the Commander of the Aviation Center, to develop an aviation branch proposal. Merryman contacted the commander of the Training and Doctrine Command, Gen. Glen K. Otis, for assistance. Otis directed a Training and Doctrine Command Review of Army aviation that conducted more than 600 interviews, 39 of which were with general officers, and reviewed 22 different major studies done on Army aviation. After the exhaustive review, Training and Doctrine Command recommended that an aviation branch be established. Meyer approved the recommendation on 27 January 1983 and forwarded it to Secretary Marsh, who concurred and signed the enabling documents.

Meyer, in his approval, also directed the Deputy Chief of Staff for Personnel to determine the branch composition in coordination with several other directorates and commands, to include the Surgeon General. This led to some spirited debates because many within the MEDEVAC community believed that this was another attempt by the aviation community to absorb MEDEVAC under their control.

Include MEDEVAC?

Scofield, who served as the Aviation Consultant on staff of the Office of The Surgeon General, attended an Aviation Branch Composition meeting in the office of Maj. Gen. Norman Schwarzkopf, the acting Deputy Chief of Staff for Personnel, on 7 April. After the meeting, he noted in a Memorandum for Record that "...all aviators (SC15, 67J and 71s) [will] be included in the Aviation Branch."[22]

In support of this position, Lt. Gen. Fred K. Mahaffey, Deputy Chief of Staff for Operations and Plans, argued that "Aviation effectiveness can be better realized if every mission element comes under the umbrella of coordinated doctrine, tactics, training, and personnel management. I believe this to be the overriding issue in this controversy."[23]

Lt. Gen. Bernard Mittemeyer, The Surgeon General, who passionately nonconcurred, did not object to the creation of an aviation branch, but he did object to the inclusion of the 67Js. Mittemeyer and Scofield had some very earnest discussions about it. They concurred that it would bode ill for the 67Js from a career progression perspective. They also felt that the pure aviators did not understand the imperative of immediate response to wounded soldiers.[24]

Mittemeyer also had strong personal feelings about MEDEVAC based on his own experiences. In 1968–1969, he commanded the 326th Medical Battalion, 101st Airborne Division, in Vietnam when the 50th Med Det (RA) inactivated and became the air ambulance platoon of his battalion. In a response to Lt. Gen. Mahaffey, he said:

> I do not believe the Army staff fully understands the working relationship that exists between the medical and aviation communities. ...The basic flying skills are common among all aviators, regardless of branch. In addition, many of the tactical concepts are essentially the same, e.g., Nap-of-the-earth flight, Night Vision Goggle operations...What is different is the fact that the aeromedical [67J] is an integral part of a medical evacuation system just as is the ground ambulance. The Aeromedical evacuation officer is more than a flyer. His training, both medical and aviation, professional career development, and experience, combine to provide the AMEDD [Army Medical Department] with a highly qualified officer who is an integral part of the finely tuned equation of evacuation, treatment, hospitalization, and command and control. What we are asking is to be allowed to continue a proud, combat proven, and highly efficient system that supports our soldiers the way they deserve to be supported.[25]

Decision

Schwarzkopf carefully reviewed all of the opinions offered. In his response to the Army Chief of Staff he wrote:

> I am satisfied that the recommendation of the [Surgeon General] is in the best interests of the Army and will best ensure continued satisfaction of the aeromedical mission. The [Surgeon General] argues persuasively that the commissioned officers assigned to aeromedical units must be professionally developed consistent with AMEDD career programs. Further, the creation of an Aviation Branch will help us correct deficiencies in the conduct of combat related aviation operations. However, the medical evacuation mission is well executed. Therefore, changes to medical evacuation procedures and professional development are not warranted at this time.[26]

Gen. John Wickham, the Vice Chief of Staff, supported Schwarzkopf. On 25 April, Meyer approved the personnel composition of the branch, which excluded MSC (67J) aviators. Then, on 6 June, he signed the order directing the centralization of proponent responsibility for Army aviation at the U.S. Army Aviation Center in Fort Rucker and issued the Aviation Branch Implementation Plan.[27]

Aviation Branch Implementation

As part of the Aviation Branch Implementation Plan, the Aviation Branch developed a very comprehensive professional development plan for the aviation commissioned officer. The plan represented a challenge for the Surgeon General because he needed to ensure that his 67Js were able to maintain equivalency from an aviation standpoint while also developing his or her Army Medical Department (AMEDD) potential. To address this thorny issue, he directed the Commandant of the Academy of Health Sciences (AHS) at Fort Sam Houston, Maj. Gen. Robert H. Buker, to modify as necessary the development track for 67Js.

The Commandant formed a working group to review available training and anticipated career assignment flow and to develop a proposal. All newly commissioned MSC officers who desired to become pilots would attend the AMEDD Officer Basic course. Then they would serve in a troop leadership position in a field medical unit for a maximum of 18 months. Their next assignment would be the Initial Entry Rotary Wing Training at Fort Rucker, followed by a three-week Medical Training Course for AMEDD Aviators, also at Fort Rucker.

From there they would be posted to a MEDEVAC unit for operational duty. At about the 4–7 year point, the 67Js would then be sent to the 20-week Aviation Advanced Course, again at Fort Rucker, followed by a shorter six-week AMEDD Aviator Advanced Course at Fort Sam Houston. This educational track highlighted the obvious fact that the 67J officers were effectively dual-branched officers.[28]

Senior officers within the MEDEVAC community were pleased that they avoided consolidation. Few expected such efforts to cease. Many remembered the repeated attempts in Vietnam. One long-timer, Col. Doug Moore, then serving as the Executive Officer to the Surgeon General, believed that the weight of opinion was slowly moving toward consolidation and that eventually the MEDEVAC community would become part of Aviation.[29]

Not too long after the new branch was set up, staff officers visited the MEDEVAC units to explain the dramatic changes coming to Army aviation. Lockard served with the Flatiron Detachment at Fort Rucker then and remembered the visit. After graduating from flight training, she joined the detachment and became a well-qualified UH-1 aircraft commander with several hundred hours of flight time gained on range accident missions and MAST.

Lockard initially had some interest in transferring. She listened to the presentations carefully. The briefing officer explained the projected growth of the branch and potential opportunities, and then asked if any of the MSC pilots would like to transfer to aviation. She pondered it but declined remembering that, "I liked the Army Medical Department and the mission we were doing. I felt … [the] Medical Service Corps was an opportunity for me to be in a field that was fulfilling, saving lives, and we were unique." Instead of changing branches, she received orders to Fort Lewis, Washington, to join the 54th Med Det (RA).[30]

Medical Evacuation Battalions?

While serving as the MEDEVAC consultant to the Surgeon General, Scofield attempted to make two more significant changes. He tried to develop an interest in reactivating the medical evacuation battalions that had been created toward the end of the Vietnam War. The intent was to create a unit that provided direct command and control to the MEDEVAC detachments and companies for better coordination and medical control. He also postulated that the large 25-ship companies should be broken up and consolidated with all of the individual detachments to form 15-ship companies with a strong maintenance and logistics support package to make them self-sustaining. A predecessor in the consultant position, Lt. Col. Don Retzlaff, had tried to sell the idea back in the mid-1970s, but had been unsuccessful. While Scofield's proposals met the same fate, his ideas were heard by other rising officers and would find a more favorable reception in the not too distant future.[31]

One of the individuals who became aware of Scofield's ideas was Maj. Bill Thresher. Completing his tour at Fort Sill, Oklahoma, in 1981, he had been posted to Fort Sam Houston to work in the Military Science Division of AHS. He lectured in both the MSC basic and advanced courses, and mentored many young MEDEVAC officers as well as taught the basics of MEDEVAC to a generation of medical officers in general. On a special project he became the lead action officer for the MEDEVAC portion of a Medical System Program Review (MSPR) directed by Maj. Gen. William Winkler, the AHS commander. Winkler believed that the AMEDD was very well organized to refight World War II, but not properly organized to support the evolving Army doctrine.

Thresher attacked the project with gusto. Over a six-month period, he and a team of other specialists conducted a lot of historical research. Recalling Scofield's efforts, Thresher specifically looked at the operations of the 58th and 61st Medical Battalions during the Vietnam War. For a period of about 18 months in 1970 and 1971, both units acted as provisional medical evacuation battalions. They took operational control of several MEDEVAC units, ground ambulance units, and some specialty medical units, and operated them as an integrated evacuation system. The initiative showed promise, but both units were inactivated as part of the overall withdrawal from the war and never again activated. Based on the positive data that he found, Thresher led several small war games based on a European scenario, and concluded that the concept of a medical evacuation battalion could provide effective command and control of MEDEVAC assets in support of AirLand battle. Additionally, Thresher's studies showed that the optimum size for MEDEVAC units was 15 aircraft in a company-sized unit with unit level maintenance versus the super 25-ship companies and six-aircraft detachments currently in existence. The companies would be allocated one per division in a direct support role and two per corps in a general support role. The battalions would be allocated one per corps to control and coordinate the companies and allocated ground ambulance companies into an integrated evacuation system to perform all of the classic MEDEVAC functions.

When completed, Thresher wrote his report on a newly purchased Apple IIC computer and briefed his findings to Winkler. In July 1985, Winkler took the entire MSPR briefing to the Gen. Maxwell Thurman, the Army Vice Chief of Staff. Thresher gave the MEDEVAC portion. Thurman approved the changes. They reshaped the AMEDD's operational concept for the modern battlefield.[32]

Europe

That same summer, after being promoted to colonel and serving an advisory tour in Saudi Arabia, Col. Jim Truscott returned to Germany to command the 68th Medical Group. It was assigned to the Corps Support Command of the V Corps, then commanded by Lt. Gen. Colin Powell, who took a strong interest in his health service support.

Upon taking command, Truscott tried to have at least one of the MEDEVAC units in the theater assigned to the 68th. Their higher headquarters, the 7th MEDCOM, disagreed. Under operations contingency plans, one or more MEDEVAC units could be attached to the 68th for operational control. Frequently they worked and trained directly with the 68th. Truscott, having learned from his earlier experiences, developed contingency plans with Corps aviation support and logistics units to ensure that when the MEDEVAC units deployed to the field with the group, they would have the necessary support to operate in support of the medical mission.

Truscott also used his influence to get permission for the MEDEVAC units to use "Dustoff" as their radio call sign. He was a strong believer in the value of heritage and wanted to share that with the younger pilots. Truscott was also still a rated Army aviator. However, he had long since passed his required flight "gates" necessary to continue to get flight pay and rarely flew. As the commander of the

68th, he visited the MEDEVAC units occasionally and was usually successful in "sniveling" a flight or two where the younger officers and warrants allowed him to touch the controls. He also mentored his young officers and encouraged those who were interested and medically qualified to apply for flight school and duty as MEDEVAC pilots. One young officer serving in the 68th, 2d Lt. Randall Anderson, took his advice and became a MEDEVAC pilot.[33]

MEDEVAC Proponency

To ensure proper coordination between the AMEDD and the new Aviation Branch, the Surgeon General directed the creation of a Medical Evacuation (Air/Ground) Proponency Action Office (MEPAO) at Fort Rucker, with an MSC colonel as its director. However, the MEPAO actually was part of the overall AMEDD Proponency Office located at Fort Sam Houston. It would ensure that the AMEDD remained abreast of current aviation concepts, training, doctrine, combined arms tactics, and force structure developments. Its stated objective was to better prepare medical evacuation personnel for war as highly trained members of the combined arms team, with the clear recognition that medical evacuation was an integral part of the health care delivery system in both peacetime and combat.[34]

With the approval of the MSPR in July 1985, Col. Eldon Ideus, the initial director of the MEPAO, and his deputy, Lt. Col. Bill Kruse, were very proactive in advocating these positive changes. They took Thresher's proposals for the evacuation battalions and the standardized 15-ship MEDEVAC companies and developed the overall doctrinal concept of MEDEVAC support for AirLand Battle. In support of these changes, unit actions occurred almost immediately. The first battalion to activate for this role was the 52d Medical Battalion (Evacuation) in Korea in 1985. As it activated, it took command of the 377th Med Co (AA).[35]

The MEPAO was collocated at Fort Rucker with the U.S. Army School of Aviation Medicine. That same summer, the U.S. Army School of Aviation Medicine started a specific course (91B2F) to train the medics assigned aboard the MEDEVAC helicopters. Heretofore, all flight-specific training for the medics occurred at their units. This move relieved the units of that training requirement and standardized the training across the entire service.[36]

Within a few years, the MEPAO became the Medical Evacuation Proponency Division (still at Fort Rucker). Its director was also formally assigned the responsibility of advising the commandant of the AHS and the Surgeon General on all medical evacuation proponency matters.[37]

In August 1985, 1st Lt. Dave MacDonald arrived a few weeks early at Fort Rucker for flight school and was assigned in casual status to the MEPAO, where he met Ideus and Kruse. He performed mundane office work that also allowed him to observe some of the larger issues affecting the MEDEVAC community as Ideus and Kruse struggled with the changes sweeping the community from both the medical and aviation perspectives. He then attended the flight course and graduated in May 1986.

MacDonald's follow-on assignment took him to the 377th Med Co (AA) in Korea. That unit was now equipped with UH-60s, and MacDonald was held over at Fort Rucker for aircraft transition. While waiting for that course, he went across the base and flew UH-1s with the Flatiron detachment. When he subsequently finished his UH-60 qualification, he departed in December 1986 for Korea.[38]

Females

To reflect the increasing role that women were assuming in MEDEVAC, the 24th Med Co (AA) of the Nebraska Army National Guard claimed a first. While encamped at Fort Chaffee, Arkansas, for summer training in 1986, the unit launched an all-female crew in support of ongoing training operations. In command was the third platoon commander, 1st Lt. Jan Harrington, a student at the University of Nebraska at Omaha. She was assisted by WO1 Joanne Votipka, the only other female pilot in the unit. The crew chief was Sgt. Linda Plock from Lincoln. She had also set an individual record of sorts by becoming the first female crew chief in 1973. The medic was Sgt. Laura Mruz, also a student at the University of Nebraska at Omaha. Somewhat taken aback by the press interest in their exploit, Harrington said, "I thought it was great. We had a great flight and crew." All had flown with one another, but never all as one crew. Asked about the role that the women were playing in the unit, the commander, Maj. David Meyers said, "Any position in the company, including mine, can be filled by a woman. I see no problem with having significant numbers of women in our unit."[39]

Capt. Pauline Lockard did not find the same reception when she arrived at the 54th Med Det (RA) at Fort Lewis. She quickly adjusted to life in the beautiful northwest and loved the flying. The unit had a heavy MAST commitment, and some of the patients picked up at automobile accidents were severe. Many missions were mountain recoveries and required challenging hoist operations. The unit also manned a detachment at the large Army training center at Yakima, where soldiers were injured in field maneuvers on a regular basis.

While at the 54th, Lockard served as the operations officer. She developed a keen appreciation for what her helicopters and crews could and could not do as they responded day and night, in good weather and bad, over the mountains, plains, and bays of the area for all manner of calls. It was, she said, "an enriching experience."

She also experienced some "gender challenges," noting that:

We had a lot of Vietnam type of guys who were not used to things, used to women being in their aircraft. There is an aviator I used to fly with. He said I was the best smelling aviator he ever flew with since he's been in Vietnam. I took that as a compliment rather than take it as a sexual harassment comment.

I literally went eye to eye with anybody who just challenged me in any type of discriminatory visual type of mode. A little wink. Especially a junior enlisted or something like that; I would challenge that on the spot. ...I just did my job and if issues came up, I faced them. It was draining, but I had to get the work done, and I had to keep a level head.[40]

Acutely aware that she was one of the first females in her field, she also was quick to mentor other female soldiers, noting that:

> I spent many, many, many hours talking with other women who were either thinking about coming into the service or specifically aviation. My biggest recommendation was "Just be yourself but also maintain composure as much as possible. If you are going to break down, do it somewhere else. Wait—go for a really long run; do something, whatever. But you have to maintain your composure."[41]

It was advice that she needed many more times in the future. After two years in the 54th, she was selected to command the 423d Medical Clearing Company at Fort Lewis. This was a nonflying position, but it gave her an early opportunity to command. The unit also had a high ratio of women. Slots for women were still restricted then, and as more enlisted, they were increasingly focused in medical units. Lockard had to point out to her superiors that, in general, women did not have the same physical strength as men and her unit needed to maintain a balance of men and women to perform its wartime taskings. She took those taskings very seriously by stressing field training and physical fitness for all of her soldiers.[42]

Operations

MAST

After completing a three-year tour of duty in Hawaii where he commanded a ground medical unit, served as the flight operations officer of the 68th Med Det (RA), and flew numerous MAST missions, Capt. Dan Gower was transferred to Fort Hood to command the 3d Platoon of the 507th Med Co, equipped with six UH-1Vs.

When he reported to the platoon in August 1981, he found a very active unit that maintained three aircraft on alert at all times and received a steady call for recoveries on the huge training ranges. The collocated 1st Cavalry and 2d Armored Divisions on the base had received new M1 Abrams tanks and M2 Bradley infantry fighting vehicles. The training load was heavy, and there were many accidents.

The platoon was also a MAST unit, and those calls arrived at a steady rate. Gower was just a year into the assignment when the unit flew its 1000th MAST mission, which drew some local press coverage.

Gower also found a downside to MAST. The previous commander had allowed some of his officers to use the constant MAST commitment as an excuse not to develop a unit training plan or significant safety program. Additionally, the unit failed its last Aviation Resource Management Survey. Gower determined that changes were necessary.

Working with several of his key unit leaders, such as his safety officer CW4 Ron Crotty, he moved swiftly to correct deficiencies. He told his warrant officers, "You are in charge of this program. You have responsibility and you have authority to do your job. Let's do the best we can." Then he let them get to it, and

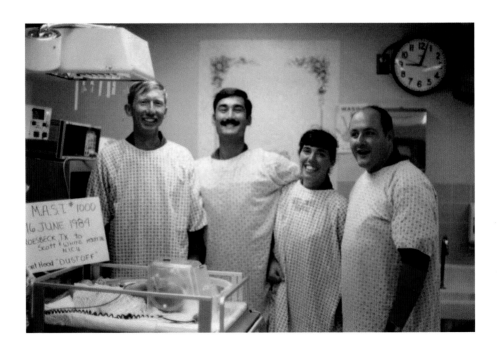

Maj. Dan Gower (left) and the crew that flew the 1000th MAST mission for Fort Hood DUSTOFF bringing a premature baby to Scott and White Hospital from Groesbeck, Texas, on 16 June 1984. Source: Dan Gower

checked that it was getting done.

Primary responsibilities previously had resided mostly with the commissioned officers, and the warrant officers were viewed merely as pilots. By expanding responsibilities among all of the officers (warrant and commissioned), Gower expanded the pool of expertise to manage and direct all of the relevant programs required to meet all of the aviation-related regulations.[43]

Gower also pushed all of his pilots to achieve and maintain instrument flight proficiency. He was impressed with the performance of one crew in particular who launched one evening under visual flight conditions to transfer a patient from Fort Hood to a hospital in Waco. Once airborne the weather closed in and the crew had to switch to instrument procedures without mishap. Other units had lost aircraft and crews under similar conditions.

Gower attended one of the first aviation risk management classes offered by the Army. None of his local superiors were aviators, and as the senior aviator responsible for flight operations, he needed to be as trained and qualified as possible. He wanted to find that best balance between mission imperative and the laws of flight physics. He also flew as much as he could, believing that leadership was also necessary in the cockpit. He established and displayed guidance and limits for his crews, and later remembered that:

I saw that in the accidents that happened in the '80s ...the drive to save a life overshadowed the skill necessary to accomplish it under the conditions that the aviators were facing. We overcame that to a certain extent with this cockpit resource management concept... My safety officer and I took this opportunity to instill in the pilots what the commander thought so that they knew where their limits were and were comfortable turning around, rather than overstepping those limitations.[44]

Also concerned that his troops were using MAST to avoid significant tactical training, he held local tactical training exercises and directed his troops to organize and run a field exercise at Fort Hood, which included elements from all of the platoons in the 507th.

Gower served three years with the platoon and oversaw a total turnaround in the unit. The unit passed its next Aviation Resource Management Survey, and by the end of this tour, were the recipients of the Army Forces Command Commander's Aviation Safety Award. He left the 507th in 1984 for duty at Fort Rucker with the U.S. Army Aviation Research Lab. He never returned to MEDEVAC duty. He later fondly remembered his time with the 507th, recalling that:

During the '70s and '80s we fought the battle of the MAST program. For those who captured it, it was good crew training. For those who wanted to hide behind it, it was a way to just do your mission and not prepare for war. And I saw both of those. I saw that in the unit I took over at Fort Hood; I saw that a little bit in the unit in Hawaii. You could hide behind the MAST mission, do lots of good stuff, get lots of press, but you weren't really ready to go to war. And you really had to do both, but all through that, we also learned during those times that bravery without skill and thought process often was the difference between being a hero and being a martyr.[45]

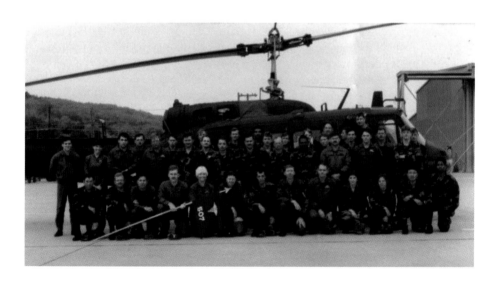

The 3rd Flight Platoon, 507th Med Co at Fort Hood, Texas, in 1984.
Source: Dan Gower

Like most from his generation of MEDEVAC crewmembers, Gower knew that MAST was their war. They engaged it with the same determination and professionalism that was the hallmark of their predecessors in Korea and Vietnam.

Another young trooper who flew his share of MAST missions was 1st Lt. Scott Heintz. After graduating from flight school in late 1981, he reported to the 498th Med Co (AA) at Fort Benning, Georgia. Assigned as a flight platoon leader, he began his mission checkout and immediately realized how much he had to learn about flying. Again, he encountered stalwart mentors who had the patience necessary to mold a promising young officer. CW2 Huey Driggers and CW2 Bryant Harp took him through his required qualification syllabus, gave him his tactical training, and taught him the nuances of flying the UH-1. The unit had a continuing requirement to cover training sites for the Ranger School in northern Georgia and the panhandle of Florida.

The 498th was also heavily committed to MAST, and Heintz sat alert for and launched on numerous missions. They covered the gamut from patient transfers to point-of-injury recoveries at automobile crashes. He saw the value of the training for his troops.

In 1984, Heintz completed his assignment with the 498th and returned to Fort Sam Houston for the MSC advanced course. He encountered another group of MEDEVAC veterans who again provided him with timely and valuable mentoring. His class received a presentation on the establishment of the Aviation Branch. The briefing officer extolled the virtues of the change and the assignment opportunities that would develop. His pitch included an implicit invitation for the MEDEVAC pilots to switch over. Maj. Frank Novier and Maj. Merle Snyder were serving as instructors and patiently helped the young officers like Heintz to work through the issues and realize that they needed to stay where they were.[46]

WO1 Bob Mitchell was another young pilot who logged many MAST missions. He had entered the Army through the warrant officer program in late 1982 after playing football for four years at the University of Toledo in Ohio. Mitchell already had his pilot's license and wanted to learn to fly helicopters. After attending the flight course at Fort Rucker, he went to the 82d Combat Aviation Battalion at Fort Bragg, where he flew OH-58s as a scout pilot for two years.

In 1985, his unit transitioned its lift company to UH-60s, and Mitchell was one of the first to retrain for it. After he was qualified, he received a call from Capt. Ken Crook, the commander of the 57th Med Det. The 57th had also recently converted to UH-60s, and it needed pilots. Crook recruited him for 60 days of MEDEVAC duty.[47]

Mitchell was immediately on the flight schedule, flying MAST and training range recovery missions. After a few weeks, Crook saw that the young warrant was a very capable soldier and made him the assistant operations officer. Crook also encouraged him to apply for a direct commission into the MSC. Mitchell did so. A few months later when he received his commission, he also received orders assigning him to the 57th. He subsequently served in the unit for three years, qualifying as a pilot in command, and then served as a section leader and assistant operations officer. He also qualified as an instructor pilot on the UH-60, which was a rare accomplishment for a detachment-level MSC pilot.

Leaving the 57th in 1989, Mitchell then attended the aviation officer's advanced course at Fort Rucker. He met many officers with whom he would later serve on subsequent tours. After completing that course, his experience as both a warrant and commissioned officer pilot led to him staying at Fort Rucker and serving as the Chief of the Utility Branch of the Directorate of Evaluation and Standardization at the Aviation Center. He was the sole MSC pilot in that organization.

Mitchell's office was responsible for worldwide standardization of Army flight procedures. Traveling to almost every flying unit that the Army possessed, he saw firsthand the strengths and weaknesses of the Army aviation and MEDEVAC communities. He also saw how much the MEDEVAC units relied on aviation units, especially on deployments. Yet the commanders seemingly refused to forge the necessary relationships at home base to facilitate coordinated operations. He sensed that many MEDEVAC officers held an elitist attitude that in some cases led to a palpable schism between the MEDEVAC and aviation communities at some bases. He remembered that:

> When I was with [the standardization and evaluation team] going around the world inspecting all of the MEDEVAC units, inspecting all of the lift units, inspecting all of the Chinook units, … there was a common theme out there. "MEDEVAC? Yeah, they are on the other side of the ramp and we don't know who they are. …They don't want to play."[48]

Mitchell concluded that it only made intuitive sense for MEDEVAC to eventually become part of aviation. He saw the reasons on his inspection trips. When he expressed those opinions, though, he received a lot of negative feedback from other MEDEVAC guys, who felt that he was a maverick and "smoking dope."[49]

MAST Continues to Expand

In the summer of 1986, another MEDEVAC unit, the 229th Med Det (RA), was activated at Fort Drum, New York. It had an area mission and supported both the tactical units and the garrison in general. In addition, its commander immediately began scripting the paperwork necessary to provide MAST service for the local community.[50]

In October 1987, the 229th's MAST request was approved, and it assumed MAST alert duties as the 25th unit to do so. Since operations had begun in 1970, the combined units had flown more than 78,000 hours on more than 35,000 missions that had transported more than 37,000 patients, medical personnel and equipment, blood, and organs for transplant. More than one-third of the sorties had been at night, and almost one-half of the missions involved moving patients from the point of the accident or injury to a major medical facility. MAST was proving to be one of the most successful and durable programs of military and civilian cooperation. Each community benefited in so many ways from the service. However, the missions allowed the MEDEVAC units locally to practice their military purpose. Except for the added exigencies of combat, the needed skill sets were the same. De facto, MAST was a full-time training program for the military crews, just as Spurgeon Neel had foreseen many years earlier.

Strong bonds developed between the units and the communities they supported. MAST now covered parts of 19 states and constantly received favorable press coverage. It was a public relations gold mine for the Army. Perhaps more importantly, it allowed the people to see the tangible results produced at no extra cost to the taxpayers. Yet it was the soldiers who made it happen. Their selflessness and dedication was visible to all.[51]

The concept also spread into the civilian side of aviation, just as originally planned. By 1988, private companies supplied air ambulances at 45 hospitals nationwide. One of the chief protagonists of this spread was Craig Honaman. A former MEDEVAC pilot with the 57th Med Det (RA) in Vietnam, Honaman had been awarded the Distinguished Flying Cross and 21 Air Medals for his service there. After leaving the Army, he became a hospital administrator and was deeply involved in the development of aeromedical standards and safety programs at both the state and federal level. Honaman also directly led efforts at two different hospitals to establish air ambulance services for each. In recognition of his accomplishments, he received the MBB Golden Hour Award presented by the MBB (Messerschmitt-Boelkow-Blohm) Helicopter Corporation in 1988.[52]

Tactical Training – Operation BRIGHT STAR

In June 1982, Maj. Art Hapner arrived at Fort Bragg to take command of the 57th Med Det (RG). The unit was beginning its transition to the new UH-60A, and he attended upgrade school en route. As the unit worked through the transition, he was notified that they would deploy to Egypt in the spring of 1983 with elements of the 82d Airborne Division to participate in Operation BRIGHT STAR, a large combined training exercise there.

Hapner was impressed with the Black Hawk, and in combination with other MEDEVAC and aviation unit officers, he formulated a plan to self-deploy their aircraft from Fort Bragg to Egypt. They devised a concept of operations and supporting training plan and briefed it all the way up to the Vice Chief of Staff of the Army. The plan called for the helicopters to fly up the east coast of the United States, to Newfoundland, over to Greenland, Iceland, Scotland, down through Germany, Austria, Italy, Greece, and then across the Mediterranean to their deployment bases in Egypt. The challenging part was crossing the Mediterranean. It was the longest leg of the journey and appeared to be just too far. They approached the U.S. Navy Staff for support and were told that an aircraft carrier would position itself so that it could be used as a mid-point refueling stop.

The total plan was approved, and Hapner readied his unit. Literally within hours of departure, the commander of the XVIII Airborne Corps informed him that a tense situation was developing with Libya and the self-deployment mission had to be cancelled. However, the deployment to BRIGHT STAR was still on, so Hapner had to get his aircraft up to Dover Air Force Base (AFB), Delaware, for packing and shipment to Egypt.

The 57th flew in support of the exercise until August, and then it returned home to Fort Bragg. Subsequently, it took three more weeks before all of their aircraft were returned. The desert environment was hard on the new aircraft, and all needed repair. The maintenance troops worked overtime to make necessary repairs because of events occurring in the Caribbean that were being watched very closely by U.S. leaders.[53]

Grenada – Operation URGENT FURY

In October 1983, for the first time since Vietnam, a sizable U.S. Army task force departed home shores for a major contingency operation to the Caribbean island of Grenada, located approximately 1,200 miles southeast of Miami, at the southern end of the Lesser Antilles.

A communist style dictatorship had taken over the nation. It had established a strong relationship with Cuba, and a contingent of Cuban military advisors and an engineering unit were dispatched to build a 12,000-foot runway and airfield that would be used by Soviet long-range aircraft. Grenada was also home to St. George's Medical Center, a prominent medical school that enrolled more than 800 American students. In early October, leftist opponents killed the Prime Minister.

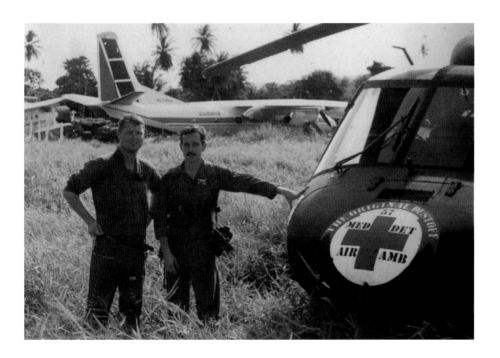

Maj. Art Hapner (left), Commander, and Capt. Kevin Swenie, Operations Officer of the 57th Med Det in Grenada.
Source: Office of the Chief, Medical Service Corps.

President Ronald Reagan and his senior leaders watched the situation closely. Reagan had taken office on the heels of the nightmare experienced by his predecessor, President Jimmy Carter, when the Iranians had seized 52 American hostages in November 1979. He wanted no replay of that debacle. Sensing that the American students were at risk of becoming hostages, he directed that American forces invade.

On the early morning of 25 October, the American joint task force descended upon the island. Two battalions from the 75th Ranger Regiment jumped onto the Point Salines Airfield followed shortly by soldiers from the 82d Airborne Division. Concurrently, special operations forces and U.S. Marines from the 2d Marine Division assaulted other island locations. Their assigned tasks were to evacuate U.S. citizens, neutralize any resistance, stabilize the situation, and maintain the peace. An aviation task force from the 82d Airborne Division also deployed to the island of Barbados, 160 miles to the northeast, and supported the operation from there. Combat operations only lasted a few days. All of the medical students were evacuated. An estimated 70 Cubans and Grenadians were killed and 394 were wounded. Of the U.S. forces 19 were killed and 115 were wounded.[54]

In support of the operation, the 57th Med Det (RG) was alerted for deployment. Hapner received the phone call on the evening of the 24th. He recalled his unit, and by early the next morning, he had three of his aircraft at Pope AFB, next door to Fort Bragg, ready for deployment aboard Air Force cargo aircraft. That day, the aircraft, equipment, and a detachment of unit personnel were loaded and flown to Barbados, where they joined up with the division's 82d Combat Aviation Battalion.

The next morning, all three aircraft were ready, and the unit detachment flew forward to Point Salines Airfield, linked up with the 307th Medical Battalion, and initiated MEDEVAC operations. Within an hour, their first task was to pick up a wounded Marine. Fortunately, MEDEVAC calls were few, and in the first month, the 57th only flew about 25 missions. They supported recovery operations for two downed aircraft and recovered 12 injured from a fratricide incident when a U.S. Navy A-7 strafed a friendly position. Missions were also flown to support the local populace. Several pregnant Grenadians were delivered to hospitals. One young boy, injured by a grenade, was MEDEVACed.[55]

When Hapner and his troops landed at Point Salines, there was no fuel available so he had his helicopters land aboard the two U.S. Navy helicopter carriers deployed for the operation. They also delivered several patients to the *USS Guam,* and overall, provided the bulk of MEDEVAC capability because no ground MEDEVAC units were deployed. The total medical package deployed was not sufficient for the operation. Fortunately, the crews in the 57th were trained to land aboard ships and were able to move the wounded to those facilities.[56]

The single biggest problem was the lack of communications connectivity between the different parts of the joint task force. When the 57th arrived at Point Salines, it had to coordinate *ad hoc* with local units to develop a crude communications plan.[57]

The 57th element stayed until February, supporting the stabilization operations. Then the detachment and its aircraft and equipment were returned to Fort Bragg.[58]

Europe

In Europe, the MEDEVAC units were mostly still in their previous locations. The 421st Med Co (AA) was still at Nellingen with its 1st and 3d Platoons. Its 2d Platoon was at Schweinfurt, and its 4th was at Darmstadt. The 421st now had assigned to it a total of 49 helicopters and 321 personnel and served as the controlling headquarters for Dustoff Europe under the 7th Medical Command. It still had assigned to it the 15th Med Det (RA) at the Grafenwöhr training complex; the 63d Med Det (RA) at Landstuhl and primarily performing intratheater transfers; the 159th Med Det (RA), which had relocated north to Garlstedt to provide MEDEVAC support for a growing U.S. Army presence in that area; and the 236th Med Det (RA), still at Augsburg. Effectively, the 421st functioned as a battalion.

During 1982, 421st units flew more than 8,000 mission flight hours performing MEDEVAC duties to include support for the annual REFORGER exercises. Starting in 1983, the 421st and subordinate units began to transition to the new UH-60 helicopters. The conversion presented the unit with a huge training challenge, yet the units maintained crews on continuous alert to provide all weather support to the soldiers and dependents in the theater and their German neighbors.[59]

They also maintained a forward operating location at the large Hohenfels maneuver complex southeast of Nürnberg. Crews from the various units rotated through for periods of up to a week to provide 24-hour coverage for troops on the field. Crews prepared their own meals or would occasionally order pizza or other fast food from local franchises. By tradition, new troops paid when they had their first patient mission. Scrambles were rare. Occasionally their efforts would save a life. Capt. Randy Maschek and his crew were launched one evening to recover a soldier who had fallen asleep in a tank. The soldier had been sleeping next to a leaking battery and breathed in hydrogen sulfide fumes from it. They delivered him to a hospital before any permanent damage was done. Another crew picked up a pregnant woman who had gone into labor. She was full-term and had some complications that required her movement to a specific hospital. As they flew her to it, she went into labor. The baby came rapidly. As they approached the hospital landing pad, the head appeared. As they touched down the baby was delivered. Medics were waiting and quickly took the mother and child into the delivery room. The crew shut down the aircraft and went into the hospital to check on them both. Mother and daughter were fine, and the MEDEVAC crew toasted them with coffee poured into urine sample cups.

However, real "keeper" missions were actually the exception. Most tours consisted of reading, sleeping, exercise, videos, or the random scribbling of notes and missives on any manner of subjects, all recorded in the totally unofficial *Dustoff Follies Notebook*, never destined to leave the alert facility at Hohenfels.[60]

Central America

In response to the Panama Canal Treaty signed between the United States and Panama in September 1977, the U.S. Army assumed responsibility for health care within the former Panama Canal Zone. The Panama Canal Zone had a Medical Department Activity (MEDDAC) with two hospitals: (1) the Gorgas Hospital on the Pacific side, and (2) the Coco Solo Hospital on the Atlantic side. To allow for more expeditious evacuation to or between the two sites, an air ambulance section was created with three UH-1V aircraft and crews on duty at all times to perform the classic MEDEVAC duties of patient movement, and the transport of whole blood, and essential medical personnel and equipment. They could also provide crash rescue support to Howard AFB, also in the Canal Zone.

Secondarily, the unit supplied local support in many forms. It provided support similar to MAST for local civilians or injured sailors aboard ships using the Panama Canal. The 210th Aviation Battalion at Howard AFB provided maintenance, logistical, and aviation support. The 210th had been in Panama since 1973 and had on many occasions performed casualty evacuation missions as needed.[61]

In June 1984, the 214th Med Det (RG) was reactivated with UH-60s at Fort Kobbe, Panama Canal Zone. It replaced the air ambulance section and provided direct support to the MEDDAC. The 210th Aviation Battalion also supported the 214th Med Det.[62]

At about the same time, Joint Task Force Bravo was activated at Palmerola Air Base in Honduras. The United States had maintained a steady presence in Central America, and it was the latest and largest in a series of task forces formed in that area of Central America at the request of local governments in response to developing internal and external threats. It served as the basis for the deployment of larger forces of any variety, and it also supported civic action operations over a wide area.[63]

The next November, two aircraft and crews from the 214th were deployed to Colombia as part of Task Force 210 to provide humanitarian relief for the victims of a volcano eruption. The ensuing mud slides and flooding caused by the rapid melting of snow pack inundated 14 villages and towns. An estimated 23,000 were killed, and another 22,000 were left homeless. Because of the high trees in the area, many of the recoveries were by hoist.[64]

In October 1987, the 210th Aviation Battalion was inactivated, and the 1st Battalion, 228th Aviation Regiment, was activated at Fort Kobbe, as part of the 128th Aviation Brigade. The 214th Med Det (RG) was attached to the 1st Battalion, 228th Regiment. Its missions were varied including providing general support to local units—both on post and in the field for training—and also supporting civic action missions in Panama and other Central America nations. The 214th crews would fly medical teams out to local villages to provide on-site medical care.[65]

In the summer of 1989, Joint Task Force Bravo activated the 4th Battalion, 228th Aviation Regiment, at the Soto Cano Air Base (formerly Palmerola) in Honduras. It had a MEDEVAC detachment assigned to it. While still forming, it provided support to operations conducted in Panama, later that year.[66]

Preparing for War on the Plains of Europe

Doctrine

Field Circular (FC) 8-45, Medical Evacuation in the Combat Zone, October 1986

With a third revision of its keystone warfighting doctrinal publication, Field Manual (FM) 100-5, ultimately published in 1986, the Army finally crystallized its concept of AirLand Battle. This version integrated the use of intelligence assets to "see deep" into the enemy's rear areas to further facilitate the deep battle. It emphasized the "operational art" of synthesizing all facets of military operations to fight and win the right battle at the right place and time.

This iteration stimulated a rewrite of medical doctrine to support it. Incorporating the concepts laid out in the earlier MSPR, the AHS at Fort Sam Houston published its new concept, now titled "Health Service Support for AirLand Battle," in April 1986. Reflecting the earnest work and advocacy of Lt. Col. Tom Scofield and Maj. Bill Thresher, and with the hearty support of Col. Eldon Ideus, still serving as the chief of the MEDEVAC Proponency Office, the AHS also published FC 8-45, *Medical Evacuation in the Combat Zone,* in October 1986, which defined how MEDEVAC would support Health Service Support for AirLand Battle with its evacuation battalions and 15-ship companies. This FC was intended as an interim change, subject to comments and recommendations from the field. As such, it would expire in 1989, if not subsumed earlier by an overriding FM.[67]

With AirLand Battle as its basis, the rewrite acknowledged that the extension of the battlefield stretched theater HSS to its limits. Medical commanders needed to understand the objectives and intent of their superior maneuver commanders. They had to be prepared proactively to maintain the initiative, agility, and synchronization necessary to preserve fighting strength, evacuate the wounded in an expeditious and efficient manner, and handle mass casualty-type operations that could occur in the expected intense combat operations or use of weapons of mass destruction. Moreover, medical commanders had to have command and control of medical assets to maximize care and to locate medical units so that casualties could be evacuated as quickly as possible.[68]

The FC also postulated that the principal threat was the forces of the Union of Soviet Socialist Republics, with that threat most dramatically arrayed in Europe or southwest Asia. Medical evacuation units with forces opposing these in any scenario faced a variety of lethal threats from air defense weapons; field artillery; the guns of massed armored vehicles and tanks; tactical aircraft, both rotary and fixed-wing; nuclear, biological, and chemical weapons; and even unconventional warfare, across the depth of the battlefield. Yet, the air ambulance units had to operate in all areas and make maximum utilization of passive countermeasures, nap-of-the-earth flight techniques, and overall threat avoidance, and make sure that the Red Cross marking was always clearly visible.[69]

The FC validated the reestablishment of the Vietnam era medical evacuation battalions and defined their role. Within a theater of operations, such a battalion

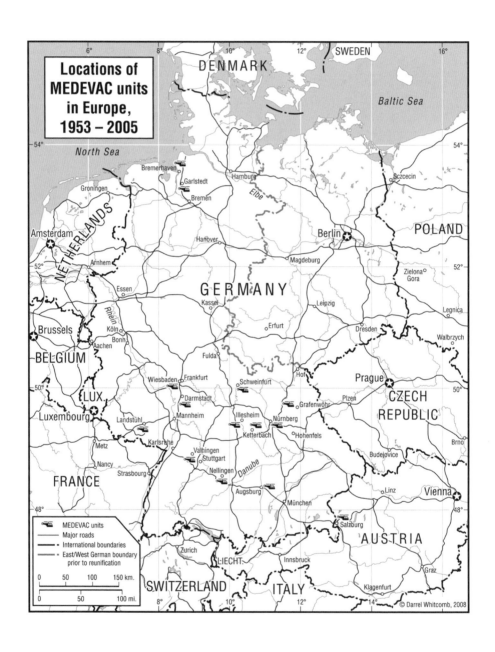

was assigned to the medical command or to a medical brigade. Its function was to serve as a central manager of ground and air evacuation assets as part of the overall HSS plan. Three to seven ambulance companies (air or ground) for command and control were attached to the battalion, which was best located where it provided such command and control. Its staff was organized with a headquarters section, an S1 section, and S2/3 section, and an S4 section. Air ambulance medical companies were assigned to it on the basis of one company in direct support of a division or equivalent force, and one air ambulance company in general support of the corps for each two divisions assigned or fraction thereof.

The MEDEVAC companies were capable of around-the-clock operations with 15 air ambulances, each with a flight medic capable of providing treatment and surveillance of patients. The companies were manned with an aviation unit maintenance section that performed organizational maintenance on all aircraft, avionics, and organic equipment, except specialized medical items. The company also provided air crash rescue support (less fire suppression) and up to three forward support MEDEVAC teams of three aircraft and crews each. A forward support MEDEVAC team was designed directly to support a maneuver brigade. The remaining aircraft performed area support MEDEVAC. In the field, the company relied on other units for higher levels of support, in particular, aviation intermediate maintenance.[70]

These changes were designed to reorganize the air ambulance MEDEVAC assets more efficiently to support the dynamic nature of AirLand Battle. FC 8-45 pointed out that:

> The increase in the speed and lethality of combat formations has served to increase the importance of evacuation as the key link in the continuum of care….The AirLand Battle will be conducted day and night under all weather conditions….The evacuation system must be prepared to operate in the added dimension of the integrated battlefield.[71]

The newly designed medical evacuation battalion was the key to the theater evacuation system and operated as per the following principles:

1. The purpose of evacuation is to rapidly transport the sick and wounded soldiers to a medical treatment facility to minimize fatalities and speed their return to duty by:
   a. Clearing the battlefield to allow the commander to continue his mission.
   b. Building the morale of soldiers by demonstrating that care is quickly available.
2. Evacuation is performed by the higher echelon of medical care going forward and evacuation from the lower level.
3. Evacuation assets must have the same mobility as the units supported.
4. The medical commander responsible for evacuation is the primary manager of medical evacuation assets. There must be one single dedicated medical command authority to manage all assets. The evacuation mode is based on:
   a. Patient's condition.
   b. Availability of resources.

c. Destination medical treatment facility.
5. On-board care of casualties is essential for optimum success.
6. Bypassing echelons of care is detrimental to the medical support system and wounded soldier. It causes over-evacuation of less critically wounded soldiers, delaying their return to duty, and removing evacuation assets from critical areas for longer periods of time.[72]

Overall, FC 8-45 was a significant change for the MEDEVAC units. If followed to fruition, it would require a complete reorganization of MEDEVAC assets as part of ultimately a larger reorganization of medical units so that all had a go-to-war mission. Eventually, the entire restructuring effort for all of the medical units would be renamed the Medical Force 2000.[73]

Organization

New Aircraft

Parallel to the changes in doctrine was consideration of a new aircraft for MEDEVAC. Since the early 1950s, aircraft designers had worked on the concept of tilt rotor aircraft that could combine the best features of both rotary-wing and fixed-wing design. Sensing the military potential for such a vehicle, Army designers conceptualized such an aircraft in 1982 and labeled it JVX. In 1985, the Joint Chiefs of Staff published a Joint Services Operational Requirement for the JVX called the Advanced Vertical Lift Aircraft. This aircraft provided the various services the ability to conduct combat, combat support, and combat service support utilizing vertical take-off and landing capabilities. The JVX replaced a number of aging and near obsolescent aircraft and provided for expanded mission capabilities. For the Army, this aircraft was well fitted for medium cargo lift and medical evacuation. In the MEDEVAC configuration, the aircraft was capable of functioning on a high-threat battlefield with an 80% mission capability rate, while incorporating the latest developments in survivability and crashworthiness improvements, operating continuously (day/night operations) in all weather, utilizing a cruise speed of 250 knots, and carrying 12 patients and two medics in the cabin with the latest comfort and load convenience items.[74]

The prime candidate for this aircraft was the V-22, which was produced by Boeing Aircraft in Philadelphia, Pennsylvania. The Army was well represented on the various working groups established to bring the aircraft to fruition as the JVX. By 1986, the Army had developed a plan for acquisition and utilization of the aircraft. The Army wanted 231 V-22s, of which 64 would be assigned to MEDEVAC to equip eight companies. This released 135 UH-1s and UH-60s for retirement or shift to other missions. Like the helicopters it replaced, the aircraft could be loaded onto C-5s for deployment. However, the aircraft could also self-deploy. It could be flown to Europe in about 30 hours, needing only one stop for fuel and crew change. This capability was something that MEDEVAC crews had desired for a long time.[75]

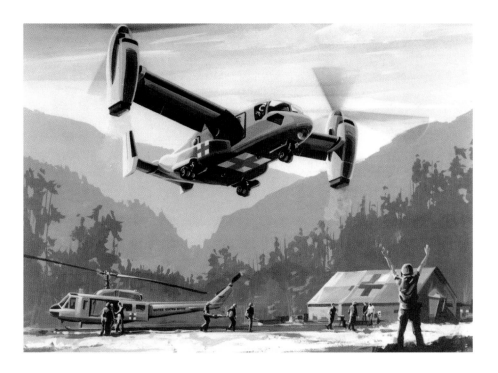

Proposed V-22 in its MEDEVAC configuration.
Source: Office of Medical History Files

The acquisition plan forecast that the aircraft would be delivered between 1994 and 2001. Potential MEDEVAC modifications to the cabin included a scheme for racking 18 litters with plenty of room remaining for medical equipment. However, in a progress review in 1988, Army leaders withdrew from the program, ostensibly to use the money for upgrades for the CH-47, UH-60, and AH-64, and the development of a new light helicopter (LHX). The UH-60 became the standard and primary MEDEVAC helicopter, although the LHX did have a MEDEVAC variant. The next year, the Secretary of Defense reviewed the entire V-22 program. With the departure of the Army from the project, the only service still interested was the Marine Corps. However, at $32.8 million per aircraft, the Secretary could not justify the cost of the planned fleet "for the narrow mission of moving marines from ship to shore" and suspended the program.[76]

Europe

In the summer of 1985, Maj. Frank Novier had completed two nonflying assignments and the Armed Forces Staff College, and he reported to Landstuhl, Germany, to command the 63d Med Det (RA). His first assigned duty was to convert the unit to UH-60s. Unfortunately, just after he arrived, the entire Army

Black Hawk fleet was grounded for a mechanical problem with a key component. To meet its mission taskings, the unit kept its old UH-1s. Known as "International Dustoff," the unit pilots regularly flew patient transfer to hospitals all over Europe or picked up sick or injured for movement to the huge hospital at Landstuhl. The unit also trained for its wartime mission in support of the 3d Armored Division and its requirement to defend the Fulda Gap. Unlike his earlier tour in Europe in the 1970s, Novier's unit and troops had real defined missions to which they regularly trained, were aware of the changes in warfighting doctrine, and had watched the arrival of new and superior equipment—like their own Black Hawks. Novier could clearly see the difference it made in their cohesion, sense of purpose, and morale.

When the Black Hawk fleet was released for flight duty, Novier literally had to reconvert his unit, and do it quickly. Fortunately, he had great troops like Capt. Scott Heintz, who had also joined the unit not long after Novier arrived. Novier took his best pilots and made them pilots in command on the Black Hawks because he was not given any extra crewmembers to make the transition. Then he assigned them to missions and never missed any tasking. It was a risky move. Yet he trusted his crews, and they did not let him down. After 18 months, his tour as the detachment commander ended and he was transferred to the 7th MEDCOM headquarters at Heidelberg to serve as the aviation staff officer.[77]

Novier arrived at a propitious time. The European MEDEVAC units were reorganizing under the concepts laid out in FC 8-45. By the end of the year, the 421st Med Co (AA) was reorganized as the 421st Medical Battalion (Evacuation). In a poignant ceremony, Company Commander Lt. Col. Merle Snyder passed command to Lt. Col. Art Hapner as the Battalion Commander in October 1987.[78]

The 421st had three companies and three detachments assigned to it: (1) the newly reactivated 45th Med Co (AA) [last active in Vietnam], which was formed from the 1st, 2d, and 3d Platoons of the 421st Med Co (AA), and was co-located at Nellingen; (2) the 159th Med Co (AA), formed from the 159th Med Det (RG) and the 4th Platoon of the 421st Med Co (AA), relocated to Darmstadt; and (3) the original 15th, 63d, and 236th Med Dets (RG), which were still separate. This streamlined overall evacuation command and control, and provided for more efficient unit level training. Hapner commanded the 421st until July 1990, when he passed command to Lt. Col. Ray Keith, a former unit mate from the 57th at Fort Bragg.[79]

Disaster at Ramstein Air Base, Germany

As the European units went through their realignments, their community was struck with tragedy in a most unexpected way. Every summer, the huge U.S. Air Force Base at Ramstein, located just three miles from the large medical center at Landstuhl, hosted a tremendous international airshow. It was a favorite with the local community and drew massive crowds. More than 300,000 visitors crowded onto the base on 28 August 1988 to watch flying demonstrations put on by teams from all over the world. It was a beautifully clear day as 10 jets from the Italian Air Force acrobatic team, *Frecce Tricolori,* took off to perform their amazing

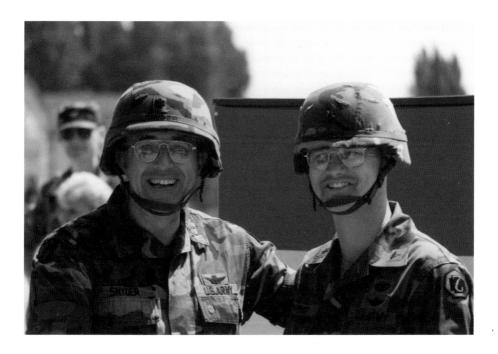

Lt. Col. Merle Snyder passes command of the 421st Med Co (AA) to Lt. Col. Art Hapner as the unit is upgraded to a battalion in October 1987.
Source: 421st Medical Battalion (Evacuation) Historical Files

maneuvers that culminated with their signature event, the "pierced heart." The maneuver required the team to do a steep vertical climb and then separate so that two groups traced a heart with their smoke trails. When this was done, another member flew through the smoke to pierce it. The maneuver required split second timing. The team had done it many times and it was always a crowd pleaser. Unfortunately on this day, the solo pilot mis-timed his piercing maneuver and collided with two of the aircraft. Some of the flaming wreckage fell on the crowd. Chaos swept them as they tried to scramble to avoid the wreckage and falling flaming fuel. A MEDEVAC UH-60 from the 63d Med Det (RG) was on alert at the air show. Tragically, some of the wreckage slammed into the helicopter, severely damaging it and killing one of the pilots, Capt. Kim Strader.

Medical personnel immediately sprang into action. Within minutes, other MEDEVAC helicopters from Landstuhl and Wiesbaden were en route, and German aircraft also responded. All totaled, 72 spectators were killed as well as three performing pilots. Additionally, 346 were seriously wounded. Over the next few hours, 120 were evacuated to Landstuhl. Others were moved to additional local hospitals. More were dispatched to other medical facilities spread across Germany or even MEDEVACed to other countries. Crews from all of the MEDEVAC units were busy transporting the patients.[80]

Two years later, the 236th Med Co (AA) was formed from the 15th, 63d, and 236th Med Dets, and consolidated at Landstuhl, also under the control of the 421st. The European MEDEVAC units had now completely reorganized under FC 8-45.[81]

Capt. Scott Heintz had finished his tour with the 63d Med Det (RG) at Landstuhl, just prior to the horrible accident at Ramstein, and was at Fort Sam Houston when he heard the terrible news that his unit buddies had been killed and injured in the ensuing fire. He was now assigned to instructor duties with the Military Science Division at the AHS, where he taught the career basic and advanced courses for all of AMEDD. Primarily, he taught basic subjects to company grade officers such as map reading, physical fitness, and even marching. He also flew as an attached pilot with the co-located 507th Med Co (AA), and initiated some rudimentary MEDEVAC field demonstrations for the classes.

While instructing at Fort Sam Houston, one of Heintz's students was newly commissioned MSC 2d Lt. John Lamoureux, who had attended Embry Riddle Aeronautical University in Florida and was interested in a career in aviation. His mother spent many years working in hospitals, and Lamoureux wanted to see if he could find a career that would combine aviation and medicine. Heintz took

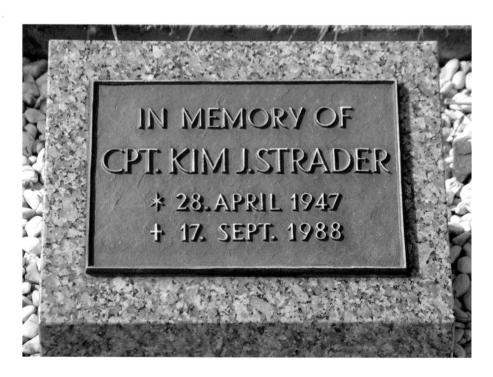

Marker at the 236th Med Co (AA), Landstuhl, Germany, commemorating Capt. Kim Strader, killed at the Ramstein Air Base Airshow in 1988.
Source: Author

Lamoureux under his wing. Acting as an advisor and mentor, Heintz convinced him to consider MEDEVAC. Flight school slots were few then, but Lamoureux had a solid record and was selected. He started flight school at Fort Rucker in September 1989.[82]

On 1 April 1990, Heintz was promoted to the rank of Major. With the promotion came a new assignment to command Delta Company, 326th Medical Battalion, 101st Division at Fort Campbell. He arrived at Fort Campbell in late June and took command of "Eagle Dustoff" on 12 July 1990.[83]

Operations

Korea

After his tour at Fort Sam Houston, Maj. Bill Thresher reported to the Eighth U.S. Army in Korea to command the 377th Med Co (AA), located at the Army Air Base just south of Seoul. It was one of the large 25-aircraft units recently re-equipped with new Black Hawks and under the direct control of the 52nd Medical Battalion (Evacuation).

The Eighth Army had designated the 377th as a top priority unit. Thresher had more than 50 pilots assigned to the company, including 16 MSC officers and three test pilots. With more than 190 enlisted troops assigned, unit operational readiness never fell below 80%. The unit was also issued ANVIS-6 NVGs, and all pilots trained on them, including Thresher, who logged almost 800 flight hours while he was in the 377th.

The aviation maintenance section was particularly robust—very similar to an aviation battalion—and could handle almost any aircraft problem. The maintenance troops were dedicated and worked extra hours when necessary to support the mission. They all shared that sense of urgency that Thresher had learned many years before at Fort Bragg.

Unit elements were scattered across four locations to provide coverage to the entire peninsula. They routinely supported the 2nd Infantry Division at Camp Humphreys and flew to locations within the Demilitarized Zone. Special flight procedures were necessary to do so, and all unit pilots were required to maintain the qualification to fly in there night and day and under any weather condition. The 377th crews also flew transfer missions for soldiers needing medical movement anywhere on the peninsula.[84]

Finishing his tour as a scout pilot in Germany in 1985 with more than 1,500 hours of flight time, CW2 Pete Smart received orders to Fort Rucker to attend the Warrant Officer Advanced Course and attend transition training to become a fixed-wing pilot flying the OV-1 Mohawk. Once qualified, he stayed at Rucker flying the Mohawk and he met some MEDEVAC pilots. When he mentioned that he always had a desire to fly MEDEVAC, they encouraged him to apply for a direct commission into the MSC. The next MSC board selected him so he traded in his warrant officer bars for his 2d Lt. rank, went through UH-60 transition and main-

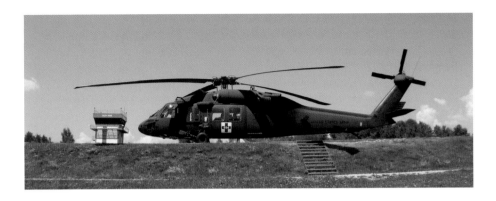

A 159th Med Co UH-60A on alert at the Hohenfels, Germany Airfield.
Source: Author

tenance officer's school, and then received orders to the 377th Med Co in Korea.

New 2d Lt. Smart arrived at the 377th in the summer of 1987. Thresher made him the unit maintenance officer for the 25-aircraft unit with those machines spread out at four different sites, and a flying authorization for almost 7,000 hours a year.

Smart was immediately consumed with the myriad details of keeping those aircraft air worthy. He flew mostly on maintenance test flights, but would occasionally pair up with Thresher and go to one of the sites to sit MEDEVAC alert.

The pressure to keep the aircraft mission-ready was constant and almost all consuming. Smart remembered that:

> There is a tremendous amount of pressure—not pressure, but a sense of urgency that exists to keep the aircraft up. And when they do go down, you can't send everybody home and say, "Well, we'll get it Monday; it can wait." ... [MEDEVAC] guys can get their missions any time...[85]

On many occasions when a maintenance crew was sent to one of the remote sites to fix an aircraft, Smart would fly it regardless of the weather or time of day. Consequently, he became very proficient at flying instrument procedures. Maintenance officers were generally not noted for their instrument proficiency, and Smart took special delight in that, especially when one of the flight examiners told him, "You know you are a pretty darned good instrument pilot for a maintenance guy." But it was more than ego that drove him. He had been a warrant officer and remembered several commissioned officers who were not good pilots. He knew how much the warrants resented that and resolved that he would always maintain his pilot skills as he expected them to do. It was a matter of professional pride.[86]

Also serving with Thresher in the 377th, 1st Lt. Dave MacDonald served as the 2d platoon leader at Camp Humphreys. Compared to southeast Alabama, flying in Korea was a bit more challenging, and MacDonald learned quickly from his warrant officer pilots, crew chiefs, and medics. He also latched on to Thresher's sense of urgency remembering that, "Every mission you go out on is real and there is always a sense of accomplishment … that you have actually been saving a life." He finished his tour there in February 1988 and returned to Fort Rucker for the Aviation Advanced Course, learning early that:

> "We have to know and understand the aviation business and what Army Aviation is all about as well as to know and understand the medical business and what the Army Medical Department is all about, and to be able to marry those two [to] effect the mission."[87]

Thresher also ensured that his unit was prepared to carry out its wartime missions. In addition to supporting the 2nd Division, the unit built transportable containers that could be sling-load carried by the helicopters. All necessary equipment and parts could be loaded into these containers so that the unit could move at relatively short notice. For one exercise, the majority of the unit did deploy to a field site. When they were settled at their assigned location, Thresher was almost overtaken with pride to see 22 of his aircraft arrayed in a large field and ready to receive taskings.

His unit responded when a U.S. Marine CH-53 helicopter crashed on a mountain side with 32 personnel onboard. The unit had just finished participating in a mass casualty exercise and launched recovery aircraft from three sites to support the disaster. Thresher's crews recovered 16 badly injured marines and flew them to hospital ships. Several of his troops received air medals for that action, and the unit was awarded a Navy Meritorious Unit Commendation.[88]

As a commissioned officer, Smart also had unit supervisory briefing and release authorities. For guidance, Thresher provided very specific procedures for handling launch authority. He explained:

> In Korea, the Army had instituted … mission briefing requirements. The way we handled it was …we would do a day mission. We would go out and assess the worst conditions that were anticipated to be met that day, and then we would conduct essentially a mission brief that talked about the high temperature, the weather, whatever it was going to be, and then the various mission modes that somebody could find himself. And then I authorized launch under those conditions up to a certain level of risk. And so they didn't have to sit around and punch buttons and figure all stuff out .… And then we would try to maximize those conditions under which the aircraft commander or the pilot in command could self-authorize. Above that, I was the authorization authority. If it was a high risk, then the battalion commander became the authorization.[89]

He also spent a lot of time and effort teaching his troops the proper focus on risk management. He said:

> I was able to help instill what MEDEVAC ought to really be about and why training was so important; why risk management—not avoidance of difficult jobs and dangerous flying environments—but risk management of difficult jobs and dangerous flying environments was the right way to go.[90]

He also harkened back to his own training as a young officer when he was mentored by a MEDEVAC legend, Maj. Gen. Pat Brady, who told him:

"You can't train people to do unsafe things by avoiding them. You have to manage the risk with which you train people to do those dangerous things…you have got to be able to mitigate the risks so you…are approaching it professionally."[91]

That focus on risk management and a sense of urgency were the hallmarks of his style of leadership and his younger officers benefited from it. Smart found his tour with the 377th so rewarding that he stayed for a second year.[92]

Thresher was immensely proud of his unit and very pleased with his tour in Korea. He departed the 377th in August 1989 for another tour with the AMEDD Center and School at Fort Sam Houston. He would never again be directly associated with MEDEVAC units. He had developed a fine appreciation for the young troops that he had trained and mentored, so he took a behind-the-scenes but active role in trying to encourage them and find ways to further their careers and develop their skills for higher levels of responsibility and command. However, he always told them that "There is no job security out there except your ability to achieve."[93]

Growing Conflict in Central America

Operations

Panama – Operation JUST CAUSE

In 1989, events in Panama drew the attention of the American leaders. For decades, Panama had been a backwater as the United States focused on other threats overseas. After a military coup in 1968 overthrew the last elected government, a series of military dictators had ruled the country. The latest was General Manuel Noriega, an intelligence officer, who eventually seized power.

Noriega assisted the United States through the Central Intelligence Agency when it conducted covert operations against Nicaraguan and El Salvadorian leftists. However, Noriega's operations eventually became so extreme that he was indicted in a Florida court for involvement in the drug trade, the smuggling of weapons to antigovernment rebels in Colombia, and collusion with Cuba to evade U.S. economic sanctions. Within Panama, he also conducted a bloody and brutal campaign against any and all opposition. He used his power to nullify national elections and survived a coup attempt, declaring himself "Maximum Leader for life."[94]

As Noriega consolidated his power, relations between the Panamanians and U.S. personnel soured. Missions to other nations in the region stopped as the military shifted focus to the political situation within Panama. Life slowly deteriorated, as businesses closed and public services fell into disrepair.

When American leaders questioned Noriega's harsh tactics, he ordered his heavily armed Panama Defense Force and paramilitary forces to harass U.S. troops. All military personnel and dependents were ordered to move on base, and in many cases they had to double up with other families in on-base housing.

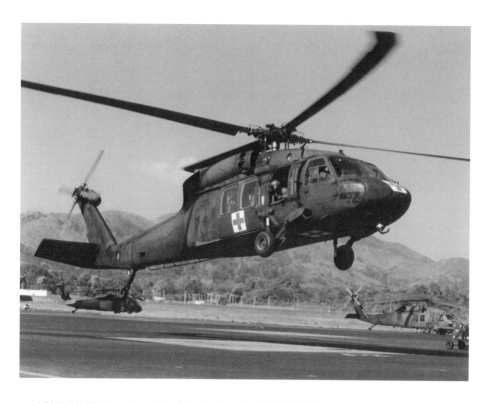

A 214th Med Det (RG) Black Hawk during Operation JUST CAUSE.
Source: United Technologies Corporation

When several Americans were detained and killed, and one man literally had to fight his way out of a possible hostage situation, President George H.W. Bush decided to take action.[95]

Panama was within the area of responsibility of Southern Command. Its commander, Gen. Maxwell Thurman, had watched these developments with growing unease and had directed increasingly more detailed planning for military intervention. He slowly but steadily moved more military combat units into the country. When directed by President Bush to act, he initiated Operation JUST CAUSE. Its stated purposes were to secure the Panama Canal, protect U.S. personnel, restore the Panamanian government to its elected officials, and take Noriega into custody to stand trial on drug-trafficking charges.[96]

As part of a joint task force, the XVIII Airborne Corps deployed 13,000 soldiers from the 82d and 7th Divisions, the 75th Ranger Regiment, several other special operations units, and the 44th Medical Brigade, which was commanded by Col. Jerry Foust. After commanding the 326th Medical Battalion, Foust attended the Army War College and did another tour in the Headquarters, Health Services Command, at Fort Sam Houston, before reporting to the brigade in June 1989. His and the other units were airlifted into Panama to join locally assigned forces and 13,000 more soldiers from other units and marines who had quietly moved there in the preceding months.[97]

The 128th Aviation Brigade at Fort Kobbe formed Task Force Aviation directly to support the operation with all of its assigned and attached units. It provided all of them the necessary intelligence, weather information, air traffic control coordination, and intermediate maintenance necessary to operate in the theater. It also had attached to it, the 4th Battalion, 228th Aviation Regiment, which self-deployed from Soto Cano Air Base, Honduras. This was the battalion's first significant event since forming that summer, and they adopted the motto "Born Under Fire."[98]

The 214th Med Det (RG) was directed to provide MEDEVAC support. Like all local units, it had planned and trained for such an operation for almost a year. As the reinforcing units arrived, the 214th dispatched its officers out to them to meet the commanders and perform any pre-coordination at the tactical level. The tempo of operations increased, both to get the new units acclimatized and familiar with the area and to desensitize the Panamanians to the movement of U.S. forces. Serving in Panama with the 214th Med Det (RG) at the time was Capt. Vinny Carnazza. He had joined the unit right out of flight school in 1987, and he was now well familiar with the area.[99]

However, the 214th Med Det (RG) only had five helicopters because one had been destroyed in a water crash in September, killing the medic, S.Sgt. Adrian Rosato. For projected operations, it quietly established refueling points at several locations and established operational procedures and communications with all local medical facilities.[100]

In the early morning hours of 20 December, U.S. forces attacked the Panamanian Defense Forces and "Dignity Battalions" of street thugs at locations and facilities across the country. They overwhelmed the Panamanian forces in the attacks that only lasted five days before all objectives were met and Noriega was captured. Most of the intense combat only occurred within the first eight hours. But there were casualties, and the medical warriors of the 44th Medical Brigade immediately went into action to care for the wounded soldiers, sailors, airmen, and marines.

During the operation, the 214th Med Det (RG) was attached to the 44th or the 142d Medical Battalion, also subordinate to the 44th. The 214th was augmented with two complete crews from the 57th Med Det (RG) at Fort Bragg. However, during JUST CAUSE, it was the only MEDEVAC unit in theater.

The pace of MEDEVAC missions reflected the intensity of the fighting. At one point, Capt. Carnazza brought out a load of 12 wounded but ambulatory soldiers. Foust authorized the 214th to take the patient litter carousels out of their aircraft to accommodate quicker loading and provide room for more wounded. The crews had to be sure to wash out the blood that stained the aircraft cabins between missions so that it did not affect the morale of the fighting soldiers.[101]

With only five aircraft, the 214th was very busy providing area support for all units and transporting patients who were soldiers, marines, dependents, Panama

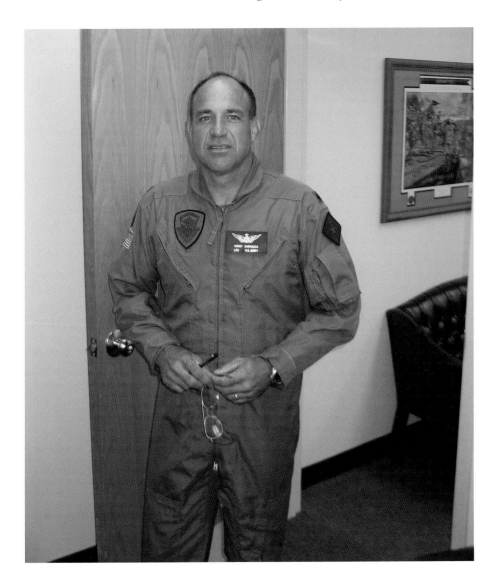

Lt. Col. Vinny Carnazza in 2006.
Source: Author

Canal Commission and Department of Defense employees, local Panamanian nationals, and enemy prisoners. The 214th also moved medical personnel and equipment, and delivered whole blood, biologicals, and medical supplies.[102]

The unit was also on call to support aircraft crash and rescue operations and search and rescue operations in low threat environments. They provided humanitarian assistance to the Panamanian Government to help the 5,000+ refugees who either fled the fighting or lost their homes in the melee.

For three weeks, the 214th provided two aircraft in direct support of Special Forces elements from the Joint Special Operations Command. Capt. Vinny Carnazza was the team leader for that effort and went to work in the hangar commandeered by the Special Forces Task Force as its command center. His crews then answered specific calls from those forces and supported several intense operations, including the rescue effort for Kurt Muse, an American civilian who had been imprisoned by Noriega for running a clandestine antigovernment radio station. One of Carnazza's crews MEDEVACed eight wounded Navy SEALs from the ill-fated attack on the Paitilla Airfield.[103]

Another detachment of one aircraft and crew was also assigned in direct support of the 2d Brigade 7th Infantry Division for operations at Fort Sherman, Rio Hato, and Santa Fe. Overall, casualties were light with 26 Americans killed and 325 wounded. The Panamanians had 314 killed and thousands wounded or captured.[104]

The 214th suffered from personnel shortages and limitations during the conflict. The pilots, overall, were inexperienced, with a flight time average of 750 total hours and 380 in the UH-60. One instructor pilot position and the safety officer position had been unfilled since September. Two of 12 unit pilots were readiness level (RL) 3 and had only been in the unit for two weeks. Of the five medics assigned to the unit, one was on leave and two were newly graduated from the flight medic's course. Six crew chiefs were available, but two were directly from the basic aircraft mechanics course. Most, but not all, crewmembers were qualified with NVGs. However, they met all taskings and logged 283 missions in the campaign, carrying 470 patients. The 142d Medical Battalion evacuated another 233 patients by ground evacuation. The 214th crews also transported 146 medical personnel, and 17,740 lbs of medical supplies. A majority of missions were flown at night with NVGs. Probably as a consequence, only three aircraft sustained damage, with all being repaired within 24 hours.[105]

The 214th Med Det (RG) wrote a detailed after-action report that was consolidated into overall medical lessons learned by the AHS at Fort Sam Houston. Several MEDEVAC observations were listed:

1. MEDEVAC must be integrated into operations in the pre-mission planning.
   a. Medical units were not given dedicated frequencies in the communications electronics operating instructions.
   b. The 82d Airborne Division lost a pallet of retransmission communications equipment during an airdrop.
   c. MEDEVAC units must have access to planned flight routes for flight plan coordination.
   d. No plans were made for armed escort of MEDEVAC helicopters into areas where enemy fire was a possibility.
2. The command and control structure for MEDEVAC must be clear, and there must be one central agency to collect and disseminate medical evacuation information.

    a. The air ambulances coordinated through the joint operating center.

    b. Ground ambulance coordinated through the forward casualty collection points and the joint casualty collection point.

3. Accurate mission information must be passed for the most efficient utilization of MEDEVAC assets.

4. Ground units only have limited knowledge of MEDEVAC procedures and limitations under hostile fire.

5. Some troops do not understand that helicopters displaying the Red Cross cannot be used for utility or combat purposes.

6. MEDEVAC helicopters do not have defensive weapons capability and may require fire suppression in hostile environments.

7. The UH-60s need more Kevlar floor protection or armor around the crewmembers.

8. The 214th Med Det should have been augmented with more personnel and aircraft.

    a. Lack of aircraft required the use of ground vehicles.

    b. Many casualties were brought in by nonmedical vehicles.

9. The new UH-60 casualty carousels were removed to provide more room for wounded.

10. NVGs were effective and made night flight more safe and practical.

11. Medics and AMEDD officers in direct support of infantry units engaged in combat should be awarded the Combat Medical Badge.

12. Fixed facility medical (TDA) facilities were not equipped with tactical radios necessary for field MEDEVAC operations.[106]

One last point was noted. Unlike most MEDEVAC units, this unit performed its combat mission from its home station. The crews were there with their families and knew that while they were out flying their missions, their families were at risk. Family support was critical to making this mission work.

Residual operations in Panama quickly shifted to peacekeeping as the legitimately elected government was restored to power. In most quarters, the American forces were welcomed as liberators, which greatly facilitated the restoration of law and order. Those forces dispatched for the operation were soon sent home, and the locally assigned units returned to normal operations tempo. Within the next few years, all would leave as the Canal Zone finally reverted to Panamanian control.

One month after the termination of hostilities, Carnazza transferred to the 498th Med Co (AA), at Fort Benning. He was dispatched as a team leader to take three aircraft, crews, and a small maintenance team to reinforce the 4th Battalion, 228th Aviation Regiment, at Soto Cano Air Base, Honduras. One of their aircraft and crew further deployed as a support package for Vice President Dan Quayle, his wife, Marilyn, and entourage as they visited Managua, Nicaragua, for the inauguration of the freely elected new President, Violeta Barrios de Chamorro, as she assumed power from José Daniel Ortega Saavedra. That MEDEVAC helicopter was one of the first U.S. military aircraft allowed back into that country in 14 years.[107]

Tactical Training at the National Training Center

At the National Training Center at Fort Irwin, California, the combat maneuver battalions and task forces regularly cycled through to train under the AirLand Battle concept. MEDEVAC elements from the various units supported each rotation, as combat teams from all continental U.S. divisions and brigades waged battle with the 32d Guards Motorized Regiment, the notional "opposition force," clearly structured and equipped as per Soviet standards, in the hot, dry valleys of the high desert. It was as realistic and intense as modern training could be without actually exchanging live rounds.[108]

The 247th Med Det (RG) was still stationed at Fort Irwin to support the National Training Center. Its purpose was not to train, but to provide MEDEVAC for any soldiers actually hurt in the sometimes accident-prone maneuvering of the heavy forces. Every brigade task force contained up to 4,000 soldiers, and injuries were inevitable. Operating in the summer temperatures as high as 120 degrees, the helicopters and crews were on call as necessary to cover the training. The terrain varied from a few hundred feet to higher than 6,000 feet and the hot temperatures could drive the density altitude much higher. Originally, the unit had been given single-engine UH-1 helicopters. However, they were grossly underpowered for these conditions and the winds through the valleys could regularly exceed their 15-knot limit. To provide better capability, the unit was given UH-60s in 1987. With two powerful engines, this machine was more suited to the conditions and averaged more than 400 missions a year.

The 247th was a good assignment for new pilots because they could accumulate flying time quickly in a tactical environment during both day operations and at night with NVGs. However, the base was remote and afforded little social life. However, the harsh environment took its toll on the helicopters. The unit, which had no local battalion to provide intermediate maintenance or parts support, relied on a support base 50 miles away, which meant that the aircraft were frequently not flyable.[109]

The training for the combat brigades in the high desert was intense and realistic. The Army began collecting and disseminating lessons learned based on what the units experienced. In November 1989, the Army Center for Lessons Learned at Fort Leavenworth, Kansas, published an edition focused on the tactical view of medical evacuations. The report highlighted several key points:

1. Violent high-tempo combat often results in areas of heavier combat action with resulting heavy casualties.
2. As areas of casualty density move away from hospital/aid station locations, routes of casualty evacuation lengthen.
3. Units should task organize and allocate evacuation assets in relation to projected casualties.
4. Units conducting the main effort will have the highest casualty load. Weigh the main effort.[110]

Such precise tactical focus showed that even tactical commanders were now thinking about MEDEVAC. Since the publication of FC 8-45 in October 1986, the MEDEVAC units themselves reorganized to provide that support if needed. However, a Medical System Program Review held at Fort Sam Houston in January 1989 showed that progress was slow. While the AHS had published a White Paper that captured the necessary changes specified in FC 8-45, the modernization of the MEDEVAC fleet languished. The Aviation Materiel Modernization Plan allocated 528 aircraft (430 UH-60s and 98 UH-1s) for MEDEVAC. At that point, only 121 UH-60s had been received with only 36 more slated for the fiscal year 1993–1997 time period. MEDEVAC UH-60s were assigned to overseas locations and to units identified for early deployment for contingencies. The additional aircraft were clearly needed to replace the aging UH-1 fleet.[111]

The Middle East

As the decade entered its later years, the Army was involved in almost continuous BRIGHT STAR exercises in Egypt and now NIGHTHAWK exercises in Jordan. MEDEVAC detachments supported both deployments. The 36th Med Det (RG) from Fort Polk, Louisiana, which was newly equipped with UH-60A aircraft, supported both in the fall of 1989 and logged 120 flight hours. However, even though both were training exercises, the unit did carry 16 actual patients who had been injured in the maneuvers.[112]

Domestic Disaster Relief

MEDEVAC units also received requests and orders to support domestic relief operations. One of the largest and most dramatic was the response to the grounding of the oil tanker *Exxon Valdez* on a reef in the Prince William Sound, Alaska, in March 1989. The estimated fuel spill was 11 million gallons of crude oil. It was a huge ecological disaster, and the nation responded on many levels. All U.S. military services supported the cleanup operation. The Army task force included MEDEVAC support. Within two days of the grounding, C-5s loaded three helicopters and crews from the 498th Med Co (AA) from Fort Benning for the long flight to Alaska. For the next 21 weeks they operated out of the Seward Airport and supported the operation of Army, Air Force, Navy, Coast Guard, and civilian contractor crews working to contain the damage. Many of the 498th crews were ship landing qualified and worked off of Navy and Coast Guard ships. They flew more than 70 medical missions and also provided VIP support for many politicians who came to review the effort.[113]

* * * *

It was a busy decade and period of change. The U.S. Army had completely rewritten its battle doctrine and begun reequipping and reorganizing to fulfill it. The MEDEVAC force, which had encountered those same challenges, avoided becoming consumed by the newly formed Aviation Branch and deployed units to support short combat operations in Grenada and Panama.

Thankfully, the requirement to fight the AirLand Battle against the Warsaw Pact on the Plains of Europe never arose. On 9 November 1989, the world was treated to the spectacle of ecstatic East Germans breeching the Berlin Wall. That structure—so long the symbol of division of Europe, and even the world between the United States and its allies and the Soviet Union and its allies—fell as the communist governments of Eastern Europe and then the Soviet Union itself collapsed. Two generations of American soldiers had stood watch along that dividing line. The cold war ended and the governments of the United States and its allies embraced plans for dramatic reductions in military spending, a "peace dividend" as it was labeled. Programs were almost immediately developed for wholesale reductions in force structure and manpower.[114]

During the decade, instead of AirLand Battle on the plains of Europe, the hot challenges had appeared elsewhere and in different forms. However, the Army and its MEDEVAC community met those challenges. Other challenges were about to appear, and perhaps the concept of AirLand Battle would be validated in another arena before that "peace dividend" could be claimed.

Part Three

An Angry Decade

Chapter Five
Desert Shield/Desert Storm, 1990–1991

"Nothing short of spectacular!"

Gen. Norman Schwarzkopf on the performance of Army medical units in Operations
DESERT SHIELD and STORM.[1]

Conflict in the Persian Gulf

The next challenge arose in the hot deserts of the Middle East, literally as the decade began. The soldiers who had returned from the short campaign in Panama did not get much of a break before they were needed in that arena. Subsequent events throughout the 10-year period dictated an almost continuous operations tempo. This and a new layer of joint doctrine lead to notable changes in Army MEDEVAC doctrine that reshaped the organization and utilization of MEDEVAC as the nation faced a "new world order."

Operations

Operation DESERT SHIELD/STORM/SABRE

On 2 August 1990, Saddam Hussein, the leader of Iraq, ordered his military forces to overrun Kuwait. The Hammurabi and Medina Armored Divisions and the Tawakalna Mechanized Division, which were built and equipped on the So-viet model, had hundreds of new T-72 tanks, were supported by three special operations forces brigades, and preceded by a short but violent aerial bombard-ment, overwhelmed the Kuwaiti defense forces and swept through the country to assume positions along the Saudi Arabian border. They were the vanguard of a million-man force built up in the 1980s, which was apparently intent on sweeping through Saudi Arabia and then the rest of the Persian Gulf.[2]

The attack cut off the supply of oil from Kuwait. As the shocks to the world oil market swept around the globe, U.S. President George H.W. Bush, on 7 August, decided that this force could not be allowed to continue because the loss of Saudi oil production would be disastrous for the United States and the world. Entreaties were made to the Saudis to allow a coalition of forces led by the United States to enter their country and "draw a line in the sand." The Saudi leaders disregarded a long-held antipathy for foreign troops on their soil and agreed to allow American and allied forces to enter. On 8 August, the ready brigade of the 82d Airborne Division arrived, as the U.S. Central Command (CENTCOM), under the leadership of General Norman Schwarzkopf, prepared to defend Saudi Arabia and the Persian Gulf region.[3]

On 22 August, President Bush signed Executive Order 12727, authorizing a Presidential Select Reserve Call-up of up to 200,000 Guardsmen and Reservists for a period of 90 days and extendable for another 90 days. Already thousands of Guardsmen and Reservists had volunteered for active duty, and complete units were mobilized. The orders began to flow. Unlike Vietnam, the Reserve Components were fully utilized in this conflict. The "Total Force" doctrine was fully tested. Col. Jim Truscott, who was assigned back at Fort Sam Houston as the Assistant Commandant for Force Integration at the Army Medical Department (AMEDD) Center and School, began visiting Reserve Component units to prepare them for duty in the Persian Gulf region.[4]

Combat Units Deploy

Over the next two months, the XVIII Airborne Corps headquarters, the rest of the 82d Airborne Division, the 101st Airborne Division (Air Assault), the 24th Infantry Division (Mechanized), the 1st Cavalry Division, the 3d Armored Cavalry Regiment, and portions of the 2d Armored Division arrived in the Persian Gulf. They were joined by a division plus of U.S. Marines and strong U.S. naval and air forces, special operations forces, and allied ground, air, and naval forces. Hundreds of National Guard and Army Reserve units were activated, and this was the first time since World War II for some of them. Many immediately deployed to the Persian Gulf. Others backfilled active duty units as they departed their home bases. The aggregate ground force consisted of more than 150,000 troops, 700 tanks, 1,400 armored fighting vehicles, and 600 artillery pieces. The buildup was called Operation DESERT SHIELD.[5]

The mission objective of DESERT SHIELD was purely defensive, and the dispatched force was adequate for it. But President Bush had a larger objective. He wanted Iraqi forces out of Kuwait. By November, diplomatic and economic efforts and United Nations mandates had not forced Hussein to remove his forces. President Bush assigned CENTCOM a new mission: prepare to liberate Kuwait. Such offensive action required a much larger force. For this mission, Schwarzkopf requested significant reinforcements. The VII Corps, which was located in Germany, was ordered to deploy to the Gulf, and thousands more National Guard and Reserve troops from all services were ordered to active duty.[6]

Within days, elements of the VII Corps were en route. Eventually, the 1st and 3d Armored Divisions, the 1st Infantry Division (Mechanized), and the 2d Armored Cavalry Regiment joined the forces already assembled. Another U.S. Marine Division was sent. Eventually, the allied forces from 24 nations exceeded 680,000 soldiers, sailors, marines, and airmen. The 415,000 American soldiers were equipped with 4,200 tanks, 2,800 infantry fighting vehicles, and 3,100 artillery pieces.[7]

The coalition faced an Iraqi force of 540,000 seasoned troops with 7,000 tanks and armored vehicles and 3,000 artillery pieces, and reinforced with excellent Special Forces units and a modern air defense system. Hussein was not impressed watching the buildup in Saudi Arabia. He believed that the United States had lost its will to fight in Vietnam. He scoffed at the gathering forces saying, "Yours is a nation that cannot afford to take 10,000 casualties in a single day."[8]

Medical Units

American commanders were worried about casualties. Hussein had chemical weapons and had used them against his own people and Iran during a bloody border war a few years prior. The U.S. Army sent a strong medical force of 65 hospitals and 198 individual medical units to the Persian Gulf region, more than half of which were from the National Guard and Army Reserve. Planners initially expected 3,200 casualties a day. They had enough beds for more than 13,000 patients and strategic airlift available to evacuate patients back to hospitals in Germany and the United States.[9]

The AMEDD was on the verge of implementing the new doctrine and organizational structure dictated by the Medical Force 2000 that stressed forward care in the combat zone to support the AirLand Battle concept. Some units had been restructured, but most had not.[10]

All deployed Army medical units were assigned to the 3d Medical Command (MEDCOM). Under it, the 173d Medical Group (U.S. Army Reserve [USAR]), the 202d Medical Group (Army National Guard [ARNG]), and the 244th Medical Group (ARNG) cared for those units assigned to Echelons Above Corps.

At the tactical level, the 332d Medical Brigade (USAR) directly supported the VII Corps with the 30th Medical Group (Active Duty), the 127th Medical Group (ARNG), and 341st Medical Group (USAR). The 39,000 Army Reservists and 37,000 Army National Guardsmen who were activated for the war by Presidential authority primarily manned these units.[11]

The XVIII Airborne Corps was directly supported by its 44th Medical Brigade, still commanded by Col. Jerome Foust, the Vietnam era MEDEVAC pilot who had taken the brigade to Panama the previous year. The 44th had assigned to it the 1st Medical Group (Active Duty), commanded by Col. Eldon Ideus, the MEDEVAC pilot who had been so instrumental in realigning MEDEVAC doctrine to support AirLand Battle, the 62d Medical Group, and the 56th Medical Battalion (Evacuation). MEDEVAC units, as they arrived, were assigned to the various medical headquarters as per evolving operational plans.[12]

The first MEDEVAC unit to deploy to the Persian Gulf region was Delta Company, 326th Medical Battalion, 101st Airborne Division (Air Assault). Maj. Scott Heintz, who had taken over just one month prior, was the commander. He and the first three aircraft and crews arrived on 20 August and immediately assumed MEDEVAC alert. The operations officer was Capt. Dave MacDonald, who had joined Delta Company the previous summer after returning from his tour in Korea. He and the rest of the unit arrived by early September. Initially, they provided general support to all forces flowing into the country until other MEDEVAC units arrived. Almost immediately, they dispatched crews to pick up solders hurt in training accidents or vehicular accidents as the combat and support units arrived and moved to their assigned areas. At all times, they also directly supported the 101st Airborne Division.[13]

When the 326th received its deployment orders, it had one Forward Surgical MEDEVAC Team (FSMT) of three aircraft on temporary duty with the Joint Task Force Bravo in Honduras. Heintz received permission to recall those aircraft. With operations still ongoing in Central America, the 571st Med Det (RA) at Fort Carson, Colorado, was directed to self-deploy three UH-1Vs to Honduras. 1st Lt. Brad Pecor, one of the 571st pilots who deployed, had entered the Army in 1984 in the aviation warrant officer program after graduating from Plattsburgh State University in New York. He flew AH-1s for four years and then took a direct commission into the Medical Service Corps (MSC) and became a MEDEVAC pilot with posting to the 571st. He flew his share of Military Assistance to Safety and Traffic (MAST) missions and became very proficient at mountain operations.

The 571st deployment took five days, with stops in San Antonio and Brownsville, Texas; Vera Cruz, Mexico; Belize City, Belize; and then into Soto Cano Air Base in Honduras. The crews flew at 90 knots and logged 26 flight hours en route. At Soto Cano, they assumed MEDEVAC duties for the next three months until replaced by another group of 571st pilots and then eventually crews from the 54th Med Det (RA) from Fort Lewis, Washington, and the 126th Med Co (AA) from the California ARNG.[14]

Lt. Col. Tom Mayes, another MEDEVAC pilot, commanded the 326th Medical Battalion. However, just before the hostilities began—in accordance with long-standing AMEDD policy—the Division Commander Maj. Gen. Binford Peay replaced him with a Medical Corps officer, and Mayes served as his executive officer. All of the company commanders within the battalion were also replaced. The policy directed that MSC officers could command medical units in peacetime, but when they were actively receiving patients, the units had to be under the command of a Medical Corps officer. All of the MSC ground company officers within the battalion were also replaced with Medical Corps officers. Heintz retained command of Delta Company. MSC officers in the battalion did not like this policy, and other divisions in the XVIII Airborne Corps did not act on it. Mayes made all operational decisions, and in a very awkward and challenging situation, he was an exceptional and inspirational leader. Mayes and his company commanders reassumed their command positions when the unit returned from the war.[15]

Another MEDEVAC unit identified to deploy immediately to Saudi Arabia was

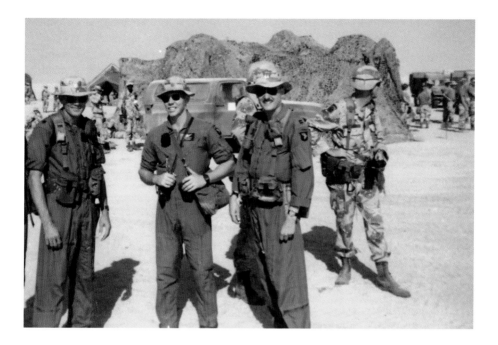

Lt. Col. Tommy Mayes, Maj. Scott Heintz, and Capt. Dennis Doyle, with the 326th Medical Battalion in DESERT STORM.
Source: Scott Heintz.

the 45th Med Co (AA) in Germany. On 12 August, the commander, Maj. Richard Ellenberger, was called to the 421st Medical Battalion (Evacuation) headquarters. Lt. Col. Ray Keith told him that the company would self-deploy its helicopters, thus minimizing the amount of strategic airlift necessary to move it, a commodity then in very high demand as heavy cargo aircraft moved combat units into the Persian Gulf. The 159th and 236th Medical Companies provided augmentation of personnel as necessary. The Company First Sergeant Jeff Mankoff took charge of the packing and shipment of all unit gear for the deployment. He and his personnel prepared 13 pallets and three trucks that were loaded aboard C-141s for almost immediate movement to Saudi Arabia. They flew to the King Abdul Aziz Air Base near Dhahran and had their company tactical operations center and area set up just 17 days after the invasion of Kuwait and awaiting the arrival of their aircraft and crews. Mankoff was a trained and qualified flight medic and fully intended to fly his share of missions because—to him—that defined leadership.[16]

The self-deployment of the 45th was the fruition of the initial plan developed by then Maj. Art Hapner back at the 57th Med Det (RG) in 1982 to support the BRIGHT STAR deployments. That one had been cancelled. This one would go.

The plan called for the movement of 12 aircraft in sections of six aircraft each and a 20 August departure date. This provided for four three-aircraft FSMTs. The selected aircraft were modified with tactical air navigation and global positioning systems and received extra maintenance support to clear all discrepancies. Two of the aircraft were also modified with External Stores Support System equipment that allowed for the carrying of external fuel tanks.

Deployment was delayed for one day because of problems acquiring the necessary diplomatic clearances. The first section was airborne on the morning of 21 August. They logged 7.5 hours of flight time before reaching Brindisi, Italy. On the next day, they flew to Athens, Greece, for an overnight rest, and onward with a refueling stop on the Island of Rhodes, Greece, and then to Paphos, Cyprus.

After another overnight stop and some maintenance, they took off on the long flight to Egypt. The intended destination was the Cairo West Airfield, but two of the non-External Stores Support System equipped aircraft barely made the Egyptian coastline before fuel exhaustion. The External Stores Support System aircraft landed next to them on the beach and transferred enough fuel to them so that they could continue on to Cairo West. After more problems with diplomatic clearances, the entire flight departed the next day for Tabuk, Saudi Arabia, where Saudi Army personnel greeted them. On the following day, the entire group took off and logged another 7 hours as they flew to Riyadh.

The scene was one of mass chaos as they arrived. They set up on one of the few unoccupied areas on the airfield and maintenance crews immediately attended to deferred write-ups. Two days later, they were ordered to proceed on to Dhahran, where they finally arrived on 27 August. Three hours after arriving, they launched a crew on a MEDEVAC mission to pick up a soldier in one of the combat units who had an inflamed appendix. Several of their pilots were qualified to land on ships, and they immediately began receiving taskings to deliver patients to the hospital ships now in the Persian Gulf.

The second element of six aircraft departed on 27 August. They modified their route of flight somewhat based on the first group's experience. They had significantly more maintenance problems, with one aircraft requiring a main rotor blade replacement. However, they arrived at Dhahran in early September, and immediately joined their predecessors who were already performing MEDEVAC missions in general support of arriving ground units.[17]

Capt. Pete Smart flew with the second element on that deployment. After he finished his tour with the 377th in Korea, he was assigned to the 159th Med Co in Germany as the maintenance platoon commander. He was selected to be one of the augmentees to make the long flight to Saudi Arabia and particularly remembered the long leg from Cyprus to Cairo as being the dividing point between two very different worlds.[18]

The next MEDEVAC unit to deploy was the 57th Med Det (RG) from Fort Bragg, North Carolina. Arriving on 9 September, it located at what later became the Medicine Warrior Heliport near King Khalid Military City (KKMC), and was initially under the control of the 56th Medical Battalion (Evacuation). The heliport eventually grew to a facility supporting 400 soldiers and 70 aircraft.

The 57th was joined a few days later by the 229th Med Det (RA) from Fort

Drum, New York, and the 431st Med Det (RA), from Fort Knox, Kentucky. Their six UH-1Vs each and personnel joined the growing fleet. The 229th was given the initial duty of establishing and building the heliport.

The 229th's unit helicopters were unique because they were the only ones equipped with LORAN-C long-range navigation systems. These systems worked so well in the hot desert environment that more were ordered for other MEDE-VAC units.[19]

Serving with the 431st was 1st Lt. Jon Fristoe. Commissioned into the MSC in 1987, the 431st was his first assignment directly out of flight school. In addition to his flight duties, he was the unit movement officer and played a major part in getting his unit to Saudi Arabia.[20]

In early October, the 82d Med Det (RA) from Fort Riley, Kansas, deployed with its six UH-1Vs and crews. It was assigned to the 34th Medical Battalion, now commanded by Lt. Col. Frank Novier, with another MEDEVAC veteran, Maj. Johnny West, as the operations officer. Novier had taken command of the battalion a month before the invasion. The battalion provided direct support at different times to the 1st Cavalry Division, the 24th Infantry Division, and the 82d Airborne Division.[21]

The 82d Med Det was followed by the 498th Med Co (AA), from Fort Benning, Georgia, with 13 UH-60s and 12 UH-1V aircraft, spread over three different Army posts. The commander was Maj. Randy Maschek. A small detachment of its helicopters also supported the Army Ranger training camp near Dahlonega, Georgia. Capt. Vinny Carnazza worked there with the Rangers when Maschek told him to get the detachment back to Fort Benning. When he did he found the entire company preparing for deployment. They delivered their helicopters to Savannah, Georgia, for surface shipment in September and received them in Dhahran in October. The unit also located at Medicine Warrior Heliport.[22]

In early December, the remainder of the Germany-based 236th Med Co (AA) deployed to Saudi Arabia. At almost the same time, the 507th Med Co (AA) from Fort Hood, Texas, arrived with its 25 UH-1V helicopters. Commanded by Maj. Greg Griffin, this was the first time that the unit had been consolidated at one place since the Vietnam era. That was no small feat. Garrison commanders of the bases where the platoons were located were unhappy about losing their MEDE-VAC assets, and they had to be directly ordered to release them.[23]

Reserve Component Units

As active duty units deployed into the theater, both USAR and ARNG units were rapidly activated to fill in at Army garrisons in the United States and Europe. The 126th Med Co (AA), California ARNG, was activated and sent to Fort Bliss, Texas, and Fort Sam Houston, Texas, assuming the home missions of the 507th. It also deployed three aircraft to Soto Cano Air Base in Honduras. On that deployment, a 126th crew was lost while flying a night rescue mission on 13 May 1991, and Capt. Sashai Dawn, 1st Lt. Vicki Boyd, and S.Sgt. Linda Simonds were killed. The crewchief survived and was recovered by rescue forces the next morning. An extensive investigation determined that the crew inadvertently flew the aircraft into a cliff while traversing the mountains on a very dark night. The accident report recommended that a MEDEVAC unit should be permanently assigned to the base instead of relying on constantly rotating continental United States-based units.[24]

The 1133d Med Co (AA), Alabama ARNG, provided backfill at Fort Bragg. The 1159th Med Co (AA), New Hampshire ARNG, went to Fort Campbell, Kentucky. The 1187th Med Co (AA), Iowa ARNG, was posted to Fort Riley, Fort Sill, Fort Knox, and Fort Hood. At those bases, its crews flew 162 MEDEVAC missions and 71 missions in support of the MAST program. The 199th Med Co (AA), Florida ARNG, was called up and provided backfill at Fort Bragg; Fort Stewart, Georgia; Fort Pickett, Virginia; Charleston Air Force Base, South Carolina; and Cherry Point Marine Corps Air Station, North Carolina.

The USAR's 145th Med Det (RA) from Atlanta, Georgia, and the 364th Med Det (RA) from Vicksburg, Mississippi, were sent to Fort Benning and Fort Polk, Louisiana, respectively. During its year of activation, the 145th flew 1,300 accident-free hours, carrying 232 patients on 221 medical missions, of which 94 were neonatal transfers, and nine were immediate response taskings under the MAST program.

The 989th Med Det (RA), USAR, from Des Moines, Iowa was activated and sent to Fort McCoy, Wisconsin, and Fort Riley. The 991st Med Det (RA), USAR, from Birmingham, Alabama, was posted to Fort Campbell. The 412th Med Det (RA), USAR, was initially dispatched to Fort Bragg for backfill before being recalled to augment other deploying USAR units. The 423d Med Det (RA) USAR, from Syracuse, New York, was called to active duty and performed backfill at Fort Bragg, Fort Drum, and Camp Atterbery, Indiana. The 112th Med Co (AA), Maine ARNG, was also activated in December and deployed to Germany to support the units and garrisons there when the 45th Med Co, the 236th Med Co, and the 159th Med Co elements were deployed to the Persian Gulf. The plan for the 112th was critical but simple. As casualties flowed into Germany from the Persian Gulf region, crews from the 112th picked up the patients at the Rhein-Main Air Base near Frankfurt and transported them to Landstuhl and other medical facilities throughout Germany. The 112th also supported training operations at the large maneuver areas at Hohenfels, Grafenwöhr, and Wildflecken, which significantly reduced ambulance reaction time at those facilities as they provided training for units designated to deploy to DESERT SHIELD/STORM. Gen. Crosby E. Saint, the United States Army Europe commander, specifically cited the 112th after the conflict: "The 112th Med Co has established an outstanding reputation providing MEDEVAC support for the theater. The staff at the Combat Maneuver Training Center has made several unsolicited compliments to the 112th because of their significant reduction of response time to maneuver units in a field environment as well as providing superior medical care."[25]

The 112th was also assisted in its MEDEVAC duties by helicopters from the military services of the Federal Republic of Germany. Under the North Atlantic Treaty Organization Status of Forces Agreement signed in 1951 and the Wartime Host Nation Support Agreement signed in 1982, Germany made available medical evacuation assets and medical facilities for casualties from the Persian Gulf War.[26]

Subsequently, many other units were also activated and dispatched to the combat theater. From the Army Reserve, the following units were called to active duty:

273d Med Det (RA)
316th Med Det (RA)
321st Med Det (RA)
336th Med Det (RA)
343d Med Det (RA)
347th Med Det (RA)
348th Med Det (RA)
374th Med Det (RA)
872d Med Det (RA) backfill to several locations, then to CENTCOM[27]

The various State National Guards provided the following units:

24th Med Co (AA) Nebraska
986th Med Co (AA) Virginia, backfill in the continental United States, then
  to CENTCOM
1267th Med Co (AA) Missouri
146th Med Det (RA) West Virginia
812th Med Det (RA) Louisiana, Backfill in continental United States, then
  to CENTCOM
1022d Med Det (RA) Wyoming

Arriving in theater, the MEDEVAC units fell in under the medical command structure as the various units organized and consolidated. Some units were transferred as necessary because of the changing tactical considerations. By the beginning of combat operations in January 1991, the structure was very robust.

Echelons Above Corps

3d MEDCOM Headquarters

173d Medical Group
- 120 Medical Battalion
  - 45th Med Co (AA) Active Duty
  - 348th Med Det (RA) USAR
  - 872d Med Det (RA) USAR

202d Medical Group
No MEDEVAC units assigned

244th Medical Group
- 92d Medical Battalion
  - 336th Med Det (RA) USAR

803d Medical Group
- 108th Medical Battalion
  - 812th Med Co (AA) Louisiana ARNG
  - 343d Med Det (RA) USAR
  - 986th Med Det (RA) Virginia ARNG

VII Corps

332d Medical Brigade
No MEDEVAC units directly assigned

30th Medical Group
No MEDEVAC units directly assigned

127th Medical Group
- 217th Medical Battalion
  - 273d Med Det (RA) USAR
- 429th Medical Battalion
  - 507th Med Co (AA) Active Duty

341st Medical Group
- 328th Medical Battalion
  - 146th Med Co (AA) West Virginia ARNG
  - 1267th Med Co (AA) Missouri ARNG
  - 316th Med Det (RA) USAR
  - 321st Med Det (RA) USAR
  - 1022d Med Co (AA) Wyoming ARNG
- 818th Medical Battalion
  Directly assigned
  - 236th Med Co (AA) Active Duty

XVIII Airborne Corps

44th Medical Brigade

1st Medical Group
- 34th Medical Battalion
  - 498th Med Co (AA) Active Duty
  - 36th Med Det (RG) Active Duty
  - 57th Med Det (RG) Active Duty
  - 82d Med Det (RG) Active Duty
  - 374th Med Det (RA) USAR

62d Medical Group
- 36th Medical Battalion
  - No MEDEVAC units
- 56th Medical Battalion (Evacuation)
  - 24th Med Co (AA) Nebraska ARNG
  - 229th Med Det (RA) Active Duty
  - 431st Med Det (RA) Active Duty
  - 347th Med Det (RA) USAR[28]

The 101st Airborne Division had its own Delta Company, 326th Medical Battalion, with its 12 UH-60s.[29] The 25 MEDEVAC units deployed possessed approximately 250 aircraft—predominantly still UH-1Vs—available to support the warfighters.

Combat Operations

After endless diplomatic efforts to force Hussein to remove his forces from Kuwait failed, combat operations designated Operation DESERT STORM commenced in the early hours of 17 January 1991. Hundreds of allied attack and bomber aircraft entered Iraq after U.S. Army Apache helicopters destroyed two Iraqi early warning radars, and dozens of decoy drones and specially equipped fighter aircraft destroyed many Iraqi air defense guns and missile batteries.[30]

Day and night, for the next five weeks, the allied armada destroyed strategic targets across the country before focusing on Iraqi forces in Kuwait and southern Iraq, especially the elite Republican Guard divisions located between Kuwait City and Al Basrah. As the air campaign progressed, U.S. and allied ground forces prepared and positioned for the necessary ground campaign designed to destroy the Iraqi occupation forces and liberate Kuwait. The combat units deployed along the Saudi border with Kuwait and Iraq, and the support units moved up to a major highway called the "Tap Line Road." It was located on-average 15 miles south of and ran parallel to the borders.

That campaign, Operation DESERT SABRE, started at 0400 local time on 24 February. Across the broad front, soldiers and marines from 37 nations attacked the defending Iraqi force. The ground campaign only lasted four days as this massive force ground its way through the Iraqi force of 30+ divisions. Arab forces attacked along the coast into Kuwait. To their left, the 1st Marine Expeditionary Force with two divisions and a U.S. Army heavy brigade drove directly through Kuwait to cut off all eastern Iraqi forces, and forces from Egypt and Syria to their left assisted. Farther to the west the VII Corps with five heavy divisions and an armored cavalry regiment prepared to attack the forces of the Republican Guard by forcing them back to the sea and then destroying them.

Next to them, the XVIII Airborne Corps on the far western flank attacked north with the French 6th Light Division on the west flank and the 82d Airborne Division in reserve. The 101st Airborne Division (Air Assault) seized a forward operating base 100 kilometers inside Iraq from which it could then launch air assault

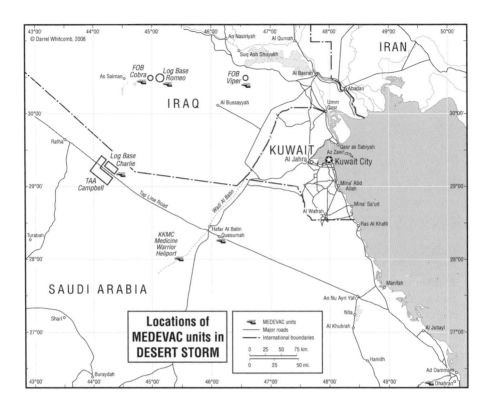

operations across a wide area. Also assigned to the corps was the 24th Infantry Division (Mechanized), which passed through the lines of the 101st and attacked east along a major highway south of the swamps along the Euphrates River toward Al Basrah.

Over the next four days, the combined force, with massive air support above, drove Iraqi forces out of Kuwait. The XVIII Airborne Corps drove 200 kilometers into Iraq before pivoting 90 degrees to the east and pushing almost to Basrah. The VII Corps attacked 100 kilometers into Iraq before also swinging to the east to maul the forces of the Republican Guard along the Iraq–Kuwait border. The U.S. Marine and Arab forces swept through Kuwait and liberated its people from the Iraqi forces. After 100 hours of ground combat, the coalition declared a ceasefire on 28 February. Considering the intensity of combat, the number of casualties was very low, at least for the coalition. Of the American forces, 145 were killed and 357 were injured. Iraqi losses were estimated in the tens of thousands.[31]

MEDEVAC Operations

XVIII Airborne Corps. The 44th Medical Brigade supported the XVIII Airborne Corps. Its attached 1st and 62d Medical Groups controlled the 34th Medical Battalion and the 56th Medical Battalion (Evacuation), respectively. Each controlled several MEDEVAC units.

Deployed as a traditional medical battalion, the 34th Medical Battalion began to operate as an evacuation battalion under the evolving doctrine. It needed more personnel with MEDEVAC expertise for this mission. One of the units assigned to it was the 498th Med Co (AA). Because it owned two platoons that operated at other bases in the United States, the 498th had a surfeit of just the right type of individuals that the 34th needed. Lt. Col. Frank Novier, the 34th commander, did some serious wheeling and dealing to get them assigned to his battalion. At one point, the 34th had assigned to it five different MEDEVAC units with 49 aircraft and a collateral ground ambulance company. During combat, it located and moved with the support elements of the 24th Division.[32]

The 498th Med Co (AA) provided direct support to the 24th Infantry Division throughout DESERT SHIELD, and it dispatched MEDEVAC teams to all of the division medical companies to make sure that all were proficient at requesting MEDEVAC support. Duty was relatively routine, and the pilots responded to calls. However, the division had to reposition to the west, which was deeper into Saudi Arabia for DESERT STORM, and the 498th covered the move.

Capt. Vinny Carnazza recalled, "We did a lot of MEDEVAC missions on the roads from young soldiers falling asleep as they were bringing in all the logistics going west. Folks driving off that road which was very narrow…Over and over, it was the same casualty, different face." It reminded him of flying MAST missions in the United States. The company also dispatched a team of two helicopters and four crews out far to the west to support special operations forces, just as they did in Panama for JUST CAUSE.[33]

The crews did a lot of night flying and developed proficiency flying with night vision goggles (NVGs). This was a real challenge because the terrain was so different than in the United States. At night, the desert was almost featureless, so pilots had to trust in their radar altimeters.[34]

The 498th moved with the division into DESERT SABRE, crossing the line of departure on 25 February. The division's Aviation Brigade provided the 498th with necessary higher-level maintenance for its helicopters and air traffic, weather support, and intelligence data necessary for safe flight. The 34th Medical Battalion coordinated that support for the company. The 24th Division moved the farthest during the conflict, and the increasingly longer lines of communication challenged the 498th as it staged with the division through its engagements. Its crews picked up soldiers at battalion aid stations or even point of injury and generally delivered them back to Combat Support Hospitals that remained in Saudi Arabia along Tap Line Road. The 34th moved into Iraq and located with the 24th Infantry Division. Working with his medical and aviation units, the 24th Division Support Command commander integrated the 498th directly into his division support plan.[35]

Two days into DESERT SABRE, the 498th moved forward, away from the Aviation Brigade, and left behind its air traffic, weather, and intelligence support. However, the move was necessary because the 24th Infantry Division itself was rapidly moving forward. Carnazza discovered that all of the training, planning, and pre-coordination that they had done with elements of the division now paid off. At one point, he brought his team forward and located with the medical company of one of the forward support battalions. He coordinated with 1st Lt. Scott Drennon, the executive officer of the medical company, for logistical support for his aircraft and crews. After DESERT STORM, Drennon would go to flight school, become a MEDEVAC pilot, and command a MEDEVAC unit in Operation IRAQI FREEDOM.[36]

For Carnazza and his team, the evacuation line from the combat battalion aid stations back to the hospitals on Tap Line Road stretched to 220 miles. Carnazza remembered, "The evacuation lines grew. We were taking those airframes away from the commanders for too long a time, the first night 30 miles, the second night, it's 80–90 miles; the third day, it's 120 miles. We were taking people to Tap Line Road and it cost us an hour and a half."[37]

One crew got trapped in a severe sandstorm and had to land, where they were discovered by a large group of Iraqi soldiers. The crew was armed only with their 9 mm pistols and immediately called for help. Instead of attacking the hapless helicopter crew, the Iraqis surrendered to them. The MEDEVAC crew was very relieved when a Military Police unit arrived to take charge of them.[38]

During the conflict, the 498th carried 668 patients. Many were Iraqi civilians and prisoners who were carried mostly after combat ceased. Carnazza had hauled wounded in JUST CAUSE, but noticed that the injuries in DESERT SABRE were different. In Panama, he had seen mostly small caliber injuries; in the desert, he saw soldiers injured by heavy caliber weapons that caused much more severe injuries, such as missing limbs or mangled shoulders, faces, etc.[39]

One mission in particular stood out for Carnazza. On the evening of 27 February, he flew to a casualty collection point south of Basrah. Since the 498th directly supported the field combat units, the commanders took the carousels out of their aircraft to make room for more patients if necessary because the emphasis at this level of care was to get them to a doctor as quickly as possible. The collection point was very close to the front lines, and this dictated that they needed to get in and out as quickly as possible. Carnazza had been told to expect three casualties. Just as they were about loaded, the ground unit medic indicated that they had three more. They loaded them in and then closed the helicopter door. The patients were not strapped down—only the doors protected them from falling out. As they flew to the evacuation hospital, the medic had to step over and around the patients to provide care to each, while trying not to slip on the "muck" of war. It was a dirty, grimy business. At the end of the day, the crews washed out their aircraft with soap, disinfectants, and lots of high pressure water if it was available.[40]

Carnazza was also very impressed with the way that the aircraft crew chiefs and medics learned to work together. On loads like this, the medic could quickly become overwhelmed, and the crew chief would assist. Most crew chiefs assisted and developed fairly good medical skills in their own right.

MEDEVAC days were usually long ones, especially in combat. At the end of missions for the day, the crew chief usually had maintenance chores. In a turnabout, many enlisted the help of their medic, and sometimes the pilots, too, to perform necessary chores. Carnazza saw this clearly in DESERT STORM. He recalled of his enlisted crewmembers:

> They are resilient. It's an interesting crew [relationship] that the aviation world will never know, the relationship of a medic and a crew chief. The crew chief almost becomes … like a combat life saver. [The medic] has oversight of the medical care. He is directing that crew chief what to do. A lot of times, that is being shared. It's the same thing when we are down. The crew chief has to pull a [aircraft inspection]…And the medic is assisting the crew chief. It is an absolute partnership.[41]

The 57th Med Det (RG), which was first assigned to the 56th Medical Battalion (Evacuation), was transferred to the 34th Medical Battalion to provide direct support to the 3d Armored Cavalry Regiment. That unit was one of the first to attack Iraq when DESERT SABRE started in the early morning hours of 24 February. Within just a few hours, the 57th had flown its first three missions. After the battle, the unit provided MEDEVAC support for the redeployment of the units out of Iraq and Kuwait.[42]

The 374th Med Det (RA), USAR, was activated and deployed in December. Initially under the 36th Medical Battalion, it moved over to the 34th for DESERT STORM and SABRE and worked with the 57th to support the 3d Armored Cavalry Regiment.[43]

The 82d Med Det (RA) was also under the 34th Battalion and directly supported the 1st Cavalry Division. During combat, it moved forward to support the 82d Airborne Division and also the French 6th Light Division. In one tactical move, the Detachment leapfrogged 70 miles to the east to stay linked up with the 307th Medical Battalion of the 82d Airborne Division.[44]

The 36th Med Det (RG) deployed from Fort Polk and provided direct support under the 56th Medical Battalion (Evacuation) to the 1st Cavalry Division. During DESERT STORM and SABRE, it moved over to the 34th Battalion and directly supported the 82d Airborne Division and the French 6th Light Armored Division, both of which provided medical liaison, logistical/maintenance, and air traffic control support. During the withdrawal from Iraq, they supported units on the move and evacuated Iraqi civilians wounded in the residual fighting. One of the unit's aircraft crashed on 12 March 1991, and 1st Lt. J.D. Maks, CW2 P.A. Donaldson, Sgt. M.S. Smith, and Spc. K.D. Phillips were killed. Ten aircraft crews from the 24th Med Co (AA) and the 229th and 347th Med Dets conducted a coordinated search that found their wreckage.[45]

Initially called to active duty to provide backfill at Fort Bragg, the 347th Med Det (RA), USAR, from Miami, Florida, deployed to Saudi Arabia in December. Initially locating at KKMC, south of Hafir Al-Batin, it was assigned to the 56th Battalion. One of the unit members was Capt. Randy Schwallie, an active duty officer previously assigned to the Flatiron Detachment at Fort Rucker, Alabama. As DESERT SHIELD began, he saw a message stating that the 347th needed an active duty advisor for their upcoming deployment, and he volunteered. He reported ASAP to Fort Stewart to ship out with the "Dolphin Dustoff," as they were

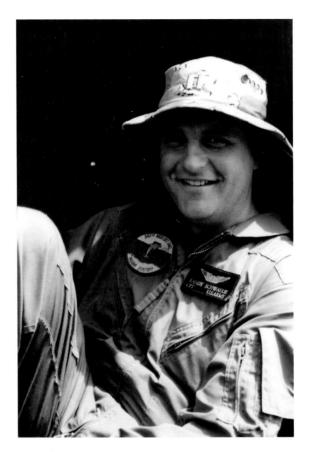

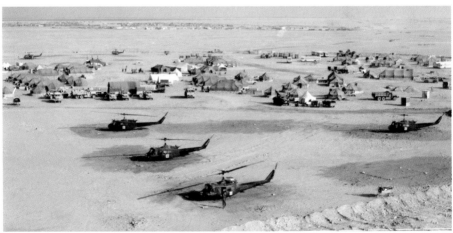

Capt. Randy Schwallie and the 347th Med Det (HA) USAR in DESERT STORM.
Source: Randy Schwallie.

known. Most Guard and Reserve units develop strong local identities. However, he was not told that the officer he replaced had recently been arrested for buying drugs in Miami, the unit's home.[46]

When Schwallie joined the unit, the first thing he learned was that he would be both the executive officer and flight operations officer. Then he noticed that the unit personnel were much older than the personnel normally found in an active duty unit. He remembered:

> My flight operations NCO was Wilhild Roessel.… Her daughter was older than me. We had twelve Vietnam veterans and seven of our warrant officers were Chief Warrant Officer Four's. Nowhere in the active Army would you find that kind of age, seniority, and experience in an operational unit.… My new commander was Maj. Russell Morris. He was an airline pilot on the Boeing 747 for United Airlines and had grown up professionally in the Georgia Army National Guard. … I trusted him and I felt like he trusted me.[47]

The 347th aircraft and personnel were loaded aboard C-5s and delivered to Dhahran as scheduled. They moved the unit to the Medicine Warrior Heliport where they were assigned to the 56th Medical Battalion. They moved patients from division area Combat Support Hospitals back to Evacuation Hospitals located in the XVIII Airborne Corps rear area. The unit had been equipped with ANVS 6 NVGs, and all crews had trained in the United States with them.

However, Schwallie had a problem with his medics. All were reservists with many having limited medical proficiency. Only two had civilian jobs in the medical field. He scrambled to get them some refresher training.[48]

Two weeks later, the unit began flight operations. All pilots received orientation flights. His first impression of the area was stark. "Depth perception is a real problem around the dunes. …Sand, sand, and more sand. It all looks the same and takes a while to get used to looking at the right things," he later noted.[49] The desert was also spotted with many towers, most of which were not marked on the outdated maps they were given for navigation.

Schwallie also arranged for the unit to receive a class on stress management. He was concerned that so few of them had actually seen a lot of "blood and guts lately" and wanted to prepare them for the inevitable shock of serious casualties.

As the aircraft accumulated flight hours in the desert, they began to break. Schwallie soon realized that getting required parts was a real challenge and that the supply system had not caught up with the flow of units into the theater. At one point, a colonel told them that they would have to find a way to fix their own aircraft. Schwallie was concerned because his unit was not organized or equipped to support itself, and it was not getting the support from above that was needed.

On 12 January the unit moved north to a spot in the desert preparatory to combat operations. They did not have maintenance kits, and there was no maintenance unit located with them. Fortunately, several of the unit personnel were masters at improvisation. They were collocated with the 24th Med Co (AA) from the Nebraska ARNG, which had a more robust maintenance capability and shared it with the 347th.[50]

All personnel were briefed on projected war plans. They received shots for anthrax and started taking pyridostigmine bromide tablets for possible exposure to chemical weapon nerve agents. All troops had full chemical suits and were required to wear them. They were awakened in the early hours of 17 January by the sound of allied aircraft overhead flying north, and a few minutes later, the sound of explosions. DESERT SHIELD had become DESERT STORM.[51]

On 26 January the unit moved to Log Base Charlie, next to tactical assembly area Campbell, and along the Tap Line Road about halfway between Hafir Al-Batin and Rafha. As the unit settled into its new location, Schwallie had some lingering concerns about its mission and organization. While immensely impressed with the magnitude of the medical force of which his units was just a small part, he recorded in his personal log the following excerpt:

> I am becoming increasingly aware of the lack of aviation support that we are receiving through our chain of command. We have not been able to get good weather reports, tactical locations of the refueling points, or information about the aviation intermediate maintenance unit that supports us. I am starting to understand the saying that "medical aviation is a step-child that no one wants to own." Our [higher headquarters] are not set up to provide the kind of support that we need. It seems odd to me that there is only one [MEDEVAC] captain on the group staff and one major on the brigade staff. Our battalion headquarters only has one aviator, the Battalion Operations Officer (S2/3). He is an excellent officer and he understands both the medical side and the aviation requirements that we need. Unfortunately, he is only one guy and has a lot more responsibilities than taking care of the aviation units. We serve two masters; the medical and aviation communities, but we don't seem to serve either one very well.[52]

Using personal connections within the aviation community, Schwallie was able to get his troops some briefings on aviation operations, airspace control, and the enemy forces arrayed to the north of them. He was not getting any of that data through the medical chain.

The 347th was located not far from the 44th Medical Brigade. Occasionally, Col. Jerome Foust, the Brigade commander, flew with the 347th. He knew some of the senior warrant officers and enjoyed sharing Vietnam Dustoff stories with them.

The members of the 347th watched as the massed formations of helicopters from the 101st, 82d, and 24th Divisions flew north into Iraq. Then they were alerted to prepare to move north to a planned Log Base Romeo, where several hospitals and medical facilities were scheduled to be moved. While most of the equipment was moved by vehicle, the helicopters and crews flew forward on the evening of the 26th, 110 miles to Log Base Romeo. It was a long flight into what had been enemy territory using NVGs through a very dark sky. The next morning, MEDEVAC helicopters from the companies and detachments assigned in direct support to the combat units began bringing in casualties. Six helicopters—both Hueys and Black Hawks—landed almost simultaneously at Romeo. They drew a crowd of helpers to unload. The scene was shocking. Several of the wounded had died in the aircraft, and several more were suffering horrific wounds.

Schwallie remembered that, "I could see one of the dead men and the horror of war suddenly became very real to me. ...One of his legs was missing and there were numbers written in big black letters across his forehead from the triage done at the aid station."[53]

A short while later, the 347th crews started receiving missions. The first carried an American soldier with two badly damaged legs and an Iraqi soldier with a broken arm and back. They flew them back to an Evacuation Hospital in Saudi Arabia. The missions steadily flowed.

A ceasefire was declared at 0800 on 28 January. After the ceasefire, most missions were to carry wounded Iraqi prisoners and civilian casualties being collected at several locations. From there they evacuated them to facilities in Saudi Arabia. Schwallie had trouble with one of the wounded Iraqi prisoners that he carried. Inflight, the man started grabbing at the medic, a young female specialist. Schwallie drew his pistol and made it very clear to the Iraqi that he had to desist.[54]

Schwallie also saw the impact of the war on the Iraqi people. He wrote:

> In the emergency tent, I saw no men among the injured. These were innocent women and children that were gunned down in cold blood during an Iraqi military raid on a town. I think it was An Nasiriyah along the Euphrates River, about 30–40 miles from our base….The Iraqi Army was retreating and went through the town on their way back to Baghdad. Since the men from that town surrendered, the Iraqis took retribution against their families…
>
> There were two women with gunshot wounds—one in the left front rib cage and one in the right thigh hip area. Also, there were many children, both at our facility and the 307th Medical Battalion. We flew one load and three other aircraft from the 24th Medical Company flew a load before the weather got really bad. It was certainly the most stressful flight I've had in a while.[55]

The 24th Med Co (AA), Nebraska ARNG, was activated and deployed to Saudi Arabia in November, where it was assigned to the 56th Medical Battalion (Evacuation). During combat, it picked up patients evacuated to the field hospitals by the front line units and moved them to theater hospitals or sites for airlift out of the theater by Air Force cargo aircraft. It evacuated 251 patients during the conflict.[56]

In addition to running the Medicine Warrior Heliport, the 229th Med Det (RA), at various times, directly supported the 82d, 101st, and 24th divisions, and evacuated 320 patients.[57]

The 431st Med Det (RA) worked closely with the 229th at Medicine Warrior. During DESERT SHIELD, it acted in general support for the 82d Airborne Division. During DESERT STORM, it moved to Logistics Base Charlie near the Iraqi border. Directly under 44th Medical Brigade's control, it provided general support to the 24th Infantry Division and backhauled 115 patients. During the ground campaign, 1st Lt. Jon Fristoe was a team leader for the 431st. At one point, Maj. Gen. Barry McCaffrey, the 24th Division commander, put his arm around Fristoe and asked him directly if there were going to be any problems with the 431st helicopters hauling out the dead. Evacuation of human remains was not a MEDEVAC task. However, Fristoe assured the division commander that it would not be a problem. Fortunately, there were few to carry, but they did haul out several dozen Iraqi bodies.[58]

As designed, Delta Company, 326th Medical Battalion, 101st Airborne Division supported the divisional brigades as they moved forward. The company flew myriad missions. Besides providing MEDEVAC capability to the division, it also served as the primary means of travel for two battalion organic surgical teams, their equipment, and medical supply. Its pilots were pushed to become proficient in NVG operations, and several qualified to land aboard ships.

During the two operations, Delta Company flew more than 400 missions and evacuated 375 patients, many of whom were Iraqi prisoners of war. It flew more than 1,900 hours with no accidents. Each infantry brigade of the division had assigned to it an FSMT of three MEDEVAC helicopters and crews. 1st Lt. Neal David led the 1st Brigade FSMT, 1st Lt. Greg Fix led the 2d Brigade FSMT, and 1st Lt. Mike Avila led the 3d Brigade FSMT. They were very effectively integrated into the operations of their combat units and collocated with their associated ground medical companies. Maj. Heintz had his crews use the "Dustoff" call sign for operations. He found it to be very effective because all soldiers knew what it meant and could expedite its approval, routing, and coordination.[59]

Before the start of the ground war, Delta Company was located just south of Tap Line Road, about midway between the 101st Division Aviation Brigade headquarters and the 326th Medical Battalion headquarters. Every day Heintz and MacDonald split up—Heintz headed to the battalion headquarters and MacDonald went to the aviation headquarters to collect intelligence from the respective sites. Once the ground war commenced, his flight sections were located forward with the combat brigades, and Heintz located the company headquarters and the support elements in close proximity to the Division Support Command headquarters and the 1st Brigade Combat Team. He accessed intelligence, A2C2, weather, and limited aviation maintenance support from the aviation element of the 1st Brigade.

There were times during Operation DESERT SHIELD where Eagle Dustoff provided MEDEVAC support to a Marine regiment in addition to the FSMTs with each of the maneuver brigades. Doctrinally, this would have required 15 aircraft but support was provided utilizing two and sometimes one-ship coverage.

This operational tempo coupled with the extremely harsh weather conditions made scheduled and unscheduled aircraft maintenance a challenge. However, the company maintenance platoon, led by Capt. Kent Brewer and CW3 Bill Rudd, kept the unit aircraft operationally ready. Heintz believed that he and his unit needed more maintenance and refueling personnel and equipment if they were to deploy forward with the medical companies supporting the maneuver brigades. Overall, Heintz felt that the unit's modified table of organization and equipment should be increased to support 15 aircraft like the Medical Force 2000 companies so that it could directly support more than three brigades or operate as an independent unit if required.[60]

VII Corps

The 332d Medical Brigade supported the VII Corps. It had assigned to it the 30th, 127th, and 341st Medical Groups. They controlled the 217th, 429th, 328th and 818th Medical Battalions that directed several MEDEVAC units.

The 507th Med Co (AA) deployed as a unit to the Persian Gulf in December as part of the buildup for offensive operations. Once assembled, it was assigned to the 429th Medical Battalion and located along the Tap Line Road, just east of Wadi Al-Batin. Upon settling in and literally building their own camp and bunkers, the crews flew night missions with NVGs and found it very challenging in the open desert.

The unit provided direct support to the 1st Infantry Division and the British 1st Armored Division. Maj. Greg Griffin, the company commander, met with the Aviation Brigade commander from the 1st Infantry Division for some pre-coordination. The first thing that the brigade commander asked was whether it was possible for his unit to have the 82d Med Det (RG) assigned versus the 507th because it was based with his unit back at Fort Riley. Griffin explained that the 82d had already been assigned and was well integrated into the XVIII Airborne Corps. Then the brigade commander wanted to assign the 507th to his general support aviation battalion. Griffin had to explain that, doctrinally, his unit could not be assigned to his unit, but would operate in direct support. As such, his division and the British unit would get the MEDEVAC support that they needed from his soldiers. Griffin then proactively integrated his operations into the operations of those units. He met with the commander of the general support aviation battalion and integrated into its operations so that his unit could have the maintenance, weather, traffic control, and operational support to operate on a modern battlefield.

Griffin later explained his rationale:

> The Oplan for Operation DESERT SABRE … began to unfold. I made the decision to co-locate the 507th with the 4th Aviation Brigade in order to better support the Operation. There was no definitive doctrine at the time that specified command and control relationships. In fact, a number of DUSTOFF units aligned themselves with hospitals and never caught up with the war. Our relationship with the 4th Brigade, [Aviation], 1st Infantry Division proved to be invaluable in keeping pace with the fast moving offensive operation and evacuating wounded soldiers from the battlefield.[61]

In early February, the 507th was ordered to move to a forward assembly area 70 miles to the northwest. While they were setting up, one of their crews was dispatched to recover wounded from a Bradley Fighting Vehicle and an M-113 damaged by friendly fire in a cross border probing action. It was a dark night, and the crew flew with NVGs, a first for the unit.[62]

A few days before the initiation of the ground battle, the MEDEVAC medical detachment assigned to support the 2d Armored Cavalry Regiment was reassigned to another unit. To fill the void, the 2d Platoon of the 507th was assigned to support them. With practically no support from the company, the 2d Platoon attached itself to the regiment and operated flawlessly with them throughout the battle.[63]

On 22 February, the remainder of the 507th moved into position with the Aviation Brigade of the 1st Infantry Division. They had also established close coordination with the 1st British Armored Division and had assigned to them a liaison team and six Puma and six Lynx helicopters, if needed, as additional evacuation assets. For operations during the breeching phase, the 236th Med Co (AA) also augmented them with three UH-60s.

Once ground combat operations started on 24 February, the 507th moved forward with the Aviation Brigade. When it was established at a forward operating base 70 miles inside Iraq, the 507th began getting steady calls for MEDEVAC.

The next day, the unit was ordered, again with the Aviation Brigade, to move 90 miles farther east. This would have extended the 507th evacuation lines beyond its fuel range. Griffin met with the operations officer from the 236th Med Co (AA) and set up an ambulance exchange point so his UH-1s could transfer their patients to the longer-range UH-60s of the 236th for recovery to the proper medical facilities in the rear areas. The ambulance exchange point—really just a designated set of coordinates in the desert—was provisioned with a fuel truck and a security team and operated throughout the rest of the campaign.

In the early morning hours of 27 February, a call came in for a MEDEVAC for a rapidly increasing number of wounded in an ongoing night battle. One of the Lonestar Dustoff birds launched but was shot down en route. More unit aircraft launched to cover the MEDEVAC request while another launched to search for any survivors. The crew chief, Spc. Nick Wright, was still alive. However, 1st Lt. Daniel Graybeal, S.Sgt. Michael Robson, WO1 Kerry Heine, and a doctor onboard, Maj. Mark Connelly, were all killed.[64]

The 507th continued to fly missions throughout the day. On one mission, several of their aircraft were assigned to assist at a rally point designated for the collection of enemy prisoners of war. Arriving at the point before infantry units from the 1st Division, the crews accepted the surrender of the enemy soldiers and "guarded" them until more heavily armed units arrived.[65]

By the afternoon, the area was blanketed with thick fog and black smoke from burning oil wells. With visibility below 50 meters, all flight operations stopped. Several calls for MEDEVAC were denied because of the unsafe conditions. However, this respite in operations did allow some of the crewmembers to grab some desperately needed rest.

When the visibility at least partially improved, the 507th helicopters resumed answering calls for MEDEVAC increasingly farther to the east as the heavy units of the VII Corps mauled their way through the Republican Guard formations. The scene was almost surreal as the crews flew between the now raging oil fires as their orange flames mixed with the hanging smoke to cast an eerie glow over the entire area. Below, the crews saw the flotsam and jetsam of battle, the burning and broken enemy equipment, and abandoned fighting positions. The ceasefire went into effect at 0800 on the next day. MEDEVAC calls still came in, mostly for soldiers involved in accidents or doing stupid things like picking up "souvenirs." There was now a steady call to transport wounded Iraqi soldiers and civilians.[66]

The 273d Med Det (RA), a USAR unit from Conroe, Texas, was called up and also deployed in December as part of the offensive buildup. It was the most highly qualified MEDEVAC unit—active or reserve—in the AMEDD. Most of its pilots were commercial aviators by trade and *averaged* 5,735 hours per pilot! After mobilization and deployment, the 273d was moved to an airfield at Qa-isumah. Under the control of the 217th Medical Battalion, it provided general support to VII Corps units as they arrived in the theater. The unit was assigned primarily to night duties because of the skill level of the high-time Reserve pilots and their training to use NVGs. The Reservists took a certain amount of pride in this, noticing that most other units required all of their pilots to land not later than 30 minutes after sunset.

The 273d crews shuttled patients from the units to the 12th and 13th Evacuation Hospitals. During DESERT SABRE, the unit was assigned in direct support of the 1st Cavalry Division as that unit mounted a feint operation into the Wadi Al-Batin and then supported the VII Corps in the main attack. Throughout its deployment, the unit flew 160 MEDEVAC missions carrying more than 240 patients, many of whom were enemy prisoners of war.[67]

The 316th Med Det (RA) was another USAR unit activated for the war. Deploying in late November from its base in Elyria, Ohio, it initially was under the control of the 328th Medical Battalion and supported the 3d Armored Division as it arrived from Germany. Transferring over to the 217th Medical Battalion in January, it found that little thought had been given to the proper support of the helicopter medical detachments in terms of the reliable provision of maintenance, logistics, intelligence support, traffic control, and weather data. It attached itself to an aviation unit to get what it needed to operate. During combat, it supported the 2d Armored Cavalry Regiment before again being assigned to the 1st Cavalry Division where it worked with the 273d Med Det (RA).[68]

Also activated for the buildup was the 321st Med Det (RA), a USAR unit from Salt Lake City, Utah. It was one of the last units to arrive in theater, not reaching Saudi Arabia until mid-January, just as the air campaign began. Upon arrival, it was assigned to the 217th Medical Battalion in direct support of the 2d Armored Cavalry Regiment as it led the 1st and 3d Armored Divisions into Iraq and Kuwait. Supporting this fast moving unit, its lines of evacuation continuously lengthened until it had to transport its patients back almost 100 miles. Missions did not end with the ceasefire. The 2d Armored Cavalry Regiment stayed forward, continuing to provide screening for the entire force, and the 321st remained in support. The 321st was directed to transport wounded Iraqi civilians when fighting broke out between anti-Hussein forces and residual Republican Guard units near Basrah. The 321st returned home in late May after transporting 424 casualties.[69]

The 1022d Med Co (AA), Wyoming ARNG, was called to active duty in late November. Its equipment was shipped by sea and was joined by unit personnel as it arrived at Dhahran in January. Initially under the control of the 429th Medical Battalion, it was transferred to the 328th for DESERT STORM and SABRE. With that battalion, it directly supported the 3d Armored Division and located with their general support aviation battalion. After the heavy battles to liberate Kuwait, it was assigned to Task Force Care and assisted in the evacuation of Iraqi civilians caught in the internecine warfare that continued near An Nasiriyah and along the Euphrates River before being shipped home in May.[70]

Another ARNG unit, the 146th Med Co (AA) from West Virginia, was activated and arrived in theater in January. It was also under the command of the 328th

Medical Battalion and was placed in direct support of the 1st Armored Division. It evacuated 439 patients, including Iraqi prisoners of war and civilians, and was sent home in May.[71]

The 1267th Med Co (AA) was a consolidated ARNG unit consisting of detachments from both Missouri and Nebraska. It was ordered to active duty in late November and arrived in Saudi Arabia in early February. It was also assigned to the 328th Medical Battalion, and it provided rear area support to VII Corps and had its aircraft disbursed among several different hospitals. The unit evacuated 375 casualties.[72]

The 236th Med Co (AA) deployed with its UH-60s as part of VII Corps. It was assigned to the 818th Medical Battalion and flew more than 900 missions, evacuating 650 patients. A medic, S.Sgt. G. Hailey, was killed in an aircraft accident on 19 January.[73]

Echelons Above Corps

Above the two Corps, the 3d MEDCOM had at its disposal several more MEDEVAC units assigned to its 108th, 92d, and 120th Medical Battalions.

The 812th Med Co (AA), Louisiana ARNG, with a detachment from the New Mexico ARNG, mobilized in November and deployed in February. It was assigned to the 108th Medical Battalion. Located at the KKMC and later, Log Base Charlie, it moved patients to and from the many hospitals in the rear area, both day and night. After hostilities ceased, it recovered soldiers wounded in vehicle accidents as the units withdrew from Iraq. In one particular incident, crews picked up several Egyptian soldiers wounded when their bus was broadsided by a large truck.[74]

The 986th Med Det (RA), Virginia ARNG, was initially called to active duty to replace the deploying 57th Med Det (RG) at Fort Bragg and the 498th Med Co (AA) detachment at Fort Stewart. It subsequently deployed to Saudi Arabia in February and reinforced the 812th at KKMC, under the 108th Medical Battalion. During the conflict, it evacuated 216 patients.[75]

Activated at its home station of Moffett Field, California, in late November, the 343d Med Det (RA), USAR, deployed to Saudi Arabia aboard C-5 aircraft. It initially located at the KKMC Airfield near the Iraqi border, also under the 108th. As soon as Kuwait City was liberated, the unit moved there and provided area general support for forces in the vicinity. It evacuated 300 patients before returning home in April.[76]

The 108th Medical Battalion was not an evacuation battalion and discovered that the command and control of MEDEVAC units was challenging. In after-action reports, it was noted that for such duty the unit needed an assistant S-3 for air operations assigned to it, a noncommissioned officer to handle air to ground communications, and an intelligence noncommissioned officer to handle the specific enemy threat data needed by the aircrews. They also suggested that on numerous occasions blowing sand and dust grounded helicopters yet ground evacuation vehicles still operated. They proposed that a unit of ambulance buses be assigned for such duty.[77]

Another subordinate 3d MEDCOM unit was the 92d Medical Battalion. The USAR 336th Med Det (RA) from New Windsor, New York, was activated in November and almost immediately deployed. Upon arrival, it was assigned to the battalion and stationed near Riyadh to provide direct support to the U.S. Air Force Mobile Aeromedical Staging Facility at King Khalid International Airport near Riyadh, Saudi Arabia. It shuttled patients from many other facilities to the Mobile Aeromedical Staging Facility, including civilians and enemy prisoners, and provided MEDEVAC training for Saudi medical units before returning home in May.[78]

The 348th Med Det (RA) from Orlando, Florida, was initially ordered to active duty to replace a deploying active duty unit. In December, the 348th was deployed to Saudi Arabia and assigned to the 120th Medical Battalion.

Capt. Pete Webb was the 348th's active duty advisor. He initially enlisted as an infantryman in 1977 and served in Hawaii with the 25th Infantry Division. After his tour, he acquired a college degree and in 1983, reenlisted in the Army National Guard of Maine who sponsored him for a commission in the Corps of Engineers, sent him to flight school, and then assigned him to an engineer unit as a UH-1 and OH-58 pilot. Maine also had a 25-aircraft MEDEVAC unit, the 112th Med Co (AA). He transferred to it and also branch transferred to the MSC. While attending a course at Fort Sam Houston, he heard that the active duty needed MSC aviators so he applied for active duty. His package was accepted, and he was assigned to the 498th Med Co (AA), at Fort Benning. After two years with that unit, he received orders to the 348th Med Det (RA), USAR, to serve as the active duty advisor. Joining the six-aircraft unit at Orlando, Florida, in the spring of 1990, like Schwallie, he found a unit with a strong local identity (it was known as "Mickey Mouse DUSTOFF" because it was located near Disney World, just outside Orlando) and full of highly experienced personnel, more than half of whom had served in Vietnam.[79]

Arriving in Saudi Arabia, the 348th aircraft were equipped with global positioning system receivers and provided general area support for the theater. They relocated several times and primarily shuttled patients between hospitals. They carried many of the 99 casualties caused by the explosion of an Iraqi Scud missile that struck a troop barracks in Dhahran on 25 February. While deployed, the unit carried more than 1,000 patients, many of whom were Iraqi prisoners of war. Webb noticed that they were always apprehensive when they were loaded aboard helicopters, but would invariably smile when they saw the unit "Mickey Mouse" patch unofficially affixed on the side of the aircraft. The 348th redeployed to the United States and demobilized in May.[80]

The 872d Med Det (RA) USAR, from New Iberia, Louisiana, was also activated early to backfill for active duty deploying units. In January, it deployed to Saudi Arabia and provided area general support under the 120th Medical Battalion before coming home in April.[81]

After its self-deployment to Saudi Arabia, the 45th Med Co (AA) initially supported the 24th Infantry Division and the 82d Airborne Division. Then it was assigned directly to the 3d MEDCOM and provided general support to all units arriving in Saudi Arabia with its FSMTs, which moved around as necessary. Several of its crews had become landing qualified aboard ships because the Navy would allow only helicopters with landing gear, like the UH-60, as opposed to aircraft with landing skids, like the UH-1, to land aboard ships. On December 15, as the buildup for offensive operations continued, the 45th was assigned as an Echelons Above Corps asset, specifically to do shore-to-ship transfers to the U.S. Naval Ships *Comfort* and *Mercy*. It then dispatched aircraft to several locations and provided hospital-to-hospital support. When DESERT SABRE commenced, the unit provided some direct support to special operations units in the west and then carried a large number of enemy prisoners of war. Capt. Pete Smart and his maintenance team were kept very busy moving aircraft around for the now well-dispersed unit and fixing aircraft damaged by the harsh desert and the heavy operations tempo.[82]

The 45th responded to the Scud missile attack in Dhahran and carried out 130 casualties. Flight medic and 1st Sgt. Jeff Mankoff was on the flying schedule that night and flew several sorties as the horribly wounded soldiers were moved to several hospitals. After casualties ceased, the 45th remained in theater and covered the withdrawal of units to Saudi Arabia for return to their home stations. In July, it responded to a mass casualty disaster when a massive fire engulfed an ammunition storage area belonging to the 11th Armored Cavalry Regiment. The 45th finally returned to Germany in August, claiming 356 days in theater, during which it had carried 1,403 patients.[83]

Return Home

With the cessation of hostilities, American forces rapidly left the theater. The mobilized Guard and Reserve units returned to their home bases and demobilized. Rotations for both active and Reserve units resumed to Central America and Africa, and units once again provided local and domestic support to natural disasters such as floods and forest fires.

Many units reassumed their MAST taskings, and soon enough the calls for assistance were received. The 3d Platoon of the 507th Med Co (AA) at Fort Hood was called out in October 1991 to support medical operations at a Libby's Restaurant in Killen, Texas, when a gunman went on a rampage and killed several patrons.[84]

Arriving back at Fort Campbell in late April, Heintz and Delta Company, 326th Medical Battalion, spent the next few months slowly receiving their equipment back from the Persian Gulf. As soon as they were again operational, they dispatched an FSMT with three aircraft back down to duty in Central America. They also reassumed alert duty to cover all of the training ranges and for MAST.

Heintz and his operations officer, MacDonald, co-authored a collection of lessons learned and tactics, techniques, and procedures based on the unit's operations in the conflict. It included the operation of an FSMT. These findings were submitted to the division and ultimately encapsulated as chapter 9 of the 101st

Airborne Division's *Gold Book,* which is the ever-evolving manual of standard procedures still used by the division.[85]

Heintz gave up command in the summer of 1992 and proceeded to Falls Church, Virginia, to serve as a mobilization plans officer for the Office of The Surgeon General staff. MacDonald left the company too, and moved up to serve as the 326th Medical Battalion operations officer, and subsequently as chief of the Division Medical Operations Center.[86]

Returning from his duty in the desert with the 45th, Smart resumed his duties as the maintenance platoon commander and also helped relocate the unit from Darmstadt to Wiesbaden. He remained in Wiesbaden as the rear detachment commander when the 159th deployed to Saudi Arabia to replace the 45th.[87]

Mission Totals

For the conflict, 25 MEDEVAC units (companies/detachments) deployed with an estimated 250 helicopters. While MEDEVAC records for DESERT SHIELD/STORM/SABRE are incomplete, available records from the individual units show that the units all totaled reported flying 19,596+ hours on 3,282+ missions and carrying 8,447+ patients. Those patients were allied soldiers, sailors, airmen, and marines, and also enemy prisoners and Iraqi civilians. In addition, the units that backfilled to posts in the United States and Europe reported flying 7,039+ hours on 1,133+ missions to transport 578+ patients. The MEDEVAC force deployed to the Persian Gulf was double the size of the MEDEVAC force sent to Vietnam. However, its length of deployment was much shorter. However, the soldiers of MEDEVAC squarely faced the unique and harsh challenges of war in the desert with the same determination and professionalism of their mentors from that earlier war. They were certainly included in Gen. Schwarzkopf's laudatory comments about the performance of the Army Medical units in the desert conflict.[88]

Chapter Six
Force Reductions, 1992–1995

"The concept of having a strong, mission ready reserve unit does not happen overnight. This unit took years to develop… that, with a stroke of a pen was taken out… all of the experience that formed the foundation of the unit is now gone."

Col. Randy Schwallie, U.S. Army Reserve (USAR)[1]

All was not quiet in the Persian Gulf region, as the huge allied forces returned to their home nations. Emboldened by the decisive defeat of the Iraqi forces, dissident groups such as the Shia in southern Iraq and the Kurds in the north began to rebel against Saddam Hussein. Fearing such a development, he had withheld some of his forces from the fight in the south to deal with any threat. The Shia were first. In March and April 1991, Iraqi infantry and helicopter gunships brutally smashed them. Some escaped into territory held by coalition forces. As noted earlier, MEDEVAC helicopter units evacuated many of them.

Operations

Operation PROVIDE COMFORT

Then Hussein turned on the Kurds in the north. When he attacked them, they feared a repeat of the brutal and indiscriminate slaughter perpetrated on them in 1988, and more than 450,000 fled to the north and assembled in the mountains along the Turkish border. Smaller numbers of Turcomans, Assyrian Christians, Chaldeans, and other Iraqi citizens fleeing for political reasons joined them. The harsh conditions created a critical and immediate need for water, food, sanitation, medical care, shelter, and security. To avert a humanitarian disaster, in early April, U.S. and allied forces—with Turkish permission—moved into the area to provide needed assistance as part of Operation PROVIDE COMFORT.[2]

U.S. Air Force and special operations forces from Europe initially led the force. They were well familiar with the area, having operated from the region against Iraq during DESERT STORM. Dealing with the magnitude of the refugees, however, required a larger effort. A combined task force with personnel from 13 nations was formed, which eventually included 21,000 personnel. They were sequestered in a security area centered on the city of Zahko, approximately 150 kilometers by 40 kilometers, with 43 separate clusters or camps. The combined task force was also augmented with numerous nongovernmental organizations. One of the major components of the combined task force was a large aviation task force composed of elements from several nations and services. In it was a U.S. Army flight detachment of 52 helicopters including a detachment of six UH-60s from the 159th Med Co (AA), which was actually located in the security zone.

Maj. Pauline Lockard now commanded the 159th. After her tour with the 54th at Fort Lewis, Washington, she transferred to Europe where she initially served on the inspector general team with the 7th Medical Command and then moved over to the 421st Medical Battalion (Evacuation) as the assistant S-3 until selected to take over the 159th. This afforded her the opportunity to return to the cockpit, and she went through a very intense checkout program with the unit instructor pilots, even getting fully qualified to use night vision goggles.[3]

Working with the medical units from almost all of the participating countries, Lockard and the troops from the 159th provided medical care to the refugees and the coalition forces until the operation was terminated in September, when Iraqi forces in the area backed away, and the majority of the refugees felt safe enough to return to their homes. Then the 159th aircraft and crews joined their unit detachment in Saudi Arabia, and eventually Kuwait, where Army MEDEVAC helicopters have maintained a presence ever since.

After-action reports from PROVIDE COMFORT indicated that the need for MEDEVAC was not identified early in the planning process and the deployment of MEDEVAC assets lagged the rest of the force flow. The main challenge for MEDEVAC was the coordination and centralization of control of all coalition assets to handle the myriad problems encountered. Civilian aid workers and medics were too quick to call for a MEDEVAC pickup when the needs of the patient did not necessarily require evacuation by air.[4]

Lessons Learned to Force XXI

In the months following their return from the Persian Gulf, all commands wrote after-action reports and lessons learned for DESERT SHIELD/STORM. More than 1,350 observations were filed on medical issues, with more than 100 directed in some form at MEDEVAC. They covered a gamut of issues including the adequacy of ground and air ambulance vehicles, Table of Organization and Equipment (TO&E) unit structures, the efficacy of the evacuation battalion, the challenges of long-range communications, challenges to operational and logistical support to MEDEVAC units, and medical equipage onboard MEDEVAC helicopters and their use to carry noncombatants.

Col. Jerry Foust, the commander of the 44th Medical Brigade, directed the collection of observations and lessons learned for his command. Several addressed MEDEVAC issues. The findings showed that Foust's medical forces were prepared to support the XVIII Airborne Corps by being able to evacuate and treat 1,600 allied casualties a day. Most of their patients were Iraqi enemy prisoners of war. Foust also saw how the long distances covered by the combat forces stretched his MEDEVAC units beyond their limits. Communication was a problem, as well as logistical support. Accordingly, he supported and encouraged assigning—where possible—MEDEVAC units to ground maneuver units, and then locating them with the aviation elements. He remembered:

> We lashed them [MEDEVAC units] up with aviation brigades. [They] had the comms. They had the involvement with the planning. That is where I see where we really, really changed because of the distances involved and because of our lack of communications. We had to depend on those aviation brigades for Intel[ligence], Ops, comms, and some maintenance, weather.[5]

As an old MEDEVAC pilot himself, he also made sure that within the 44th launch authority rested within the medical chain. He stated:

> Our job was release authority. Our job is to take care of patient. [The] individual pilot, the ops officer and the commander had release authority. …we had to release it so that the pilots and crewmembers could get enough information where the mission would be inherently safe. We didn't have the comms.[6]

The General Accounting Office did an overall effectiveness study examining the efficacy of the large medical force deployed to the Persian Gulf. The report included data from the Office of The Surgeon General and the U.S. Army Health Services Command and Academy of Health Services, both at Fort Sam Houston, Texas. The study included recommendations for improving medical effectiveness.

The report found that out of a concern for massive casualties potentially caused by modern warfare and the possible widespread use of chemical weapons, the U.S. Army deployed 23,000 medical personnel for all components and organized into 198 medical units, in addition to those units directly assigned to the maneuver forces. The deployment occurred in two phases: the first consisting of primarily active duty forces to support the defensive mission of protecting Saudi Arabia, and the second consisting of units from Europe and the Reserve Components to support offensive operations to eject the Iraqis from Kuwait.

Many deficiencies were noted including incomplete or out-of-date personnel information systems. Many personnel were nondeployable for a variety of reasons including a lack of training for wartime missions. Unit status reporting was not accurate. Some hospital units were never fully equipped or supplied. Medical supply centers in the theater could not adequately respond to the demands of in-theater units for various reasons. Some hospital units lacked the mobility to stay up with rapidly moving maneuver formations.[7]

Noting that "A prompt and well planned patient evacuation process is a key factor in saving the lives of those who suffer battlefield casualties," the report pointed out that "The Army's ability to effectively and quickly evacuate casualties from the battlefield was impeded due to rugged terrain, distances between the hospitals and the front lines, poor communications, and the lack of navigational equipment and repair parts."[8]

Several specific lessons learned for MEDEVAC were offered:

1. Ground ambulances were ineffective because of rugged terrain, a lack of navigational equipment, communication difficulties, and the long distance between units and medical treatment facilities.

2. Desert conditions degraded air ambulance capabilities. The UH-1 Huey legacy aircraft was inadequate because it lacked proper navigation capability and instrumentation for flight in bad weather and low visibility conditions; its lift capability was limited by the hot weather; its overall usefulness was limited by its low speed, short range, and maintenance requirements; and it also had trouble meeting its requirement to perform backhaul and hospital transfers because of the distances involved and lack of refueling points.

3. Communication and navigation shortfalls impeded patient evacuation and regulation. Units were severely limited because radio communication was limited in range to only 15 miles or less by the altitudes at which they flew for protection and the harshness of the desert. Before combat, the 44th Medical Brigade had reported this radio deficiency and had requested FM radio repeaters for emplacement in the desert, but did not receive them. Some air ambulance units deployed without secure radio capability, forcing them to make all calls "in the clear," thus violating Operations Security guidance.

4. Ambulance units also had difficulty getting modern navigational gear on their aircraft. Global positioning system units and LORAN were slow to arrive.

5. A lack of spare parts also affected overall aircraft sustainability.[9]

The report recommended that the Secretary of the Army should take steps to ensure that the doctrine for using ambulance units was consistent with the battlefield of the future and that these units were sufficiently resourced with equipment and support to accomplish their missions.

The Department of Defense, in its review of the findings, concurred with the assessment, and indicated that the development of new air and ground ambulance doctrine was another element of Medical Force 2000 (MF2K). However, overall Army priorities and fiscal constraints determined the upgrade of the fleet from older UH-1s to UH-60s.[10]

These noted deficiencies, the increasing sophistication of modern aircraft, and the availability of and need for advanced navigation, instrumentation, and communication gear indicated that the MEDEVAC units needed to be more closely aligned with aviation units from which they could get more constant intelligence and Army Airspace Command and Control, weather, supply, logistics, and maintenance support.

The MEDEVAC community's lessons learned collection was a part of the inclusive medical collections for the conflict. In turn, they were a part of the overall

Army process. Assuming the position of the 32d Army Chief of Staff in June 1991, Gen. Gordon Sullivan directed several boards and study groups to analyze the data and suggest force structure changes to better prepare the Army for the fast changing world. In a series of experiments and exercises called the Louisiana Maneuvers, the collected groups scoped out a plan for change called Force XXI. It took advantage of evolving technologies to develop lighter but no less lethal and strategically mobile forces capable of fighting as part of inevitable joint and/ or combined task forces for almost any mission from humanitarian assistance to conventional war. One suggested approach proposed modular units or forces that would craft organizations from discrete elements with different capabilities in combination to produce a functional military unit. These ideas developed in future years.[11]

Hurricane Andrew

The next challenge for the MEDEVAC forces occurred within the United States. The hurricane season in 1992 started off very quietly. The first named storm did not form until August, but it more than made up for its lateness by becoming a monster that slammed into Florida just south of Miami on 24 August. It was named Andrew and would forever be remembered as one of the worst storms of the century.

The storm, which first formed as a tropical depression on 17 August, steadily gained strength and was declared a hurricane on 22 August. It crossed the Bahamas the next day as a Category 4 storm and headed directly for south Florida.

Hurricane warnings were posted for the southern portion of the state and more than a million persons evacuated north. The storm came ashore near Homestead at 0500 on 24 August with peak winds of 150 knots and traversed the state in four hours. The resulting storm surge, thunderstorms, tornadoes, and heavy rain left a path of utter devastation. It then proceeded across the Gulf of Mexico and turned north into the generally less-populated areas of western Louisiana, finally dissipating over the southeast United States.[12]

Early warning of the storm allowed Florida state agencies, local governments, and National Guard units to mobilize and pre-position. However, massive federal help was also needed, and President George H.W. Bush declared Broward, Dade, and Monroe counties as major disaster areas and ordered federal assistance to include military forces.

While military units across the nation deployed, local units sprang into action. Coast Guard helicopters were airborne as soon as the winds died down, as well as helicopters from the Homestead-based 301st Rescue Squadron, U.S. Air Force Reserve. Several Florida Army National Guard (ARNG) helicopter units sent aircraft and equipment that were organized into Task Force 50. The 347th Med Det (RA) of the USAR was based in Miami and its personnel were personally affected. The pilots flew the aircraft out of the path of the storm. As soon as it was safe, they flew them back, providing opportune help to people they could see en route who could flag them down. Upon returning to home station, they volunteered their services to the Florida ARNG, but were not utilized. Then they asked their parent Army Reserve command to activate them. When they did, the unit began flight operations, eventually as the core of a larger Army Reserve task force designated Task Force 3220, which also received some augmentation from the 348th Med Det (RA) from Orlando, Florida.[13]

At first, these operations were rescue and damage survey operations. Capt. Pete Webb was still the active duty advisor to the 348th and participated in the Andrew response. He recalled:

> We were called up for Hurricane Andrew. About 80% of the people in the unit had their houses damaged or facilities damaged and we were ordered by our Army Reserve Command out of Atlanta, Georgia, the 81st ARCOM, to scramble three ships and crews and go to Hurricane Andrew and do anything we could do to assist humanitarian wise with anything we saw or happened on to. We were sent there for approximately two weeks. It was quite an amazing scene as part of the most dangerous environment I have even flown in just because there was no air structure. VORs [aviation navigational aids] were out of commission. There was every branch of service, every civilian counterpart, every type of aircraft you could think of out there flying and no one knew how to talk to anybody.... It was kind of crazy, a lot of near misses.[14]

The XVIII Airborne Corps deployed for hurricane relief. It formed Joint Task Force (JTF) Andrew, which included an aviation task force. That task force supported the 57th Med Det (RG) from Fort Bragg, North Carolina, which was commanded by the 55th Medical Group of the 44th Medical Brigade, both of whom also deployed units.

The elements of the aviation task force and medical units were in southern Florida in strength by 28 August. The aviation task force immediately commenced a much larger operation, with the earlier task forces remaining separate, but coordinating all of their actions with JTF Andrew. Within days more than 120 helicopters supported the operation.

JTF Andrew provided critical command and control to the overall operation. Within a few days, its staff put together an overall plan consisting of three phases: (1) relief, (2) recovery, and (3) reconstitution. The aviation task force also developed a rudimentary airspace control plan to coordinate the myriad operations ongoing.

Relief operations were terminated on 15 October. At that point the aviation task force dissolved and was replaced by the Aviation Brigade of the 10th Mountain Division, which continued the recovery and reconstitution support operations. Subordinate units returned to their home stations. Despite other hazards generated by the storm, occasional stormy weather, and low visibility operations, the aircraft of JTF Andrew and the other task forces logged 8,000 accident free hours. Partial records also show that they carried 6,279 passengers and 3.54 million pounds of cargo. Medical units treated more than 20,000 patients and uncounted animals, and also replenished local medical facilities so that they could operate. No specific number of MEDEVAC missions or patients carried was reported, but the two units involved provided 12 aircraft and crews, or 10% of the fleet. Hurricane Andrew was the worst natural disaster to hit the United States up to that point. The cost of rebuilding was estimated at $25 billion.[15]

Postevent lessons learned highlighted two areas of concern to MEDEVAC:

1. Joint aeromedical operations needed to be better coordinated.
2. Medical units lack adequate communications capabilities.[16]

The deficiencies in communications capabilities were a repeat complaint from the experiences in DESERT SHIELD/STORM.

Hurricane Iniki

One month later, as the cleanup for Hurricane Andrew proceeded, Hurricane Iniki struck Hawaii. The response was similar to that dispatched for Andrew, although on a smaller scale, and included Army active and Reserve Component units. For two weeks, JTF Hawaii deployed more than 5,000 troops to the island of Kauai. As part of the medical element, the 68th Med Det (RA) provided helicopters and crews that flew 41 immediate life-saving missions and transported medical personnel and supplies to many isolated locations until the roads could reopen.[17]

Doctrine

FM 8-10, Health Service Support in a Theater of Operation, March 1991

Almost coincidental with the collecting and writing of the lessons learned for DESERT STORM, the Academy of Health Sciences at Fort Sam Houston published an updated version of Field Manual (FM) 8-10, dated 1 March 1991, which replaced the October 1978 version. Released to the Army literally as its forces concluded combat operations in the Persian Gulf, the rewrite—like FC 8-45—acknowledged AirLand Battle as the warfighting doctrine of the Army. It reaffirmed that the Army Medical Department (AMEDD) played a key role in developing and maintaining combat power by accomplishing its mission to maintain the health of the Army to conserve its fighting strength. Discussing the command and control relationships in the theater communications zone, it reaffirmed the formation of medical groups to provide command and control and administrative supervision of assigned or attached medical units. Paralleling lessons learned in DESERT STORM, this included the newly redesigned medical evacuation battalions. These battalions were also assigned to the medical brigades supporting the corps.[18]

The medical evacuation battalions provided command and control, supervision of operations, training, and administration of a combination of three to seven air ambulance companies of either the 25-ship (TOE 08-137H200) or new MF2K 15-ship (TOE 08-447L100 or L200) variety, ground ambulance units, or the older six-ship medical detachments (TOE 08-660H0) with either the UH-1s or UH-60s. The basis of allocation was one battalion for three or four air or ground ambulance companies.

The battalion also provided medical supply support and limited Echelon I health service support (HSS).[19]

FM 8-10-6, Medical Evacuation in a Theater of Operations, Tactics, Techniques, and Procedures, October 1991

Published eight months later, a new manual, FM 8-10-6, was released. It devolved from the new FM 8-10, but was a more expansive and updated rewrite of the 1983 version of FM 8-35. It took the philosophy and doctrine of that FM and applied it specifically to medical evacuation in a theater of operations. Acknowledging again that evacuation is a critical link in the continuum of care, it then explained the structure and function of the evacuation battalion and subordinate 15-ship air ambulance companies and six-ship medical detachments.[20]

The manual also explained in significant detail how the medical battalion functioned to include the following:

1. A combined S2/S3 for properly coordinating MEDEVAC operations into combat operations.
2. Coordination with the Army Airspace Command and Control system.[21]

The 15-ship air ambulance companies were allotted on the basis of one in direct support per division or .33 per separate brigade or armored cavalry regiment, and one assigned in general support to a corps for every two assigned divisions or fraction thereof. The company accomplished unit-level maintenance on aircraft and equipment (less medical), and organizational maintenance on all organic avionics equipment. The unit also provided air crash rescue support and the rescue of downed aircrews. However, the companies had to rely on higher commands for other personnel, supply and security items, and aviation intermediate maintenance support. The company was organized with three forward support MEDEVAC teams that were assigned to specific brigades and generally located with the forward support medical company in the brigade support area. The company also maintained a six-aircraft area support MEDEVAC section designed to provide area support or reinforce the forward support MEDEVAC teams.[22]

The legacy six-aircraft medical detachments were tasked similarly to the companies. Although they were also capable of 24-hour operations, they could only provide two three-ship sections and needed more maintenance (unit and intermediate level) personnel and administrative, supply, logistical, and security support.[23]

Perhaps in early response to lessons learned being developed for DESERT SHIELD/STORM/SABRE, the FM stated, "Evacuation support for offensive operations must be responsive to several essential characteristics. As operations achieve success, the areas of casualty density move away from the support facilities. This causes the routes of medical evacuation to lengthen."[24] That is exactly what happened in Kuwait and Iraq.

The FM also included chapters dedicated to a revision of the evacuation precedence codes, the nine-line request, and tactics, techniques, and procedures that were repetitive of the earlier FM 8-35 manuals but updated for the newer equipment available. In essence, the evacuation battalions balanced both medical and aviation concerns to run an integrated evacuation system for the medical brigades supporting the corps.

A Contrary View

Serving as an observer/controller at the Joint Readiness Training Center at Fort Chaffee, Arkansas, Maj. Van Joy certainly was aware of the changes. His work required him to know the latest in doctrine and lessons learned to properly evaluate the MEDEVAC units coming through the center.

Joy had initially joined the Army as an enlisted soldier with the Nebraska Army National Guard in 1978. He had a college degree in environmental sciences, and the ARNG sponsored him for a commission and flight school. While at Fort Rucker, Alabama, he applied for active duty and was accepted and branched into the Medical Service Corps. Subsequent tours included the 247th Med Det (RG) at Fort Irwin, California, where he transitioned to the UH-60; Korea, where he served in the 377th Med CO (AA) with Maj. Bill Thresher, Capt. Dave MacDonald, and 2d Lt. Pete Smart; and Panama, where he served in the 214th Med Det (RG) from just after JUST CAUSE until August 1992, when he was posted to Fort Chaffee for this present job.[25]

Serving at Fort Chaffee until the summer of 1993, he evaluated numerous MEDEVAC units that deployed to the center to support brigades going through the training cycle. While serving in Panama with the 214th, Joy was impressed with the full support that the unit received from the aviation brigade. However, he noticed that most of the MEDEVAC units coming through Fort Chaffee did not receive the same degree of support he was used to seeing and their performance suffered in the exercises because of it. He remembered:

> I was the one at JRTC [Joint Readiness Training Center] when the MEDEVAC would come there and deploy with the rotational units. I saw that where they needed to be was up under the Aviation task force … The Medical community had no clue of where the MEDEVAC was on the battlefield at any one time; they never tracked them; they never did anything with them. They would a lot of times want to push them off to the Aviation brigade or the Aviation task force…But they had no control over them. We then pushed to say "When you deploy, you need to deploy up under the Aviation Task Force, not up under the Medical task force or that Charley Med out in the FSB." In doing that, in giving it up under the Aviation Task Force, now that Aviation Task Force commander has an inherent responsibility for them. He not only now has to worry about their training, but has to worry about their feeding, the fueling, the fixing: all of the life support…Doing it up under the Aviation brigade, now they are already in the pre-deployment training cycle there; they are rolled up there in everything. It is not an afterthought which MEDEVAC had always been—an afterthought for everything. They never were brought in from the very beginning for the planning all the way up through execution.[26]

Joy left Fort Chaffee in the summer of 1993, just as the Joint Readiness Training Center moved its entire operation to Fort Polk, Louisiana. His orders took him back to Panama for more duty in Central America. Regardless of how MEDEVAC doctrine was evolving, he left Fort Chaffee with a firm belief that MEDEVAC should be assigned to the aviation brigades. He would have occasion in a few years to again deal with that issue, but in a more definitive way.[27]

Reorganizing and Reducing the Forces

Organization

Active Duty

In April 1991, as the allied forces returned from the Persian Gulf, the North Atlantic Treaty Organization (NATO) Council met in Rome and formally declared that there was no longer an immediate threat of a Soviet Bloc invasion of western Europe. However, it did identify regional political instability in eastern Europe and the Balkans region as new threats to the general peace. The American people, however, were convinced that the cold war was over and wanted a "Peace Dividend," which would be paid for with large military force reductions.[28]

In the United States, calls for force cuts actually started as early as 1987, and they only accelerated with subsequent events. Some unit inactivations were planned to take place during DESERT SHIELD/STORM, but they were delayed until the units returned from the war, with many inactivating as they returned home. At one point, Secretary of Defense Dick Cheney proposed reducing the Army from 28 to 18 divisions, with commensurate cuts in the ARNG and U.S. Army Reserve (USAR), arguing that both components had grown with the active forces in response to needs and should now be so reduced. Between 1989 and 1994, total Army strength declined from 772,000 to 529,000.[29]

Other NATO nations also reduced their military forces. The alliance developed a new strategic concept based on smaller and more flexible and mobile forces. Subsequent restructuring led to the development of bi-national and multinational units and task forces that could be utilized for a variety of operations other than war.[30]

Reserve Components

Proportional reductions were also made in the two Reserve Components of the Army. Reflecting the guidance from Cheney, the Chairman of the Joint Chiefs of Staff, Army Gen. Colin Powell, pointed out that even though the Reserve Components were a robust part of the total Army, there was no longer a requirement for the current force levels. They—like the active Army—would need to be cut. Accordingly, the ARNG was reduced from 457,000 in 1989 to 375,000 in 1995, and the USAR was reduced from 319,000 in 1989 to 260,000 in 1994.[31]

No active Army MEDEVAC units were inactivated. However, the discussions of which Reserve Component units to inactivate became very heated and political, as various U.S. senators, representatives, and many veterans organizations weighed in on the issues. As the rancor built concerning the equitability of cuts between the two Reserve Components, the Army Chief of Staff, Gen. Gordon Sullivan, held an "off-site" working conference in October 1993, with the Chief of the Army Reserve, Maj. Gen. Roger Sandler, and the Director of the Army National Guard, Maj. Gen. John D'Araujo, Jr. No records exist of the discussions, but at their conclusion, the Chief of Staff announced that 14,000 USAR positions would be "transferred" to the National Guard. These positions were primarily combat arms and aviation rotary-wing positions. In return, the National Guard transferred to the USAR about 12,000 medical, signal, military police, and transportation positions. These were position swaps, not unit movements. Those affected personnel who desired to remain in drilling positions had to find billets individually. This action generated personnel turbulence that was staggering to men and women who had just recently put civilian careers on hold proudly to serve in the Persian Gulf.[32]

The rotary-wing flying units of the USAR were the most dramatically affected by this action. Before the agreement, the USAR had 44 different aviation or aviation support units, including two MEDEVAC companies and 13 detachments. Most had been activated and deployed for DESERT SHIELD/STORM. As a result of the "off-site" agreement, the USAR would be left with just four flying units: lift and attack battalions. *All* of their MEDEVAC units would be inactivated within two years.[33]

The personnel in the affected organizations were devastated. Some quit and others scrambled to find jobs in other USAR or ARNG units. The competition was keen, and many had to cross-train to stay in uniform. Capt. Randy Schwallie found a position with the 429th Medical Battalion (Evacuation) in Savannah, Georgia. However, he would not fly again as a MEDEVAC aviator. Personally, he felt the loss and sensed it, too, in larger terms:

> The concept of having a strong, mission ready reserve unit does not happen overnight. This unit took years to develop a strong flight program that, with a stroke of a pen, was taken out of the hangar and put into the history books. Before any reserve unit is disbanded, the Army must be absolutely certain those assets will not need to regenerate quickly. Unfortunately, all of the experience that formed the foundation of the unit is now gone, too.[34]

As a result of that action, the USAR got completely out of the MEDEVAC business, and the Army lost about one-third of its entire MEDEVAC force.

Capt. Bill LaChance, then serving as an active duty advisor to the 321st Med Det (RA) USAR, at Salt Lake City, Utah, also witnessed the process. He was commissioned into the Medical Service Corps through the Reserve Officers' Training Corps program at the University of Rhode Island in 1988. He was interested in hospital finance, and his first tour was with a hospital unit. The commander was an old MEDEVAC pilot, Lt. Col. Bob Romines. He entertained the young officer with tales of MEDEVAC. LaChance had given some thought to flying, and within two years, he was at pilot training. Subsequently, he flew with the 36th Med Det (RA), at Fort Polk, and then attended the Medical Service Corps advanced course at Fort Sam Houston.

While in the course, he was offered the advisor job in Salt Lake City. LaChance had no idea if such an assignment would be good or bad for career advancement. Fortuitously, Col. Bob Romines was also assigned at Fort Sam Houston, and LaChance visited him to ask his advice. Romines knew that such service could be broadening, professionally rewarding, and even enjoyable and counseled him to take the job. LaChance took the assignment and reported to the 321st in June 1994.

LaChance, who replaced someone who had been fired, fell in love with the unit and developed a deep respect for the dedication and professionalism of the reservists. As the only active duty soldier in the unit, he flew a lot, especially on mountain rescues, which was a unit specialty.

Sadly though, he was there at the unit when the announcement of the ARNG-USAR swap was released. Rumors abounded about the back room deals and sell-outs that must have occurred for such a bad decision to be made. The unit was devastated, and morale plummeted. Many of the reservists did not find slots with other units and gave up on many years of faithful service.

LaChance also found out that the unit soldiers had never received any awards for their service in DESERT SHIELD/STORM. On his own, he researched their tour in the conflict and then recreated all of the necessary paperwork for more than 70 individual awards for those reserve soldiers. They deeply appreciated his efforts. He left the unit in 1996 for a staff job at Landstuhl, Germany, just a few weeks before the unit inactivated.[35]

Active Duty Forces – MF2K

Whereas the active Army did not lose any MEDEVAC units, it did take steps to consolidate the continental United States based units under the MF2K initiative developed before DESERT SHIELD. Under a plan developed and disseminated by the U.S. Army Forces Command in April 1992, it realigned the current 25-ship companies and six-ship detachments into 15-ship companies and three residual detachments. The Delta Company of the 326th Medical Battalion assigned to the 101st Airborne Division remained as it was with 12 aircraft.

The plan dictated that the 498th Med Co (AA) at Fort Benning, Georgia, decrease to 15 aircraft and move to Fort Stewart, Georgia. The 57th Med Det (RG) at Fort Bragg gained nine aircraft and became a company. The detachments at Fort Drum, New York, Fort Polk, Louisiana, and Fort Irwin, California, remained as they were, as well as the 68th at Wheeler Army Airfield, Hawaii, and the 283d at Fort Wainwright, Alaska, both of which were assigned the U.S. Army Pacific. The 507th at Fort Hood, Texas, the 82d at Fort Riley, Kansas, the 571st at Fort Carson, Colorado, and the 54th at Fort Lewis, Washington, re-aligned as 15-aircraft equipped companies under the MF2K design. These units were assigned for C2 to the corps-assigned evacuation battalions also being created under the MF2K initiative and provided aeromedical support throughout the corps area.[36]

In the summer of 1993, the Army initiated the plan and took additional steps to consolidate some of the MEDEVAC units. The 237th Med Det (RG) at Fort Ord, California, was inactivated. Some of its personnel and assets were moved to the 54th Med Det (RG) at Fort Lewis, so it could grow to a company. The 431st Med Det (RA) at Fort Knox, Kentucky, was inactivated. The 57th Med Det (RG) at

Fort Bragg and the 571st Med Det (RA) at Fort Carson completed their transitions to Med Cos by absorbing aircraft and personnel from the inactivating MEDEVAC and some aviation units.[37]

Medical Reengineering Initiative

That same summer, the AMEDD initiated another force restructuring focused on medical units above the division level. The Medical Reengineering Initiative was designed to correct deficiencies in large medical units and hospitals that had been modified under the MF2K initiative but were too cumbersome for the post–cold war. It involved Combat Support Hospitals, area support medical units, forward surgical teams, ground evacuation units, and multifold support units. One of its goals was to push medical care forward. It also advocated enhancing the en route care available aboard the MEDEVAC helicopters by purchasing UH-60Q models as proposed by Brig. Gen. Foust and Col. Frank Novier at the Medical Evacuation Proponency Directorate (MEPD).[38]

Eagle Dustoff

At Fort Campbell, Kentucky, the 326th Medical Battalion, 101st Airborne Division, was directed to convert to the 626th Support Battalion (Forward) as part of a larger Army-wide restructuring of divisional support battalions occurring since the late 1980s. Under the restructuring, all divisional medical, supply, transportation, and maintenance battalions were combined and reorganized into a main and three forward support battalions. Most heavy divisions were converted before DESERT STORM; the 101st Airborne and 82d Airborne Divisions were converted after that conflict.

In this reorganization, the 326th lost its Delta Company MEDEVAC unit, which would be reassigned. Working with planners at Fort Campbell and Fort Sam Houston, Col. Jim Truscott, still the Assistant Commander for Force Integration at the AMEDD Center and School, Fort Sam Houston, convinced them to allow Delta Company to return to its original MEDEVAC heritage. Subsequently, Delta of the 326th was redesignated the 50th Med Co (AA) and assumed the heritage of the well-decorated 50th Med Det (HA/RA) from Korea and Vietnam. The commander at the time was Maj. Garry Atkins. For administrative purposes, it was assigned to the 8th Battalion, 101st Aviation Regiment, an aviation intermediate maintenance unit, also located at Fort Campbell. Truscott was proud of that small accomplishment, which was one of the last things that he did before he retired in 1992.[39]

Six months later the 50th was tasked under the Military Assistance to Safety and Traffic (MAST) program to support recovery efforts for communities in the vicinity of the Great Smoky Mountains National Park and the Appalachian regions of Tennessee and Kentucky in the aftermath of the "Blizzard of the Century," which dropped record amounts of snow and swept the area with severe weather conditions. For two weeks, aircrews flew missions to rescue stranded hikers caught in the woods by the fast moving storm. More than 100 persons were hoisted or recovered from the deep snow and severe conditions.

A New Blackhawk

After DESERT STORM, Foust continued to command the 44th Medical Brigade until October 1991, when he was transferred back to Fort Sam Houston again, to serve now as the Deputy Chief of Staff for Operations at the Health Services Command. The next year, he was moved over to be the Commander of the Army Garrison. Shortly thereafter, he was selected for promotion to brigadier general and became the Chief of the Medical Service Corps, the first MEDEVAC pilot selected in that position. At that rank, he could no longer be the garrison commander, so he was transferred over to serve as the deputy commander of the AMEDD Center and School. In those twin capacities, he quickly became involved in a full regimen of issues including the structure of the basic and advanced courses, force restructuring based on lessons learned from DESERT STORM, and the Army-wide downsizing.

One item particularly captured his interest. He wanted to modernize the MEDEVAC helicopter fleet and pushed for an upgraded UH-60. He pulled funding from several sources to facilitate the development of the UH-60Q variant. Reflecting deficiencies identified and lessons learned in the recent conflicts and contingency operations, the new aircraft had an improved intercom system for communications between the pilots and crewmembers in the cabin, better long-range radios, and a global positioning navigational system. It could also carry forward looking infrared for better navigation at night or in bad weather.

For enhanced patient carrying capability and comfort, the "Q Bird"—as it was subsequently called—was also extensively modified. It was provided with a litter lift system, a hoist, improved cabin lighting, improved cabin heating and cooling, upgraded intravenous bag provisions, a suction system and secure waste collection unit, an oxygen generating system, defibrillator capability, and increased medical storage capacity.[40]

One of the officers who joined Foust in the UH-60Q effort was Col. Frank Novier. After returning from his DESERT STORM service with the 34th Medical Battalion, he remained in command until the unit was inactivated in 1992. He attended the Army War College and graduated in 1993. After the War College, he was selected for duty on the Joint Staff in the Pentagon. Instead, Foust asked him to be the head of the MEPD at Fort Rucker, because he needed an aggressive officer to do battle with the Aviation Center Staff there in the fight for the new Q model. Novier accepted the assignment.

After he was briefed on the new aircraft, he quickly gave it his full support and began to do battle with the Aviation Center Staff to get it funded for MEDEVAC. Such funding came through Aviation Procurement Army dollars—not AMEDD—planned for and requested through the Aviation Branch Program Objective Memorandum submission each year.[41]

At the time, the UH-60Q was low priority for Army Aviation. None was funded for the active duty. However, the Tennessee ARNG procured a line of funding through a congressional insert. Novier continued as director of the MEPD until the fall of 1995, when he was sent to Fort Hood, to command the 1st Medical Group.[42] Foust continued to champion the UH-60Q in every forum. However, he was unable to establish steady funding for the program before he retired in October 1996.[43]

Military Operations Other Than War

Operations

Somalia

The newspaper headlines explaining the humanitarian disaster in northern Iraq had barely faded when they were replaced by equally shocking pictures and stories of an unfolding horror in the arid and pitifully impoverished country of Somalia. The United States had some interest in the country because it was located on the Horn of Africa astride the entrance to the Red Sea and thence the Suez Canal. That interest grew when Somalia was struck in 1992 with a devastating drought that destroyed most crops and precipitated a famine. For survival, local clans attacked each other to steal food supplies. Social order broke down. International relief agencies tried to intervene. They were also put upon by the armed locals, and the international press was awash with troubling pictures of Somalis starving en masse.

In August 1992, President George H.W. Bush directed the initiation of Operation PROVIDE RELIEF, and U.S. Air Force cargo aircraft flew food and other relief supplies into Somalia from neighboring Kenya. Sensing opportunity, the local warlords immediately unleashed their thugs on those disbursing the food and material. They stole the well-intended supplies and then sold them to the locals. With practically no money, the people continued to starve.[44]

As the situation steadily deteriorated, President Bush, now supported with United Nations resolutions, ordered the initiation of Operation RESTORE HOPE, and in December 1992, dispatched 13,000 airmen, soldiers, sailors, marines, and Special Forces troops to staunch the violence and restore stability to the country. This force was reinforced by 25,000 more military personnel from 22 other nations. This combined force restrained the local militias so that relief organizations could disburse more than 40,000 tons of grain and other foodstuffs. Stores reopened, commerce resumed, and new crops were planted.

The Army component from the 10th Mountain Division also included a robust medical task force consisting of the 62d Medical Group from Fort Lewis, the 86th Evacuation Hospital from Fort Campbell, several smaller specialty units and detachments, and the 159th Med Co (AA) from Germany, equipped with 15 UH-60 aircraft and still commanded by Maj. Pauline Lockard.

The 159th was attached to a larger aviation package built around the 5th Battalion, 158th Aviation Regiment, sent by V Corps under U.S Army Europe. The Task Force members self-deployed to Livorno, Italy, where they boarded their equipment aboard a fast freighter, which then delivered it to Somalia in early January 1993.

The unit initially located its aircraft at Baledogle airfield, 25 miles north of the capital of Mogadishu, and brought a small tractor and trailer and a 10-ton forklift. They were the only ones in the task force and were in high demand by all units. Lockard also packed a goodly amount of sports gear and other "comfort" items for troop morale, welfare, and recreation. Given the very austere cultural environment, these items were also well sought after by the rest of the task force. Her unit helped build a small physical fitness facility—open to all—that was well utilized and offered a "free life membership." Working under the medical task force, Lockard had launch authority for her crews and supported almost of all the different national and international task forces working in the country.[45]

Also still serving with the 159th, Capt. Pete Smart deployed again as the maintenance platoon commander. As in previous deployments, he flew few actual MEDEVAC missions, but focused instead on keeping the fleet flying. He had an outstanding crew of noncommissioned officers and young soldiers, and he infused them with that sense of urgency for mission that Bill Thresher had instilled in him in Korea. He later said of them:

> They understand that they have a real world mission; it's not play; this is not a drill…You make a difference in someone's life every day and whether you are going out there and actually flying that mission or you are the guy who's fixing a broken airplane that needs to get fixed so it can be used for the next mission.

> I can remember nights when a bird would come flying in at 2 o'clock… It had a problem. And the guys would hear it come in. I didn't even have to get them out of the rack. We would hear the bird coming and we'd say, "Probably something wrong." So people would just get up on their own and head out to the flight line and wait for it to shut down and find out what was wrong.[46]

Like most of his fellow soldiers, Smart was shocked by what he saw in Somalia, remembering:

> It was a mess… At that point in time, it was such a huge humanitarian crisis, there was very little in-fighting going on. The militias had pretty much pulled back, established their lines; it was trench warfare going on in the city. There was just very little activity. The place was in very bad condition. I have never been in a place in the world that was in worse condition than what I saw in Mogadishu at that time. There wasn't a piece of glass that wasn't broken; the utility lines were all ripped out of the ground. Anything that was salvageable was torn down, ripped out. …That was the mission of the task force: to go in there and restore the supply lines, to get the food moving, because it was all being held up at the ports and being used as barter. There was no currency exchange; food was power.[47]

The U.S. Navy had several major ships off shore with extensive medical capability. Unfortunately, none of the 159th pilots was qualified to land aboard the ships. A quick training program solved that problem, and this deficiency was

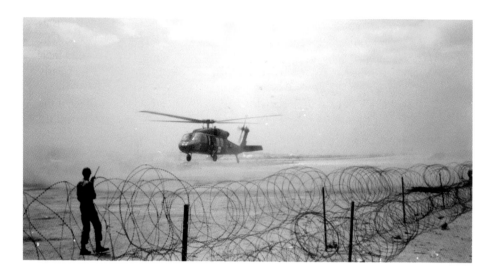

A MEDEVAC helicopter from the 159th Med Co (AA) landing at the 86th Evacuation Hospital deployed to Somalia.
Source: Lt. Col. Rich Prior.

logged as a noted lessons learned for inclusion in postconflict doctrinal revision efforts. The MEDEVAC aircraft and crews were disbursed to four other fields for duty. Casualties were rare, and few actual MEDEVAC missions were needed.[48]

Operation RESTORE HOPE was terminated in May 1993 and replaced by a smaller United Nations operation labeled UNOSOM II. The initial medical task force was simultaneously replaced by a smaller force that consisted primarily of the 42d Field Hospital from Fort Knox, several smaller supporting units, and the 45th Med Co (AA) also from Germany, which replaced the 159th.[49]

The aircraft and crews of the 45th were also spread out over several locations to provide wider coverage. Although they were joined by helicopters and crews from France, Italy, Germany, and Malaysia, the crews of the 45th flew more than 75% of the total MEDEVAC missions. They all supported deployments of medical teams into villages to provide desperately needed medical support to the civilian populace. The 82d Med Co (AA) from Fort Riley, which deployed with six UH-1Vs, replaced the 45th at the end of August.[50]

However, the relief effort did not bring political and social stability. In June, a local clan leader, Muhammed Aideed, led a force that ambushed a United Nations Pakistani unit, killing 24 of their soldiers and causing 122 casualties overall. As the fighting increased, more MEDEVAC missions were requested.

The United States reacted to the increase in violence by dispatching a large special operations task force to capture Aideed and his supporters. In a series of hard-hitting raids in August through October of 1993, they slowly captured his troops. Unfortunately, the seventh raid failed when Aideed's supporters surrounded the raiding force and shot down two American helicopters. The ensuing

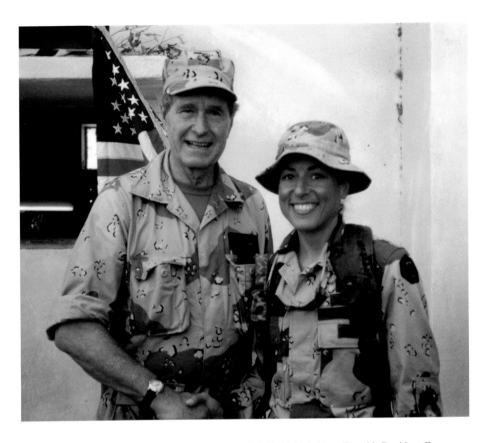

Maj. Pauline Lockard, commander of the 159th Med Co (AA) in Somalia, with President George H.W. Bush.
Source: Col. (ret) Pauline Lockard.

battle and rescue operation lasted into the next day before a relief column from the 10th Mountain Division recovered the force from the middle of the city. The 82d flew many missions recovering the wounded from this operation.[51]

As a result, the medical task force was reinforced with several specialist physicians and support personnel, and two more UH-1Vs from the 82d joined their unit in Somalia. However, the news of the horrible battle in Mogadishu shocked the American people. They thought that the mission to Somalia was a humanitarian effort and had not closely followed the steady rise in violence. When presented with scenes showing American bodies being dragged through the streets of Mogadishu, they quickly turned against the operation and demanded that American troops be brought home.

President Bill Clinton concurred and ordered American forces to return to their bases. They were out by the following March, with two 82d Med Co UH-1Vs and crews among the last to return home. The larger United Nations operation slowly withered away over the next year.[52]

Doctrine

The recent experience in Operations PROVIDE COMFORT and RESTORE HOPE in northern Iraq and Somalia reflected a changing philosophy in the United States concerning the use of military force for armed intervention both unilaterally and as part of a coalition. During the cold war, the United States had been only a minimal participant in such operations. As these two events showed, the nation was now prepared to consider the use of military forces in traditional peacekeeping missions, in particular, with others in broad-based coalitions or as party to existing international agreements to deal with lingering problems not dealt with while the world was engaged in the cold war.

FM 100-5, Operations, June 1993

These real world changes were reflected in the next rewrite of FM 100-5, as American troops sweltered in the blazing heat of Somalia. While reaffirming the basic tenets of AirLand Battle, it redefined thinking in a new strategic era. The cold war was over, and the threats had changed, driving a new strategy for the United States. That strategy now focused on stronger joint operations, as directed by the landmark *Goldwater-Nichols Act of 1986*, whereby Congress mandated integrated operations, and the Chairman of the Joint Chiefs of Staff was directed to publish doctrine for joint operations. AirLand Battle evolved into a series of choices for a battlefield framework and a wider interservice area and allowed for the increased incidence of combined operations, recognizing that Army forces could operate across the range of military operations. It became a manual offering a doctrine for full-dimension operations and focused more on the strategic versus operational level of war. In a chapter devoted to "operations other than war," commanders were encouraged to act to control the environment rather than let the environment control events and then have to devise imaginative methods of applying their resources as the circumstances changed.[53]

The Army would not fight alone. It integrated its operations within the theater commander's unified operations with the other services, other national agencies, and perhaps allied and coalition forces. In any given situation, HSS forces could be the first deployed into a contingency operation if they possessed the capabilities necessary to handle that unique situation. This was partly the case in Operation PROVIDE COMFORT in northern Iraq.[54]

The rewrite included an updated chapter on joint operations, pointing out that, "Army doctrine is compatible with and supports joint doctrine...." It also defined joint command relationships and the utilization of JTFs, and suggested a standard structure for a theater of war.[55]

A chapter dedicated to combined operations was also inserted. It discussed the inherent challenges of bringing together military units from different nations with different languages, organizational structures, and cultures to achieve common goals and objectives.[56]

The manual also included for the first time an inclusive section on HSS. While reiterating that the purpose of the HSS was to ensure a medical presence with the soldier and provide state-of-the-art medical and surgical treatment, it also stated:

> HSS requirements will surface in support of operations other than war. Typical operations will include disaster relief, nation assistance, support to domestic civil authorities, and peacekeeping activities...HSS is based on ... standardized air and ground medical evacuation units using air evacuation as the primary means of medical evacuation; flexible and responsive hospitals ...[57]

In a chapter defining and describing operations other than war, the manual explained that it may include a variety of operations that could generate a need for humanitarian assistance and/or disaster relief. These operations would "use DOD personnel, equipment, and supplies to promote human welfare, to reduce pain and suffering, to prevent loss of life or destruction of property from the aftermath of natural or man-made disasters... The Army's global reach, its ability to deploy rapidly, and its ability to operate in the most austere environments make it ideally suited for these missions."[58]

This was a dramatic change for FM 100-5, a manual classically designed to describe how the Army intended to *fight*. Now it was vastly broadening its scope and explicitly reaching out into missions beyond combat. While it reaffirmed the Army's primary focus was still to fight and win, it acknowledged a far more complex world where operations other than war would require Army services. They were services that the MEDEVAC force—as a key component of the HSS community—had been providing since its creation in Korea, domestically and overseas, in both war and peace. This suggested a larger mission for MEDEVAC, beyond the recovery of American soldiers, and possibly as a key instrument in operations other than war.

FM 8-55, Planning for Health Service Support, September 1994

As the actions in Somalia were winding down, medical staff officers were busy revising medical doctrine to reflect the changes presented in FM 100-5. In September 1994, they published an updated FM 8-55. It acknowledged the increased emphasis on operations other than war as an evolution, not a revolution. Such operations included missions such as disaster relief, nation-building assistance, security and advisory assistance, counter-drug operations, arms control, treaty verification, support to domestic civil authorities, and peacekeeping. They required an HSS that was flexible enough to support a diversity of operations.[59]

Reflecting the emphasis placed on joint operations in the new FM 100-5, this revision of FM 8-55 incorporated a section on joint HSS planning. It pointed out that joint force commanders could choose the capabilities they needed for any tasking from the air, land, sea, and special operations forces at their disposal. It also specified that the JTF surgeon could be directed to plan for civil-military, civic-action, or peacekeeping operations support.[60]

The manual included a discussion of the role that the medical evacuation battalions play in the HSS as the C2 headquarters for air and ground evacuation companies. It listed the post-MF2K MEDEVAC companies, showing the same classic capabilities as in previous FMs, with allocation of one per division supported in direct support and one per two divisions supported in general support. Reflecting the recent events in Somalia, it also specifically directed that one company should be assigned to an active theater directly in support of hospital ships if they were deployed. However, no consideration was given to any larger patient group in terms of assignment of MEDEVAC companies. All allocations were still based on division sets.[61]

Joint Doctrine

As a result of the *Goldwater-Nichols Act of 1986*, the Chairman of the Joint Chiefs of Staff directed that the Joint Staff publish joint doctrine that would be applicable to all of the services. It would be specifically directive to commanders of combatant commands and subordinate components of those commands. The guidance provided was to be considered authoritative and to be followed except when—in the judgment of the commander—exceptional circumstances dictated otherwise.

Joint Publication 1 was published on 11 November 1991. As the initial and keystone document, the Chairman of the Joint Chiefs of Staff, Gen. Colin Powell signed it. The document was designed to guide the joint action of the Armed Forces of the United States so that they could fight as one joint team. Recognizing that individual service skills form the core of combat capability, it did not seek to lessen service traditions, expertise, or cohesion, but rather to present a common perspective from which to plan, operate, and fundamentally shape the way U.S. forces think about and train for war. All commanders were directed to integrate the values and concepts presented in this publication into the operations of the U.S. armed forces. From it would spring a full panoply of doctrine across the broad spectrum of military operations.[62]

Joint Publication 4-02, Doctrine for Health Service Support in Joint Operations, April 1995

The first joint medical doctrine was published in Joint Publication 4-02. Clearly structured similarly to the FM 8 series of manuals, it reiterated that the primary objective of HSS was to conserve the commander's fighting strength of land, sea, air, and special operations forces through continuous planning, coordination, and training to ensure a prompt, effective, and unified health care effort. It also reiterated the classic five echelon levels of care.[63]

The document highlighted the critical role that timely patient evacuation played in the design of the treatment sequence from front to rear. It also included a large section on military operations other than war, stating:

> Military operations other than war are usually joint operations, often performed in concert with other government agencies, nongovernmental organizations and private volunteer organizations. HSS policies during military operations for operations other than war may be substantially different from the policies associated with general war... Humanitarian and civic

assistance (HCA) programs operate in conjunction with U.S. military operations or exercises. HCAs serve the local populace by furnishing assistance that the local government is not capable of providing. HSS is often provided within a larger military involvement. A significant number of humanitarian assistance programs involve disaster relief operations. The military can provide assistance to help ease the effects of natural disasters and manmade events.[64]

Within a combatant command, the joint force surgeon would have the responsibility of identifying HSS requirements and assigning cross-service support where practical. The surgeon was also responsible for identifying other medical factors that could affect operations and advising the joint force commander. All planning should be done through the Joint Operation Planning and Execution System. Timely patient evacuation was a key part of that plan. Patient estimates should be calculated for numbers distribution, areas of density, possible mass casualty events, and evacuation. These estimates should reflect the entire potential patient population at risk.[65]

This was potentially a dramatic change for MEDEVAC forces. The evolving doctrine seemed to suggest that while the allocation of MEDEVAC assets was based on a purely Army-designated ratio of MEDEVAC companies to combat divisions allocated to an operation, actual need could be driven by a potential patient base that—in a joint operation or operation other than war—could be much larger.

Operations

Disaster on the Green Ramp, Fort Bragg

On 23 March 1994, as the last few Americans were leaving Somalia, an F-16 and C-130 collided while trying to land at Pope Air Force Base, North Carolina. The C-130 landed safely. The F-16 crashed on the loading or "Green" ramp where more than 500 paratroopers were marshaled to board a C-141 for a training jump. Dozens of soldiers were immediately killed or severely burned by the wreckage and flaming aviation fuel.

As horrendous as the event was, its occurrence at such a high-density and high-training tempo base dictated that—fortuitously—significant medical assets and facilities were nearby. Based on well-written and rehearsed contingency plans, the men and women of the 44th Medical Brigade and its subordinate units sprang into action. The 57th Med Co (RG) located at the smaller helicopter airfield about four miles to the southeast had two aircraft on alert for MAST duty or base support, and both were immediately launched, arriving at the disaster site about 20 minutes after the F-16 crashed. They were rapidly loaded with wounded and took off for the Womack Army Medical Center at adjoining Fort Bragg.[66]

The 57th immediately generated six more crews and aircraft that then joined the recovery effort as other medical personnel from all base units responded. Ultimately, there were 130 casualties, of which 24 died. Later, in addressing the outstanding effort by all to care for those hurt, the commanding officer of the XVIII

Airborne Corps, Lt. Gen. Hugh Shelton, said of the responders, "No one shied away…It's the kind of phenomenal response that allowed us to get all the injured to the hospitals within 40 to 45 minutes."[67]

Haiti – Operation UPHOLD DEMOCRACY

The new Army strategy laid out in the latest iteration of FM 100-5 was put on vivid display a year later when a large Army task force consisting primarily of soldiers from the 10th Mountain Division landed at the Port-au-Prince Airport in Haiti in September 1994. They were part of a larger JTF whose objective was to reestablish a democratically elected government deposed by a military coup. During the cold war, such transgressions were—in many cases—ignored. However, the coup had disrupted the stability of Haitian society and generated a massive refugee migration. Thousands of Haitians fled on flimsy boats to brave the passage to the United States. For the most part, they were economic refugees. Democracy needed to be reestablished in that country so that the economy could revive and provide jobs for the disaffected. The United Nations initially tried to introduce a small task force of "blue hats" to resolve the issue. In response, the coup leaders called their thugs into the streets and blocked the arrival of the United Nations forces. When the Secretary General of the United Nations acknowledged the failure of a peaceful resolution of the dilemma and the General Assembly passed a resolution authorizing the "application of all necessary means to restore democracy to Haiti," President Bill Clinton directed the military to act.[68]

Troops from the 10th Mountain Division initially led the way, and then joined with a large U.S. Marine contingent to reestablish peace. A Special Forces task force of 1,200 who spread into the countryside augmented the division. There was some violence initially, but a show of strength by a Marine team, which killed 10 rebels and conducted active street patrolling by the 1,000 military police, quickly restored order among a very grateful populous.

Eventually, the force exceeded 20,000 with a battalion-size element supplied by other Caribbean nations. The 44th Medical Brigade from Fort Bragg deployed a supporting medical task force that included an element from the 56th Medical Battalion (Evacuation) and a combined package of six UH-60s, crews, and support personnel from the 57th Med Co (AA) and the 498th Med Co (AA). However, there was little business for them. Most patients were soldiers who were sickened with tropical diseases or civilians caught in sporadic violence. The crews had all been trained for shore-to-ship transfers and flew many sorties ferrying the patients out to the USNS *Comfort*.[69]

Serving with the 57th as a flight platoon leader on that deployment was Capt. Greg Gentry, who had entered the Army in 1988 and was commissioned into the Medical Service Corps. His first assignment was to the 326th Medical Battalion, 101st Airborne Division, as an evacuation platoon leader. Subsequently, he served as a medical platoon leader with a 101st Division infantry battalion and deployed with it to DESERT SHIELD/STORM. That experience provided him with an excellent grounding in Army medical operations at the "retail" level. Subsequently, he went to flight school at Fort Rucker and then served a very productive tour with the 377th Med Co (AA) in Korea before reporting to the 57th at Fort Bragg in 1994.[70]

The deployment was also supported by a detachment from the 28th Combat Support Hospital from Fort Bragg. Serving with it as the Bravo Medical Company commander was Capt. Bob Mitchell. His tour with the Aviation Standardization and Evaluation Team at Fort Rucker ended in the spring of 1992, and he was then ordered to Korea for two years. He spent the first year with the 377th Med Co (AA) at K-16 Air Base serving as the company operations officer. He was able to get on the flying schedule a lot and flew over most of the country. The next year he moved over to the 52d Medical Battalion (Evacuation) and served as the S-3 operations officer. He found that job to be very challenging because the only way to learn the job was by doing it. His battalion commander, Lt. Col. Bill Nichols, had a very simple command philosophy. He directed what he wanted done and then left it to his subordinates to decide how to get it done. Mitchell had to learn fast, but it proved to be a very rewarding tour, as he learned to balance medical versus aviation issues at the unit level.[71]

He left Korea in the summer of 1994 and reported to the 28th to take command of the company. It included a forward surgical team consisting of 20 physicians and enlisted troops that directly supported the 44th Medical Brigade. That unit belonged to the XVIII Airborne Corps, which meant that the forward surgical team had to be airborne-qualified. Mitchell got the command position because he had gone through airborne training at Fort Bragg a few years prior. He made several jumps with the surgical unit, but they were not required to do so in Haiti.

In September 1994, the coup leaders fled the country and the deposed president triumphantly returned. Rebel elements were disarmed, and more than 15,000 weapons were collected. The weak Haitian Army was then reorganized and retrained as a border patrolling force. Violence rapidly subsided, and the American forces were seen as liberators as thousands who had fled the country steadily returned.

In January 1995, a brigade-sized force from the 25th Infantry Division from Hawaii replaced the troops of the 10th Mountain Division. The supporting aviation task force included helicopters and crews from the 68th Med Det (RG). Maj. Pete Webb, then serving as the medical planner for the Division Surgeon, planned the deployment.

At the time, the 68th was transitioning from UH-1s to UH-60s. Capt. Pete Smart was the unit operations officer. After leaving Germany in late 1993, he had attended the AMEDD Advanced Course and had then been sent to Hawaii to facilitate the unit's conversion to the UH-60. When the arrival of the aircraft was delayed, Smart had to requalify in the UH-1. The 68th still had a heavy commitment to MAST, and the aircraft had to be ready.

For Haiti operations, the six UH-60s were deployed, and six UH-1s remained behind to provide MAST support to the islands. Smart deployed with the detachment, but Haiti had been stabilized and there was little to do. On 31 March 1995, the U.S. forces handed over all responsibilities to a residual United Nations Mission and departed for their home stations. President Bill Clinton visited them to thank them for their effort. Before the assembled troops he said, "To every one of you who has taken part in Operation UPHOLD DEMOCRACY, on behalf of the American people, I am here to say thank you. Thank you for serving your nation. Thank you for being democracy's warriors. Thank you for helping to bring back the promise of liberty to this long troubled land. You should be very proud of what you have done."[72]

MAST

When the 68th Med Det (RG) returned to Hawaii, Webb was selected to take command of the detachment and held that position for the next two years. It was a busy time for the unit. There was no civilian MEDEVAC capability on any of the islands, and the 68th was in high demand. The unit constantly had helicopters on alert at Schofield Barracks on Oahu and also had to have aircraft available to support the maneuver and firing ranges in the Pohakuloa Training Area on the big island of Hawaii. Additionally, the 68th had to provide MAST coverage. Calls came in all the time, varying from water rescues to vehicular accidents to jungle hoist recoveries. Sometimes 30 calls were received in one 24-hour period. Webb discovered that it was the busiest MAST unit in the Army.[73]

Smart was the unit MAST coordinator who had to ensure that the 68th had two aircraft and crews available 24 hours a day. Smart himself flew more than 150 MAST missions. On one mission, Smart and his crew picked up an 18-month-old baby that had been run over by his mother when she had backed her car out of the driveway. It was the rush hour, and travel by ground ambulance would have taken hours. They picked up the mother and baby for the 10-minute flight to the hospital. As they lifted off, the mother was hysterical, but she calmed down as she saw the intensity and concern of the crew. They landed on the landing zone on top of the hospital and orderlies there took the baby immediately into intensive care. The mother thanked them profusely and then followed.

Smart was very touched by the mission. Returning to the base, he called the hospital and discovered that both the baby and mother were doing just fine. Smart was very impressed with the MAST program and felt that it was a win-win for both the Army and the nation. He said:

> I always felt like the MAST mission was such a good [public relations] vehicle not just for the Army but for the entire federal system because we are all taxpayers… And sure, we are a combat unit and our primary mission is to defend the Constitution of the United States. But, you know, there is nothing better in a peacetime environment than to be able to help your fellow citizens…We hauled a lot of retirees; we hauled a lot of people on vacation; we hauled military folks; we hauled police officers.[74]

Smart served with the 68th until June 1998, when he returned to Germany to command the 45th Med Co (AA) at Ketterbach.

In June 1995, newly promoted Maj. Dave MacDonald reported to Fort Bragg to take command of the 57th Med Co (AA). He intuitively knew that MEDEVAC was a combination of medicine and aviation. It was only when he took command of the unit that he understood what that meant. Medically, the 57th was assigned to the 56th Medical Battalion (Evacuation), 55th Medical Group, which belonged to the 44th Medical Brigade. However, those commanders neither knew nor cared much about aviation. MacDonald discovered very rapidly that he had to establish a solid working relationship with the 82d Aviation Brigade of the 82d Airborne Division to function as an aviation unit. This was a shock for him because he had gotten used to the strong aviation links that the 50th had at Fort Campbell.

He was also disheartened by the unit training plan. Forward support MEDE-VAC teams were formed and functioning, but they spent little time with the brigades that they were supposed to be supporting. Little tactical training was accomplished because of the heavy MAST commitment levied on the unit.

MacDonald attended operational planning sessions and attempted to get his unit into the operations or exercises. He discovered that the 57th was viewed as an outsider—a "bunch of cowboys"—who played loose with the rules and were not professional aviators. It was only after he developed personal relationships with some of the aviation unit commanders that he obtained access to some of the exercises. Then he found himself as a bit of a marriage broker as he balanced the demands of both his medical and aviation superiors to maintain relevance in both communities to accomplish his job.

His effort suffered a terrible setback when his unit had a tragic accident. While supporting a brigade exercise at the Joint Readiness Training Center at Fort Polk in February 1996, an attached flight surgeon was killed by the rotating blades of one of the unit's aircraft as he disregarded safety instructions and attempted to board the aircraft while the pilots were doing an engines-running refueling.

The resulting investigations stretched out for nine months. Many extenuating circumstances led to the tragedy. As the investigations played out, MacDonald concluded that their purposes were more to find a scapegoat than to determine the actual causes of the accident. Ultimately, the pilot in command, a young CW3, received blame for the accident, and proceedings were started to remove his pilot wings. MacDonald prevented that by having him transferred to a Special Operations unit on base, but the young soldier was never again promoted.

This unfortunate incident soured relations between the 57th and the 82d Aviation Brigade. As the investigations were conducted, the 57th also received several other inspections. The constant strain of all of this and mundane unit operations took a hard toll on MacDonald. As his tour concluded in June 1997, he seriously considered leaving the Army. Fortunately, his senior rater, Col. Fred Gerber, the 55th Medical Group Commander, supported his actions and encouraged him to stay. MacDonald had been selected to attend the Army Command and General Staff College at Fort Leavenworth, Kansas. That experience gave him an opportunity to shake off the hard events at Fort Bragg and prepare for bigger and better things in the future.[75]

MAST – 25 Years

During 1995, the Army celebrated 25 years of continuous support for the MAST program. In the wake of the post–DESERT STORM force reductions, MAST participation had been substantially reduced. Still, 13 active TO&E units, one Table of Distribution and Allowances unit, one USAR unit (soon to be inactivated as per the "off-site" agreement), and one U.S. Air Force unit maintained aircraft on alert and provided community support across the United States. By the end of the year, aggregate statistics showed that since its inception, 44,664 missions had been flown, lasting 95,204 flight hours and carrying 48,806 patients.[76]

One of the stalwart units in MAST, the 54th Med Det (RG) at Fort Lewis was lauded for a particular mission typical of the overall MAST effort. The unit was honored as the Thurston (Washington) County Emergency Medical Services Provider of the Year for rescuing a man severely wounded by an accidental gunshot. After the emergency call was received, a 54th helicopter launched out of Fort Lewis and flew to the site of the accident in a very remote location where rapid surface transportation was impossible. As the medic cared for the patient, the crew quickly flew him to the closest hospital, where he received immediate surgery and care that saved his life.

To the crews, it was just another mission. "Any possible way people can get hurt, we've flown missions for," said one pilot. The unit operations officer, Capt. Charles Zuber, added, "The medic and crew chief get medical training, and the pilots get combat training by flying real emergency missions." MAST was still doing exactly what it was designed to do a quarter of a century earlier.[77]

About that same time, a new ARNG MEDEVAC unit was formed, the 1042d Med Co (AA) in the Oregon ARNG. Like almost all National Guard units, it claimed a lineage that reached back through units that were at one time perhaps transportation, infantry, or aviation units. The 1042d, which was activated at the Salem Airport, was initially equipped with older UH-1V aircraft. All had hoists so that the unit could perform mountain rescue. These aircraft were replaced in 1997 with new UH-60L aircraft.

The acquisition of those new production aircraft was the result of actions taken by Senator Mark Hatfield of Oregon, serving at that time as the chairman of the Senate Appropriations Committee. One aircraft called a Firehawk was modified with special tanks so that it could carry water for forest fire duty. The unit was also licensed to assume MAST duty for its region.[78]

Europe - Partnership for Peace

In further recognition of the changes sweeping the globe, the United States military in 1993 joined NATO in establishing the Partnership for Peace program. The combined effort sought to draw heretofore neutral nations, former members of the Warsaw Pact, and even former Soviet states into multinational exercises. These exercises focused on search and rescue, humanitarian relief, and peacekeeping efforts, with initial objectives targeted to develop standard operating procedures, communications formats, and command and control protocols. NATO held a series of exercises for all who wanted to participate and extended these exercises to other areas of the world, although with less consistency. Some exercises were also held at the various training centers in the United States, such as the National Training Center at Fort Irwin. U.S. and allied soldiers, sailors, airmen, and marines developed mutual understanding and respect that was very useful in any potential coalition operations.[79]

Organization

Korea

In September 1995, the 377th Med Co (AA) in Korea was split, with one-half of its assets and personnel being used to create a new unit, the 542d Med Co (AA), commanded by Maj. Tom Bailey. Both units were assigned to the 52d Medical Battalion (Evacuation), commanded by Lt. Col. Rick Agosta, and assigned to the 18th Medical Command. The 542d assumed MEDEVAC duties in the northern part of South Korea, and was given the moniker of the "DMZ Dustoff." The 377th maintained coverage over the rest of the peninsula.[80]

Eight months later, Lt. Col. Scott Heintz arrived in Korea to take command of the 52d Medical Battalion (Evacuation). After his tour as the commander of Delta Company, 326th Medical Battalion, he served three years on the Office of The Surgeon General staff as the Deputy Director of Mobilization and later, within current operations. Then he became the medical operations officer for the Command Surgeon in the United States Special Operations Command. Although he found the tour to be interesting and challenging, he was more than glad to be back in MEDEVAC.

The 52d Battalion headquarters was at Yongsan Garrison located within Seoul. Besides the two MEDEVAC units, the battalion also commanded two ground ambulance companies: the 560th and the 568th. Heintz, who controlled all tactical evacuation assets within the theater with detachments spread all over the country, was responsible for the tactical evacuation plan and operation.

The assignment also afforded him the opportunity to return to the cockpit. He requalified in the UH-60 and then flew with pilots from both the 377th and the 542d whenever he could. On New Year's Eve of 1996, he and Maj. Tom Bailey were pulling 1st up alert at Camp Casey when they received a mission to transport two patients: a female soldier who had been diagnosed with chicken pox and a soldier who had his jaw broken in a New Year's Eve fight. As they launched out on the first mission of 1997 to transport the patients to Yongsan they encountered "moderate" turbulence. The resultant bumpy ride was uncomfortable for both patients.

Heintz also took a strong interest in the training of his medics. Calling on a few

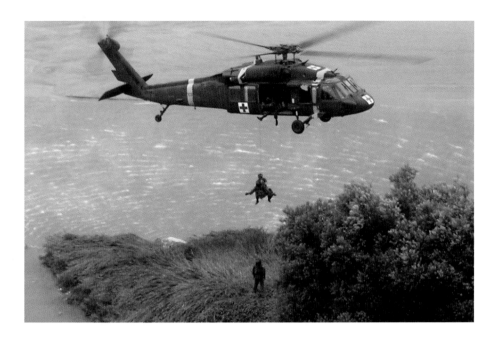

A UH-60 of the 377th Med Co (AA) in Korea. The yellow stripes (called "Bumble Bee" stripes) designated nonhostile aircraft authorized to operate in the Joint Security Area along the DMZ. Source: Lt. Col. Brian Almquist.

things he learned at the Special Operations Command, he designed a field competitive training exercise for them and then conducted it one month before their weeklong Expert Field Medical Badge evaluation.

Heintz gave up command of the 52d in June 1998. He had enjoyed the tour and the great soldiers with whom he served, especially his two executive officers, Maj. Lou Kozlowski and Maj. Dave Bitterman, his two Command Sergeant Majors, Ricky Terrell and Terry Porter, and his second 542d Medical Company Commander, Maj. Anastasia Ippolito. He felt that everything he had done as an officer before the assignment had prepared him for it, especially the mentoring he had received. More challenges were yet to come. He attended the Army War College at Carlisle Barracks, Pennsylvania, and then served at Fort Rucker as the Director of the MEPD from 1999 to 2002. He would lead the MEDEVAC community into the next century.[81]

Force Structure

In mid-decade, force structure documents showed that the following MEDEVAC units existed:

Active Duty

United States

50th Med Co (AA)	Fort Campbell, Kentucky
54th Med Co (AA)	Fort Lewis, Washington
57th Med Co (AA)	Fort Bragg, North Carolina
82d Med Co (AA)	Fort Riley, Kansas
498th Med Co (AA)	Fort Benning, Georgia
507th Med Co (AA)	Fort Hood, Texas
571st Med Co (AA)	Fort Carson, Colorado
36th Med Det (RG)	Fort Polk, Louisiana
68th Med Det (RA)	Wheeler Army Airfield, Hawaii
229th Med Det (RG)	Fort Drum, New York
247th Med Det (RG)	Fort Irwin, California
283d Med Det (RG)	Fort Wainwright, Alaska
Air Ambulance Det (Flatiron)	Fort Rucker, Alabama

Germany

45th Med Co (AA)	Ketterbach
159th Med Co (AA)	Wiesbaden
236th Med Co (AA)	Landstuhl

Other

377th Med Co (AA)	Korea
542d Med Co (AA)	Korea
214th Med Det (RG)	Panama

ARNG

24th Med Co (AA)	Nebraska/Kansas
104th Med Co (AA)	Maryland
107th Med Co (AA)	Ohio
112th Med Co (AA)	Maine
121st Med Co (AA)	Washington, DC/West Virginia
126th Med Co (AA)	California
148th Med Co (AA)	Georgia
172d Med Co (AA)	Arkansas
198th Med Co (AA)	Delaware/Pennsylvania
681st Med Co (AA)	Indiana
717th Med Co (AA)	New Mexico/Nevada
812th Med Co (AA)	Louisiana/Oklahoma
832d Med Co (AA)	Wisconsin
1022d Med Co (AA)	Wyoming/Colorado
1042d Med Co (AA)	Oregon

1059th Med Co (AA)	Massachusetts
1085th Med Co (AA)	South Dakota/Montana
1133d Med Co (AA)	Alabama
1159th Med Co (AA)	New Hampshire/ New Jersey[82]

Ongoing world events suggested that some of these units would be needed for overseas duty in the not too distant future.

Force XXI – Army After Next

Gen. Dennis Reimer followed Sullivan as the 33d Army Chief of Staff in 1995. He continued the Force XXI concept, but added another concept called "Army After Next," which attempted to define what warfare would be like in 2025. These efforts lead to the realization that the Army needed forces that could be tailored rapidly to respond to unpredictable crises. A middleweight force would be required that could "arrive at a crisis point early with sufficient combat power to deliver a critical blow to an adversary's operation." This could best be done with brigade-sized strike forces composed of modular elements tailored to the demands of each mission and using advanced digital information technologies that provided timely critical data. Reimer would not see their maturity during his time as the Army Chief of Staff. However, the seeds of technological advance and restructuring had been sown, and in time would bear fruit.[83]

Chapter Seven

The Balkans, 1992–Ongoing

"Missions would be less clear, like peace operations, … humanitarian assistance … inherently joint … multinational … with non-DOD agencies in achieving national objectives."

TRADOC Pamphlet 525-50[1]

Conflict in Southeastern Europe

While the Army struggled with the post–DESERT STORM force reductions and contingency operations in Somalia and Haiti, serious issues arose in the southeastern regions of Europe. After the collapse of the Soviet Union in the early 1990s, another communist bastion, the nation of Yugoslavia, started to disintegrate. It had been a post–World War I construct that sat on a cultural fault line between old Europe and the Ottoman Empire. It was designed to conglomerate Serbs, Slovenes, Croats, Bosnian Muslims, Albanians, Macedonians, Montenegrans, Hungarians, and other smaller ethnic groups into six republics and two provinces.

Natural and historic tensions existed among these groups and were exploited by Germany and Italy during World War II. After that conflict, Communist revolutionary/strongman Marshal Josip Broz Tito seized power and applied a heavy hand that forcefully unified this disparate group.

Tito died in 1980 with no clear and agreed upon successor. Ethnic rivalries reemerged, especially when they were inflamed by Serbian leader Slobodan Milosevic. Fearing the worst, two of the republics, Slovenia and Croatia, held free elections in 1991, which established a mandate for independence and they both declared so. Yugoslavia ceased to exist, and Serbia and Montenegro established the Federal Republic of Yugoslavia, a rump nation, with its capital in Belgrade. It also maintained control of what was left of the Yugoslav National Army (JNA).[2]

Both Slovenia and Croatia had strong ethnic majorities and immediately formed local militias that fought off primarily Serbian forces sent to squelch their efforts. Slovenian forces prevailed handily. However, the struggle in Croatia was more difficult as the JNA and local Serbians used heavy weapons for the first time to prevent the separation. The battles were hard-fought before the Croatian forces prevailed in early 1992.[3]

The next bid for independence was made by Bosnia-Herzegovina. It declared its freedom in April 1992. Several European nations immediately recognized it. However, it was more ethnically mixed. Its population was 44% Muslim, 33% Serb, and 17% Croat. The Serbian minority did not agree with the move to independence, revolted against the new government, and declared its own Serb Republic of Bosnia-Herzegovina. The JNA, which was heavily dominated by Serbs, joined with the Bosnian-Serbs and attacked the Muslims and Croats. In a brutal campaign reminiscent of the Middle Ages, they introduced the world to a new phrase — "ethnic cleansing" — as their forces used violent intimidation, murder, and rape to force the Muslims and Croats from areas that the Serbs wanted to own and control.

Operations

The Balkans

Watching the dissolution of Yugoslavia and fearing for the worst, in 1991 the United Nations (UN) passed a resolution embargoing all arms shipments to the former Yugoslavia. Alarmed at the continuously deteriorating situation in the region, the UN deployed a United Nations Protection Force (UNPROFOR) in 1992. Its mission was to guarantee the delivery of relief supplies and perform other humanitarian and peacekeeping duties. Ultimately including forces from 37 different countries and growing to 38,000 troops, it became the largest and most expensive UN peacekeeping operation to date.[4]

The United States supported UNPROFOR with a medical task force. In November 1992, U.S. Army Europe deployed the 212th Mobile Army Surgical Hospital to Zagreb, Croatia, and numerous personnel to act as liaison on several staffs. A MEDEVAC unit was not assigned to accompany it. The 502d Mobile Army Surgical Hospital replaced the 212th in April 1993. The 502d remained in place until October, when a hospital unit from the U.S. Air Forces in Europe replaced it. The 212th and 502d treated more than 9,700 UNPROFOR and civilian casualties from 31 countries.[5]

UNPROFOR's relatively lightly armed forces operating under tightly restricted rules of engagement were no match for the more heavily armed JNA and Bosnian Serbs. After several egregious attacks on UN Safe Areas, both the North Atlantic Treaty Organization (NATO) and the United States provided UNPROFOR naval and air support to enforce the arms embargo at sea and in the air. NATO imposed and enforced a no-fly zone over Bosnia. When Serbian attack aircraft challenged this restriction, U.S. Air Force F-16s shot down four of the six aircraft.

Tensions heightened as Bosnian-Serbs and JNA units seized UNPROFOR peacekeepers to use as human shields and besieged Muslim areas and the city of Sarajevo. When a Serbian mortar round killed 37 people in a crowded market square in Sarajevo, NATO retaliated with a three-week air campaign to destroy the enemy guns arrayed around that city and eliminate other key JNA elements and forces. A total of 3,515 air sorties were flown, and only one allied aircraft—a French Mirage—was shot down. The crew was captured but eventually released.[6]

Almost simultaneously, strong Croatian forces joined the fight against the Bosnian Serbs and JNA. These two bold strokes convinced Serbian President Milosevic to begin peace negotiations at Wright-Patterson Air Force Base near Dayton, Ohio, in the fall of 1995.

In September, the foreign ministers of Bosnia-Herzegovina, Croatia, and Serbia met and agreed to the basic principles of a cease-fire and peace agreement in Bosnia. The document titled the General Framework Agreement for Peace was finalized and signed on 14 December 1995. It called for a military cease-fire and a confirmation of the existence of the independent state of Bosnia and Herzegovina. The country would be a multiethnic federal body with two political "entities": (1) the Federation of Bosnia and Herzegovina and (2) the Serb Republic. A zone of separation divided the two entities. Within days, the UN approved this agreement, and NATO was authorized to implement the peace agreement with an Implementation Force, Bosnia (IFOR). Five days later, IFOR replaced UNPROFOR and assumed responsibility for enforcing the zone of separation. The mission was expected to last one year.[7]

NATO had anticipated such an outcome and had developed several contingency plans. The chosen plan called for a multinational force of 60,000 troops from several countries. It was more heavily armed than UNPROFOR and was deployed with more robust rules of engagement. The force was subdivided into three multinational divisions (MNDs). MND North (MND-N) was a U.S.-led force. Its core was the 1st Armored Division from Germany, under Operation JOINT ENDEAVOR. Maj. Gen. William L. Nash, the 1st Armored Division commander, also served as the commander of MND-N, which was augmented with forces from other nations.

Starting in late December, the 1st Armored Division, as Task Force Eagle, began to move its units to Bosnia through Hungary and was joined there by brigades from Poland, Turkey, Russia, and smaller elements from nine other nations. U.S. Army Europe pre-positioned a National Support Element at Taszar to support the movement that included elements from the 30th Medical Brigade, which contained the 212th Mobile Army Surgical Hospital. They would form the core of Task Force Medical Eagle (TFME). Also supporting the 1st Armored Division was the 236th Med Co (AA), which was attached to the Aviation Brigade of the 1st Armored Division. It had been reinforced with a Forward Support MEDEVAC Team (FSMT) from both the 159th and 45th Med Cos. All 145 aircraft of the brigade team flew from their home bases in Germany to their deployment sites in Bosnia.[8]

Capt. John Lamoureux served with the 1st Armored Division and then as the medical planner in the Division Medical Operations Center (DMOC). Using his

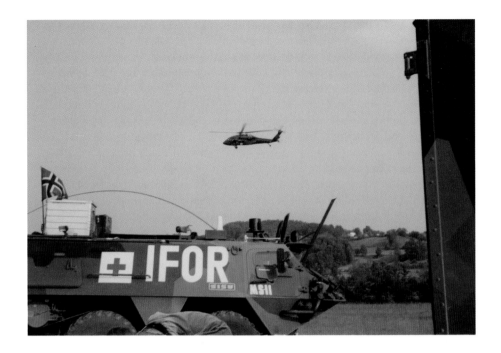

A MEDEVAC crew from the 236th Med Co (AA) supported the IFOR in Bosnia in July 1996. Source: 421st Medical Battalion (Evacuation) Historical Files.

accumulated medical and aviation skills, he became heavily involved in establishing the medical infrastructure for the operation. After he graduated from pilot training at Fort Rucker, Alabama, in August 1990, Lamoureux had served a short tour at the U.S. Army Aeromedical Research Laboratory—also at Fort Rucker—where he participated in several projects concerning aviation issues that arose in Saudi Arabia during DESERT SHIELD and STORM. Then he did a three-year tour with the 377th Med Co (AA) in Korea, where he served as a section leader supporting the 2d Infantry Division. He logged many sorties flying along the Korean DMZ, doing nap-of-the-earth navigation, and night patient pickups using night vision goggles (NVGs). He also deployed to Thailand for annual Operation COBRA GOLD exercises with Army Special Forces teams and Thai military units.[9]

Lamoureux returned to the United States in 1993 and attended the Medical Service Corps advanced course. He was then posted to a ground job as the medical company commander in the 501st Forward Support Battalion assigned to the 1st Armored Division in Germany. Serving directly with combat soldiers, he quickly came to appreciate what MEDEVAC meant to the front-line troops. He used personal connections to establish a strong relationship with the 421st Medical Battalion (Evacuation) and its three air ambulance companies. Lamoureux also called upon his MEDEVAC experiences to establish procedures within his unit to provide support for FSMTs so that they would have the logistical items necessary to co-locate in the field with his medical company. Those procedures became standard throughout the division.

In the Army just six years, Lamoureux already had the opportunity to see both the aviation and medical sides of MEDEVAC. Juxtaposing his assignments in Korea and Germany, he recalled:

> My first assignment was in Korea and I felt that I had a good firm grip on the aviation piece. You fly a lot and do great things. Being a forward support medical commander allowed me to get my foot firmly planted in the medical community because I was clearly writing plans for the maneuver brigade, I was briefing at the DISCOM level, I was in lockstep with the medical planners at the Division Medical Operations Center. It really gave me a great foundation to match my aviation experience.[10]

It was also the perfect preparation for him to assume the medical planner duties in the DMOC. A few weeks later, the chief of the DMOC was needed for another assignment, and Lamoureux was given the job of chief of the DMOC as the 1st Armored Division moved south into Bosnia. He stayed with the DMOC until September 1996, when he was moved to Wiesbaden to serve as the S-3 of the 421st Medical Battalion (Evacuation), commanded by Lt. Col. Ken Crook.[11]

Moving briskly and purposefully into Bosnia, the IFOR handled its mission fairly handily. The local people were tired of the war and respectful of the NATO forces. They readily identified weapons caches and the location of land mines. De-mining operations were extensive and always dangerous. Civilian contractors hired local workers to build the necessary base camps. The wages stimulated the local economies.

Initially locating at the U.S. air base at Tuzla, the 236th—as part of TFME—subsequently deployed FSMTs to remote locations as necessary to support the MND-N units. Its first MEDEVAC mission occurred on 30 December when two aircraft were launched to a site where an American vehicle was damaged by an anti-tank mine. Only one soldier was seriously injured, and he was MEDEVACed through a snowstorm to the 212th. In early February, two soldiers on foot patrol were injured by a land mine. Crews from the 236th again answered the call and MEDEVACed them to the 212th. In another encounter with a landmine, medic Spc. Chad Blair of the 236th had to be inserted and extracted by hoist as he tried to help a Lithuanian team who had driven into a minefield. At one point, he had to freeze when the soldiers saw that he was dangerously near a live mine. Some very delicate flying by Maj. Tim Hartnett and outstanding hoist work by crew chief Spc. Courtney Cypert made it possible for Blair to recover four wounded troops.[12]

There was really little call for MEDEVAC. The people were tired of fighting. However, that did not mean that there was an end to strife. Emotions were still relatively raw, and the intricate process of undoing so much wrong was very time consuming. Crime was rampant, and drugs and prostitution proliferated. The absence of a credible and respected police force meant that allied forces had to fill the void. As one commander noted in a press conference, as the clock ran out on the IFOR deployment, it did not appear that conclusive peace could be ensured in one year.[13]

Doctrine

TRADOC Pamphlet 525-50, Operational Concept for Combat Health Support, October 1996

As Army units became deeply involved in the Balkans, the Army Training and Doctrine Command (TRADOC) published TRADOC Pamphlet 525-50. Applicable to all Army Medical Department and TRADOC activities that covered doctrine and training development, leader development, organization, materiel, and soldier requirements, it acknowledged the post–cold war international environment that presented the nation with new security challenges unprecedented in ambiguity, diversity, risk, and opportunity. Whereas in the cold war, the enemy was clear and present; in the "new world order," old forces of adventurism, nationalism, and separatism had reappeared with sometimes violent and unpredictable consequences.[14]

The new pamphlet proposed an operational concept for combat health support (CHS) required to support the Army into the 21st century. Missions were less clear, like peace operations, force protection, humanitarian assistance, and operations in aid of civil authorities. All operations were inherently joint, many were multinational, and frequently, Army forces had to work with non-Department of Defense agencies in achieving national objectives.[15]

The CHS system needed to take advantage of evolving technologies. Modern ground and air evacuation systems with enhanced en route medical support capabilities were required along with better communications capabilities over longer ranges, both for command and control (C2) reasons and to provide the medics with access to physician guidance.

These concepts were based on the recent doctrinal guidance in the 1994 version of Field Manual (FM) 8-55. The CHS system had to project support worldwide to help preserve U.S. global interests in operations from forced or unforced entry to humanitarian/nation assistance missions to multiple-corps operations requiring long-term sustainment. Evacuation forces still had to be capable of rapid clearing of the battlefield and the movement of sick or injured soldiers into the CHS system. Air evacuation remained the primary means, and all evacuation vehicles needed to be capable of providing enhanced en route medical care and monitoring capabilities.

The pamphlet also stated that future medical doctrine had to continue to underscore the joint and multinational nature of future operations. Synchronization of all available medical assets should not have duplicated the capabilities of other services and needed to be established in doctrine. This requirement dictated revision or rewrite of all FM 8 series manuals.[16]

The pamphlet also addressed the training of medics and combat lifesavers. Continuous emphasis was needed on their training and sustainment of medical proficiency in the multitude of environments in which Army operations took place.[17]

Although only directly applicable to the TRADOC and the Army Medical Department, this pamphlet was far reaching in its message. The cold war was over, and Army medicine had to be prepared for the new joint, combined, and possibly intergovernmental mission sets arising while supporting large combat operations if they improbably arose.

Joint Doctrine – Joint Publication (JP) 4-02.2, Joint Tactics, Techniques, and Procedures for Patient Movement in Joint Operations, December 1996

In December 1996, the Joint Staff released another doctrinal document, JP 4-02.2. It was designed to delineate the requirements and considerations for joint patient movement within the health service support (HSS) system as well as the HSS aspects of joint patient movement planning and military operations other than war. It did not present specific tactics, techniques, and procedures, but it did emphasize that they could be found in service documents.[18]

The publication highlighted the role that patient movement played within the HSS. Service components were given the responsibility to provide for patient movement from point of injury to Echelon III facilities. The Army was given specific responsibility for providing medical rotary-wing support to ship-to-shore and shore-to-ship patient transport operations on an area support basis for all services operating within assigned grid coordinates.[19]

Reflecting evolving doctrine and the reality of recent events, JP 4-02.2 also included a chapter on military operations other than war such as: noncombatant evacuation operations, peace operations, terrorism, and combat zones enforcement. In these operations the medical forces were tailored to meet the HSS requirements for the specific type of operation being supported. Planning also had to consider the need to move local civilians or coalition personnel and their ability to provide their own medical support. Their capabilities or host nation support could make up a significant portion of the overall medical and possibly evacuation effort. Essentially, the overall joint guidance provided in this new JP reflected the tried-and-true MEDEVAC procedures developed by the Army but expanded to a joint and theater perspective.[20]

Operations

The Balkans

The mandate for the IFOR ended on 20 December 1996. It was abundantly clear to all that the UN and NATO forces could not leave. The ethnic hatred and strife were just too strong. The parties involved in the effort agreed to continue the mission with a NATO-led stabilization force (SFOR). However, reflecting some progress in the overall effort, it numbered 31,000 troops versus the 60,000+ force of the IFOR, and was expected to last for 18 months.

The force continued to include a sizable U.S. contingent built around a division. The 1st Infantry Division replaced the 1st Armored Division as Task Force Eagle under Operation JOINT GUARD.

Subsequently, several divisions served as the lead command of Task Force

Eagle. It also always had a medical subcomponent known as the TFME. It was manned by various U.S. Army medical elements such as the 44th Medical Command and the 56th Medical Battalion (Evacuation) from Fort Bragg, North Carolina, the 249th General Hospital from Fort Gordon, Georgia, the 334th Medical Group (USAR) from Grand Rapids, Michigan, and the 115th Field Hospital from Fort Polk, Louisiana. MEDEVAC units were assigned to all of them. The following divisions and MEDEVAC units deployed to Bosnia for SFOR/JOINT GUARD:

SFOR – SFOR1: 1st Infantry Division, November 1996 – October 1997. 45th Med Co (AA). The unit, commanded by Maj. John Cook, replaced the 236th. The 45th provided general support to the MND-N and operated 13 aircraft from Tuzla, Kaposjulak, Hungary, and Slavonski Brod, Croatia. Its crews received few calls for support as the number of U.S. forces steadily dropped from 8,500 to 5,300. An element from the 1st Medical Group commanded by Col. Frank Novier led TFME. Novier had his medical teams spread over the same three locations. As a former MEDEVAC pilot, he took particular interest in the preparation of the MEDEVAC crews. He insisted that as part of the training for the deployments, all crews should be trained in proper snow-landing techniques. He also requested that the crews have access to the tactical command centers so that they could get up-to-date intelligence for their flights. He worked very closely with the MND-N aviation staff officer to ensure that his crews were authorized to fly at lower weather minimums than the aviation task force pilots so that they could be more responsive to MEDEVAC calls.[21]

The 498th Med Co (AA) replaced the 45th Med Co (AA) in April 1997. The unit deployed from its home station at Fort Benning, Georgia, to join TFME, now led by the 61st Area Support Medical Battalion. The 498th was located at Tuzla where it worked closely with a Norwegian Medical Company. It was also in general support of the MND-N and kept aircraft on alert at the same locations.

While the 498th was deployed, four helicopters and 27 soldiers were activated from the 812th Med Co (AA) from the Louisiana Army National Guard (ARNG) to backfill for the unit at Fort Benning. They joined Wisconsin Guardsmen from the 832d Med Co (AA), which was also activated for backfill duties. The combined units covered MEDEVAC duties and Military Assistance to Safety and Traffic (MAST) commitments at Fort Benning and Fort Stewart, Georgia, and they deployed with several XVIII Airborne Corps units to major training activities at the Joint Readiness Training Center at Fort Polk.[22]

SFOR2 – SFOR3: 1st Armored Division, October 1997 – October 1998. Operation JOINT GUARD was terminated on 20 June 1998. The follow-on operation was JOINT FORGE, an open-ended commitment to support NATO in its assigned peace enforcement mission in Bosnia-Herzegovina.

The 159th Med Co (AA) supported this operation from October 1997 to June 1998. Upon arriving, this Germany-based unit scattered its 13 aircraft and crews essentially as the previous units had done, while accomplishing the same general support mission. The unit worked closely with Norwegian medical teams and carried them to remote villages for civic action projects. Its crews also worked directly with Swedish explosive ordnance demolition teams and dogs to clear out minefields.[23]

In June 1998, the 236th made its second deployment to Bosnia and replaced its fellow Germany-based unit with nine aircraft and 78 troops. Six aircraft were sent to a landing area called the Blue Factory, where they sat alert. The other three rotated between various forward locations and Taszar, Hungary. There were few calls for MEDEVAC and the unit logged mostly training missions.[24]

SFOR4 – SFOR5: 1st Cavalry Division, October 1998 – August 1999. The 126th Med Co (AA), California ARNG mobilized and deployed with 10 aircraft and 81 soldiers in August for an October handover. As a Reserve Component unit, the 126th had some problems getting all necessary equipment because it was not a priority unit. Additionally, the late arrival of orders caused problems for some of the unit soldiers. More lead time was needed to do all of the actions necessary to activate, mobilize, and deploy. Arriving at Tuzla, they were assigned to the 41st Combat Support Hospital. The crews received orientation rides from the pilots of the 236th, who then returned to Germany. The unit placed seven aircraft and crews at Tuzla and three aircraft and crews at Taszar, Hungary. Many of the crewmembers were veterans of duty in Vietnam. All agreed that duty in Bosnia was better where the facilities were nicer and the operations tempo was much lower. Most of the Guardsmen were "M-Day soldiers," who willingly volunteered for the activation and deployment, which required stepping away from their civilian professions. When briefed on the potential threats to flying in the theater, most agreed that it was less dangerous than many of the missions that they flew at home to fight forest fires or rescue lost mountain hikers.[25]

The 24th Med Co (AA) Nebraska ARNG, with 77 soldiers of the unit and its sister detachment from Kansas, mobilized and deployed to support the 1st Cavalry Division in March. Personnel took five aircraft from Nebraska and four from Kansas. Aircraft and crews sat alert at both Tuzla and Camp McGovern. On one particularly notable mission two crews rescued a team of NATO soldiers who had wandered into a minefield. They remained in place to support the next rotation when the 1st Cavalry Division returned home in August and performed 35 air evacuations.[26]

SFOR6: 10th (Mountain) Infantry Division, August 1999 – March 2000. The 24th Med Co (AA) was replaced by the 112th Med Co (AA) Maine ARNG, which also deployed with five aircraft and 77 personnel. In February 2000, the 1042d Med Co (AA) Oregon ARNG replaced the 112th. When the 1042d arrived, the TFME was led by an element of the 115th Field Hospital from Fort Polk. The 1042d deployed under the command of Maj. Mathew Brady. Brady, a classic Guardsman, had initially joined the Oregon ARNG in 1984 as an enlisted soldier and was subsequently sent through the state officer candidate program and commissioned as an infantry officer in 1986. Within two years he was branch transferred to aviation and attended pilot training. After attaining his flight wings, he was transferred to the 1st Battalion, 108th Aviation Regiment, and rose to command B Company of that unit. He also started a career with the Oregon Department of Corrections. When the 1042d Med Co (AA) was activated, he transferred to its parent command, the 641st Medical Battalion (Evacuation), also an Oregon unit. When the 1042d transitioned to the UH-60Ls, he completed the conversion training, applied for a branch transfer to the Medical Service Corps, and was accepted. He then attended the aeromedical evacuation course and the medical officer advanced course to qualify as a 67J.[27]

In 1999, he was given command of the 1042d. He took a leave of absence from his civilian job and went on active duty to prepare the unit for its scheduled rotation to Bosnia.

The unit deployed with six aircraft and 90 troops and arrived at Tuzla in the dead of winter. Traumatic injuries were few, and the unit flew only 25 actual MEDEVAC missions during the tour. Most missions involved patients with broken bones from automobile accidents. The unit participated in a mass casualty drill with the other TFME elements and other coalition medical units.

The aircraft were divided with three maintained at Tuzla and three farther north at Camp McGovern. The maintenance crews were outstanding and kept the aircraft mission ready 97% of the time.[28]

SFOR7: 49th Armored Division Texas ARNG, March 2000 – October 2000. This was the first time that a Reserve Component division-sized unit had deployed out of the United States since the Korean War, and it was a significant shift in use of the Guard commands. Traditionally, the units had been trained and organized to fight in "the big war." But with the reductions that had occurred since DESERT STORM, they were used increasingly for peacekeeping operations. While in SFOR, the 49th commanded active duty units and established a paradigm that became increasingly common in future operations. The 1042d Med Co supported the 49th Armored Division during the rotation and returned home shortly after it.[29]

SFOR8 – SFOR9: 3d Infantry Division, October 2000 – September 2001. The 57th Med Co (AA) supported the 3d Infantry Division for SFOR8. The unit deployed from Fort Bragg with six helicopters and 59 troops. It was assigned to TFME, then under the control of the 56th Medical Battalion (Evacuation), also from Fort Bragg, and commanded by Lt. Col. Pauline Lockard.

Lockard had taken command of the battalion in the fall of 1998, after attending the Army Command and General Staff College and then serving in staff assignments. The position authorized her to requalify in the UH-60, and while in Bosnia she flew several MEDEVAC missions. Returning with her headquarters element to Fort Bragg in April 2001, she subsequently gave up command of the battalion in July and reported for more staff duty with the Office of The Surgeon General in Falls Church, Virginia.[30]

On 1 November, the 57th was called to launch an aircraft to pick up a U.S. Navy sailor who had been badly injured when he fell off a high wall while on shore leave in Dubrovnik, Croatia. This area was not under the coverage of TFME. However, medical authorities determined that the sailor needed to be evacuated to Germany. The best way to do that was to move him to Tuzla where he could then be cross-loaded to a C-130 that could transport him to Ramstein Air Base. TFME assigned the mission to the 57th.

The second up crew of CW2 Michael Philips, CW2 Kevin Smelser, S.Sgt.

Richard Rigsby, and medic Sfc. Donald McMillon received the call to go, but an early winter storm moved in with low clouds and visibility, and heavy precipitation. The crew took off anyway. They were in the weather most of the time but flew into Dubrovnik where the sailor was taken care of by Navy personnel.

When he was safely loaded, the crew took off for the return flight. Again facing terrible weather, they made a refueling stop at Mostar to ensure that they had plenty of fuel to divert in case they could not get into Tuzla. Thankfully, the weather improved as they flew north and arrival at Tuzla was not a problem. As they landed, the C-130 was waiting. The patient was quickly transferred and then flown to Germany for treatment. The entire mission was a great demonstration of teamwork.[31]

For SFOR9, the 1022d Med Co (AA), Wyoming ARNG, which was attached to the 2d Battalion, 3d Aviation Regiment, 3d Infantry Division, supported the 3d Infantry Division. The Wyoming guardsmen deployed with four aircraft and 54 personnel and maintained alert at two locations. In May, the division surgeon held a mass casualty exercise. It had been a while since anything like this had happened, and the exercise highlighted several procedural shortcomings and provided excellent training for all participants. Overall, the rotation was relatively quiet, and only six air evacuations were made.[32]

SFOR10: 29th Infantry Division, Virginia ARNG, September 2001 – April 2002. The 498th Med Co (AA) supported an element from the 28th Combat Support Hospital from Fort Bragg, which led the TFME. Maj. Greg Gentry commanded the 498th and deployed four aircraft and crews and 39 support personnel. He was new to the unit. After his tour with the 57th at Fort Bragg, he served with the 56th Medical Battalion (Evacuation)—also at Fort Bragg—and then at Fort Sam Houston, Texas, as a combat developer before taking command of the 498th in May 2001.[33]

While in Bosnia, the 498th performed 10 MEDEVAC missions, carrying 10 patients. Most missions were relatively routine with a mix of civilian and military patients. On one occasion, the "patient" was a military working dog who was carried from Camp McGovern to Eagle Base. The task force veterinarian rode along to provide expert en route care.

The unit also took part in three larger operations. Two were directed at possible terrorist elements and resulted in the recovery of several weapons and significant quantities of explosives. Another mission involved an attempt to capture a known war criminal responsible for ethnic atrocities. The mission lasted two days, but the criminal was not found.[34]

SFOR11: 25th Infantry Division, April 2002 – September 2002. The 1085th Med Co (AA), South Dakota/Montana ARNG, mobilized and deployed to support the operation when the 498th departed. The unit only deployed four aircraft, six crews, and 47 soldiers. It was under the control of TFME, led by a team from the 249th General Hospital from Fort Gordon, and was attached to the 1st Battalion, 25th Aviation Regiment, 25th Infantry Division.[35]

SFOR12: 28th Infantry Division, Pennsylvania ARNG, September 2002 – March 2003. On 3 January 2003, the MND-N was redesignated the Multi-National

Brigade North, with ARNG divisions in overall command. The total U.S. force commitment was about 1,400 troops. Active duty units were initially scheduled for the subordinate roles. Because of new commitments generated by the horrible events of 11 September 2001 and subsequent Global War on Terror, they were re-tasked and ARNG units replaced them. Subsequently, almost all units and troops dispatched to JOINT FORGE were ARNG and U.S. Army Reserve troops.

The 1159th Med Co (AA) New Hampshire/New Jersey ARNG supported this rotation. The unit deployed with 35 personnel and four UH-60s. Assuming alert duties at the two main sites, the unit supported all the coalition forces and also picked up civilians hurt in the declining but still troublesome internecine violence. On numerous occasions, the unit also dispatched aircraft and crews directly to support teams performing dangerous minefield-clearing operations.[36]

SFOR13: 35th Infantry Division, Kansas ARNG, March 2003 – September 2003, and SFOR14: 34th Infantry Division, Minnesota ARNG, September 2003 – March 2004. The 86th Med Co (AA), Vermont/Massachusetts ARNG, supported these two rotations under the command of the 5th Medical Group, a U.S. Army Reserve unit from Birmingham, Alabama, commanded by Col. Dan Dire. Maj. John Johnston from Vermont commanded the 86th for the first rotation, and Maj. Dave Underwood from Massachusetts commanded the second. The combined unit deployed with two aircraft from each state that remained for the duration. Their crews performed 34 MEDEVACs, although most flying was routine training as the country continued to stabilize.[37]

SFOR15: 38th Infantry Division, Indiana ARNG, March 2004 – December 2004. In December 2004, the SFOR had shrunk to a residual force of only 7,000, of which about 1,000 were U.S. troops. At that point, Task Force Eagle was disestablished, and the U.S. base at Tuzla was turned over to European Union forces who assumed the mission under Operation ALTHEA. A Finnish element took command with a small U.S. contingent of 150 troops that remained to facilitate the transition, continue the search for war crime suspects, and ensure—that if necessary—a stronger NATO force could rapidly re-enter if the need arose. For SFOR14 and 15, an element from the 5502d U.S. Army Hospital commanded the TFME and was supported with a collage of detachments from many units that included four UH-60 helicopters and crews from the 1256th Med Co (AA) Indiana ARNG, and Det 1, 149th Med Co, Arkansas ARNG. They were both attached to the 2d Battalion, 238th Aviation Regiment, also from the Indiana ARNG. There was little to do except to train allied medical units, be ready for any calls, and shut down the operation and go home.[38]

Organization

Unit Realignments

In a larger vein, 1998 was another year of change for the MEDEVAC force and saw the completion of the Medical Force 2000 plan as units in the Pacific were realigned. The 283d Med Det (RA) at Fort Wainwright, Alaska, was inactivated.

Its personnel remained at Fort Wainwright but were now assigned to the 68th Med Det (RA), which was converted to a Med Co (AA). At the same time, the last air ambulance medical detachments, the 247th Med Det (RA) at Fort Irwin, California, the 229th Med Det (RA) at Fort Drum, New York, and the 36th Med Det (RA) at Fort Polk, were also inactivated and transitioned to U.S. Army Air Ambulance Detachments as Table of Distribution and Allowances units.[39]

In Central America, the 214th Med Det (RG), commanded by Maj. Scott Drennon, remained in Panama, although it had changed its base twice. Since the early 1990s, it had also maintained a team of three aircraft and crews at Soto Cano Air Base, Honduras, to support Joint Task Force-Bravo, where it was attached to the 4th Battalion, 228th Aviation Regiment. As part of this change, the 214th was inactivated. Its assets were moved to Soto Cano and reestablished as a U.S. Army Air Ambulance Detachment under the control of the 1st Battalion, 228th Aviation Regiment, which had also moved up from Panama. The detachment had four aircraft assigned to it and was augmented with ARNG aircraft and crews and support personnel.[40]

Literally as this change was occurring, the unit was tasked to provide support for hurricane relief operations when Hurricane Mitch swept through Central America in November 1998. Scott Drennon led a small task force of two UH-60s, two CH-47s, and two MEDEVAC UH-60s that worked directly with Nicaraguan crews to provide relief for the local inhabitants. One crew, "Witch Doctor 36," conducted 10 rescue-hoist missions in severe weather to rescue 36 Honduran civilians from raging floodwaters. The crew also delivered food and water to locals stranded by washed out roads and mudslides. Overall, the crew transported 192 injured patients in 18 days.[41]

The unit subsequently supported ongoing counter-drug operations and civic actions programs with the Joint Task Force-Bravo medical element. It was also routinely supplemented with both active and ARNG MEDEVAC units or detachments from the continental United States.

Operations

The Balkans – Albania and Kosovo

NATO's benevolent and persistent actions brought relative peace and stability to Bosnia. However, they did not completely quash the virulently nationalist enthusiasm of Serbian leader Slobodan Milosevic. He turned his attention to Kosovo, one of the few remaining Yugoslavian provinces. Located just south of Serbia, it had been a historic part of the larger nation where Serbian roots ran deep. However, by the 1990s the population was 90% Albanian, and they had been given a form of local autonomy. After the loss of Bosnia, Milosevic used his overbearing military to suppress the Albanian Kosovars. In response, they formed a guerilla-type movement called the Kosovo Liberation Army (KLA) and retaliated against the Serbs.

The Serbs stepped up their actions, and in one particularly bloody attack, killed

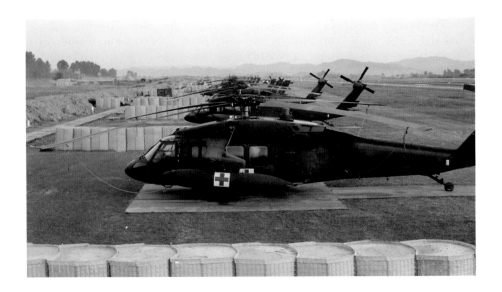

Flight Line at Rinas Airfield, Albania, showing the UH-60s of the 159th Med Co as part of Task Force Hawk.
Source: Dave Zimmerman.

45 Albanian civilians in the Kosovar village of Racak. NATO leaders then invited all involved parties to peace talks in Rambouillet, France, in February 1999.[42]

The talks were futile as Milosevic refused to accept a NATO peacekeeping force, which was vital to enabling any ceasefire and stability in that area. He unleashed his troops to conduct what had clearly been preplanned offensive operations in Kosovo. Heavily armed mechanized troops, Special Forces, and paramilitary elements ravaged both city and countryside in an orgy of arson, murder, and rape. It was a repeat of the horrible events in Bosnia—ethnic cleansing of the worst kind, all designed to drive out the Albanians and establish Serbian hegemony over the area. The casualties mounted into the thousands. Hundreds of thousands of refugees fled into the mountains or into Albania and Macedonia, threatening to overwhelm those small nations and destabilize the entire area.

Allied aircrews flew more than 500 missions hauling supplies into Albania where American engineers quickly built three camps to care for the 60,000+ refugees.

The NATO members resolved to counter the Serbian aggression with strong military actions. However, a ground campaign was ruled out and an aerial bombing campaign was initiated. For 78 days, NATO aircraft pummeled Serbian targets within Kosovo and the homeland with more than 38,000 sorties. Using primarily precision-guided weapons delivered from higher altitudes to avoid the Serbian air defenses, NATO aircraft destroyed oil refineries and reserves, bridges, command posts, and military airfields, as well as more than 100 aircraft on the ground. Ten Serbian fighters were also destroyed in air-to-air combat.

The strategic damage to Serbia was profound, but it did not deter them from terrorizing the Albanians. Additionally, the aerial attacks against Serbian targets in Kosovo were less effective because of weather conditions and the Serbian forces' skillful use of camouflage techniques and decoys. NATO countered by developing connections with the KLA. These forces began feeding targeting data for the air campaign, and the effectiveness of the airstrikes increased dramatically. The KLA coordinated its actions with the air campaign, and the two forces developed a synergy of effort. In effect, the KLA became an effective ground campaign to complement the effort from the air.[43]

Task Force Hawk

NATO could not deny the effectiveness of the KLA forces and quietly built up support ground forces in Macedonia and Albania. The U.S. Army contribution to this force was Task Force (TF) Hawk, commanded by the V Corps commander, Lt. Gen. John W. Hendrix. It included an aviation/mechanized force package commanded by the TF Hawk deputy commanding general, Brig. Gen. Richard A. Cody, and a smaller ground force called Task Force Falcon. Hawk was a brigade-sized element of 24 AH-64 attack helicopters named Task Force 11 (TF-11), joined by a force of support helicopters including MEDEVAC, designated Task Force 12 (TF-12), 27 multiple launched rocket systems, a 105 mm artillery battery, a company of M-1A tanks, a mechanized infantry battalion, an airborne infantry battalion, and a significant logistics element. However, when the Macedonian government vetoed the deployment, TF Hawk moved into Albania.[44]

The task force deployed in April and set up at the Rinas Airfield, 12 kilometers northwest of Tirana. The task force consisted of 5,000 soldiers task organized for deep aviation operations with AH-64s, long-range fires with multiple launched rocket systems, and lift operations to insert peacekeeping forces into Kosovo. Lt. Col. Alan Moloff commanded the medical support package that comprised medical personnel from the 212th Mobile Army Surgical Hospital, which headed up the Contingency Medical Force.

A six-aircraft package of MEDEVAC helicopters from the 159th Med Co (AA), under the command of Maj. Michael Avila, joined TF-12. The unit had recently returned from a humanitarian deployment to Austria where it had been part of a task force that evacuated individuals from the small town of Galtur who had been trapped by a massive avalanche.

Reflecting the recent changes in MEDEVAC doctrine, the 159th was tasked to support combat search and rescue operations as part of downed aircraft and aircrew recovery teams, in addition to its classic MEDEVAC functions. During the predeployment training, its crews practiced these procedures. The attachment of the 159th to TF-12 allowed the MEDEVAC unit to better integrate into the task force aviation supply and maintenance structure; and it afforded better access to all of the intelligence, weather, and airspace control data necessary to integrate properly into theater-wide aviation operations.[45]

Reminiscent of aviation operations for DESERT SHIELD, the majority of aircraft from TF-12 self deployed. Because of airspace restrictions the 1,100-mile flight took the aircraft and crews through France and Italy, and across the Adriatic Sea to Rinas. Arriving there in mid-April under rainy conditions and near freezing temperatures, the soldiers found an airfield awash with deep mud and engineers frantically scrambling to build proper hard stands and roads for the aircraft, ground vehicles, and troops.[46]

Once in place, the aviation and MEDEVAC crews began flying missions. Flying conditions were challenging. Low visibility and turbulence were constant factors over the mountainous region near the Kosovo border. All aircrews also had to be aware of the threat of surface-to-air missiles both along the border and within Albania from infiltrating Serbian teams.

As teams of up to eight AH-64 gunships proceeded to the border region, they were supported by CH-47 "Fat Cow" refueling aircraft and a downed aircraft and aircrew recovery team that included three aircraft:

1. A C2 helicopter;
2. A C2 helicopter with a security team onboard; and
3. A MEDEVAC aircraft.

The majority of missions were flown at night utilizing NVGs to give them the maximum protection against enemy forces. While conducting these missions, two AH-64s crashed. In both instances, the MEDEVAC crews responded as part of the downed aircraft and aircrew recovery team packages. They rescued one crew, but the second was killed in the ensuing fire.

The following personnel from the 159th crew made the unsuccessful rescue attempt:

- Pilots: 1st Lt. Dave Zimmerman and CW2 Derek Reel
- Medics: S.Sgt. Judy Mumm and Sgt. Paul Yocum
- Crew Chief: Sgt. Don Stewart

Zimmerman landed the UH-60A near the AH64 crash site, although the intensity of the light from the exploding 2.75 rockets, Hellfire missiles, and 30 mm ordnance made the crew's NVGs almost unusable. When safely on the ground, he immediately dispatched his crewmembers to search the wreckage. Col. Jeff Schloesser, the TF-12 Commander, was also on the ground and attempted to assist. Mumm saved Schloesser's life by protecting him when more ordnance exploded. The heroic efforts of the 159th crew were in vain because neither AH-64 pilot survived the crash. However, all crewmembers received Air Medals for their efforts. Additionally, Mumm, Yocum, and Stewart each received the Soldiers' Medal for their actions, and Zimmerman received the 1999 Aviator Valor Award presented by the American Legion.[47]

Aircrews from the 159th also performed four classic MEDEVAC pickups in support of TF Hawk including the evacuation of local civilians, foreign military

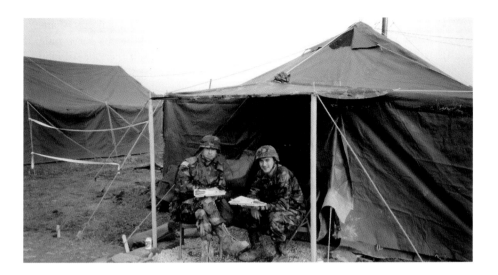

Capt. John McMahan, Flight Platoon Leader, and 1st Lt. Dave Zimmerman, FSMT Leader of the 159th Med Co, in Albania with Task Force Hawk in 1999.
Source: Dave Zimmerman.

personnel, and U.S. service members. The 159th also supported ongoing efforts of the larger humanitarian effort in Albania called Operation SHINING HOPE.[48]

As he had been trained, Avila maintained launch authority for his crews. He briefed them at the beginning of the flying day and then expected them to launch themselves unless conditions had significantly changed. On one evening, a mission came down for a MEDEVAC. The pickup site was up in the mountains, and there was a known threat. The aircraft commander asked that the quick reaction force be launched to escort him. He was told that only the brigade commander could authorize their launch. When the brigade commander was approached, he refused the use of the quick reaction force, and the wounded were eventually brought out by land evacuation. The aviation commanders questioned the handling of MEDEVAC launch authority and whether it should rest with the MEDEVAC company commander.[49]

Operations in Albania only continued until June. They were terminated when— after 78 days of continuous bombardment—the steady buildup of ground forces on his borders, and intense international diplomatic efforts, Milosevic capitulated and evacuated his forces and sycophants out of Kosovo. The Military Technical Agreement was signed on 9 June 1999. The next day, the UN Security Council signed Resolution 1244 directing NATO to establish a security presence in Kosovo so that displaced persons could return home safely, a transitional administration could be established, and humanitarian aid could be delivered. NATO established a Kosovo Force (KFOR) under Operation JOINT GUARDIAN consisting of five international brigades—one led by the United States—that divided the country into zones similar to Bosnia.[50]

Task Force Falcon

Few incidents occurred as the Serbian forces departed and the various national task forces quickly deployed. Speed was essential to prevent a power vacuum and the caching of weapons possibly left behind by the Serbs. Many of the U.S. forces were from TF Hawk. They were moved into Kosovo and joined TF Falcon, led by the 2d Brigade of the 1st Infantry Division, from Schweinfurt, Germany, which was assigned duty as the lead command for the Multi-National Brigade East (MNB-E).

As the task force moved into the region, it was initially prepared to protect the ethnic Albanians. The reality on the ground was much different. The hatred among all ethnic groups was so rife that the larger threat was general anarchy. The disparate groups were so intermixed that there was no practical way to physically separate them. One unidentified infantry battalion commander noted, "The hatred is so intense and irrational it is unbelievable." He could not believe that the internecine strife had led to the virtual destruction of all public service and utilities. Whole villages had been burned. Cemeteries were destroyed, vandalized, or mined.[51]

One of the units that moved forward to Kosovo was a detachment from the 159th Med Co (AA), still attached to the aviation task force. Its crews received all of their taskings through the maneuver brigade operations center because it was the only command node with any communications capability.

TF Falcon also had a medical element - TF Medical Falcon (TFMF). The mission of TFMF was to provide up to Echelon III combat health support to the MNB-East. It also was on call to support the larger UN Mission in Kosovo and various nongovernmental and international organization initiatives to establish a stable health care system for all Kosovars. TFMF comprised about 200 personnel from many specialties, with small detachments from many different units. A detachment from the 30th Medical Brigade from Heidelberg, Germany, provided overall command and control, with personnel from the 67th Combat Support Hospital based at Würzburg, Germany, providing critical support. The structure was essentially maintained as units and personnel from both active duty and reserve units rotated through it. The 159th detachment directly supported them.[52]

Joining the task force, the 159th sent two helicopters and crews to Camp Able Sentry, which was set up near Skopje, Macedonia. The crews provided MEDEVAC coverage for the large convoys moving all of the heavy equipment and supplies being unloaded at the Greek port of Thessaloniki for the Kosovo force. The 159th left two aircraft and crews in Albania to cover the remnants of TF Hawk until all had either moved over into Kosovo or returned to their home stations. At one point, Avila had his crews and support personnel scattered between three widely separated locations. He could only communicate with them via the Internet.[53]

For the next several weeks, as the NATO forces moved into Kosovo, 159th crews flew 55 missions to evacuate wounded soldiers and civilians, several of whom were women in labor. In July, several missions were flown to evacuate some of the 30 Serbs wounded when a bomb was detonated in an open air market in the small city of Vitina. The MEDEVAC crews also flew many medical teams on a weekly basis to remote villages to work with local medical personnel to stem the spread of diseases such as tularemia, a bacterial disease usually found in water contaminated by dead animals and spread by rodents.[54]

The TF Hawk deployment to and employment in Albania only lasted about 100 days. Yet it was eventful from a MEDEVAC perspective. The MEDEVAC lesson learned collected by the Army Center for Lessons Learned stated:

> A particularly valuable innovation involved the attachment of the Air Ambulance Company to the Aviation Brigade, instead of the Medical Command. This enabled the company commander to play an active role in the development of evacuation planning instead of working with the aviation assets externally. The commander sat in the meetings as a green-tab commander and had complete access to all information necessary for him to accomplish his mission. Access to aviation supply and maintenance was easier to attain, as well as integration into the Army Airspace Command and Control (A2C2) plan…To ensure prompt release authority is available to them, medical commanders traditionally prefer to retain aeromedical evacuation under their direct command and control. But the many benefits derived by placing the MEDEVAC units under aviation control in the field makes this a viable option for future operations.[55]

The commander of the Contingency Medical Force, Lt. Col. Alan Moloff, concurred with this assessment, stating in a post-operation interview:

> One of the conscious decisions made was to attach a rotary-winged air evac unit [the 159th Med Co (AA)] to the AV Bde, which was a very smart thing to do in this kind of operation. They have maintenance, the flight operations and…flight following. They came in with the first wave of [AH-64s].[56]

The Task Force Surgeon, Lt. Col. James Bruckart, supported this by saying in his post-operation interview that "The way we have the C2 lined up with the MEDEVAC guys attached to support AV [aviation] is the right thing to do. It allows us access to the C2 structure in the AV chain." When asked if this was doctrinal, he stated:

> It is and it isn't. There are some folks who would like to have release authority strictly with the medical folks, and it depends a lot on the unit. I think this is one area of our doctrine that you can take two different directions, depending on whom in the [medical] community you talk to. I think this is an area of our doctrine that is not as clear as it should be, and there are two ways we can get to our solution…If MEDEVAC were separate, it is much more likely that we would be used as a normal ground force, and would not follow the [AH-64] strikes in. There may be other operations, particularly peace support, where the primary mission may not be to support strikes, but rather to support the medical community. This could be where direct support to a medical [task force] commander is the right way to go as well.[57]

The 159th Med Co (AA) established itself in a semipermanent facility at Camp Bondsteel in late June as part of what was now KFOR 1A, and it was then replaced with a six-aircraft detachment from the 45th Med Co (AA). The 45th was under the command of Maj. Pete Smart, who had taken over in July 1998, after four years in Hawaii with the 68th Med Co (AA).

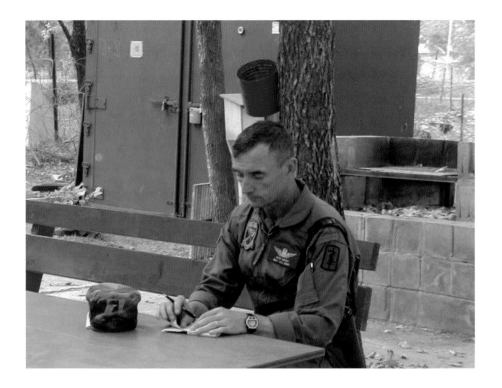

Maj. Pete Smart in Kosovo in 1999.
Source: Pete Smart.

The Bondsteel facility, which covered 955 acres with a perimeter of about 7 miles, was located in the rolling hills and farmland near the city of Ferizaj/Urosevac, about 30 kilometers south of the capital of Pristina. Missions were few as the ground forces found themselves engaged mostly in keeping the various factions separate and helping to develop a functioning government, police force, and peaceful society. Most MEDEVAC calls were for local nationals.

One of the allied elements in the area was a Russian task force. Smart fortuitously had a fluent Russian speaker in his unit who came from a most unexpected background. S.Sgt. Felix Gomez was from Nicaragua. As a young man, he had joined the Nicaraguan Air Force and had learned the language when he attended a three-year technical school in Russia. When he returned home, he defected to the United States and joined the Army. Smart appointed Gomez as an unofficial liaison with the Russians. Overall, Kosovo duty was relatively peaceful and even boring. It was a replay of Bosnia as some semblance of economic activity and civil life returned.[58]

The 45th served with KFOR until December, when six aircraft and crews from the 236th Med Co (AA) from Landstuhl, Germany, as part of KFOR1B replaced it. Maj. Jon Fristoe commanded the unit. He and the 236th detachment deployed as part of an aviation task force from the 11th Aviation Regiment from Ketterbach. They were assigned to the aviation brigade from the 1st Infantry Division. A team from the 67th Combat Support Hospital led the medical detachment. Fristoe worked directly with them on all medical issues and discovered that they knew almost nothing about aviation.[59]

Missions were relatively routine, with weather posing the biggest challenge. In early January 2000, Fristoe and his crew were called to rescue a young child who had fallen through ice into a stream. Scrambling out just ahead of lowering fog, they reached the site, but could not find the boy. They called for a second aircraft, but none could take off because the weather had moved in at both operating bases. The medic, Sgt. David Estrada, volunteered to go into the water. That was ruled out as far too dangerous. Instead, he was lowered on the hoist so that he could closely search the stream and accumulated ice. For several minutes, the medic dangled from the hoist as the crew chief carefully coordinated the movement of the aircraft with the pilots to allow Estrada to search. However, the boy was not found. Estrada had to be hoisted back into the aircraft and then cared for himself because he became dangerously chilled. The mission was unsuccessful, but showed the determination and professionalism of the MEDEVAC crew. During that rotation, the 236th crews logged 1,242 flight hours and evacuated 188 patients in support of UN forces and the civilian populace.[60]

In May, the 159th Med Co (AA) again replaced with the 236th Med Co for KFOR2A, with TFMF commanded by an element from the 30th Medical Brigade. By that June, the MEDEVAC units had flown 131 missions, carrying 71 U.S. soldiers, eight NATO troops, and 47 local nationals. One-half of them were urgent status, and 80% of the missions were conducted during the day. Given the hilly terrain and poor roads, the air ambulances accomplished most evacuations. The commanding general released a directive requiring all soldiers to be proficient in the utilization of MEDEVAC request procedures. Radio repeaters had to be placed throughout the area of responsibility so that all personnel could make radio contact to pass MEDEVAC requests.[61]

However, the overall political and security situation continued to steadily stabilize, and the size of the KFOR/JOINT GUARDIAN task force also steadily decreased. The 45th Med Co (AA) replaced the 159th in September 2000, as part of KFOR2B, and was then replaced by the 236th Med Co in early January 2001.[62]

On 16 February 2001, Serbian partisans attacked a bus filled with Albanian locals, killing 14 and injuring 32 persons. Crews from the 236th MEDEVACed 13 seriously wounded persons to Camp Bondsteel.[63]

The 50th Med Co (AA) replaced the 236th in May 2001 for KFOR3A. The unit deployed as part of a larger 101st Airborne Division package called TF Sabre. Led by the Company Commander, Maj. Steven Millward, it took six aircraft and 39 personnel. The unit kept four aircraft and personnel at Camp Bondsteel and two aircraft and crews at Camp Able Sentry. Unit crews flew 127 evacuation missions that carried 158 patients including U.S. and allied soldiers and local nationals.

The unit also took advantage of the deployment to conduct some focused NVG training using new goggles for all aircrew. CW3 Andrew Feris was on that deployment and made good use of his NVG training to make several recoveries at night. On a mission into Macedonia he and his crew picked up a badly wounded individual from a British unit and delivered him to Pristina. On another mission they picked up an Albanian who had been severely beaten by a mob. Feris also found that language could be a barrier. It was not uncommon to dispatch to a pickup location to recover a patient with a reported common problem, such as an appendicitis, and then discover that the patient had actually suffered severe gunshot wounds. The non-English speaking teams could not clearly express themselves in detailed medical terms and used a few common phrases to make their requests. For the crews, it made every mission potentially very interesting.

In general, duty in Kosovo proceeded at a more steady and leisurely pace. Newly elected President George W. Bush visited Camp Bondsteel on 24 July 2001, and the summer passed relatively benignly. Likewise, the 11th of September started out as another quiet day. However, that rapidly changed when the few televisions around the base showed the horrific scenes from New York, the Pentagon, and later, Pennsylvania. The base was immediately locked down, and all soldiers were ordered into their full combat gear, wondering—while they donned it—where events would take them in the future.[64]

For KFOR3B, in October 2001, the 717th Med Co (AA), New Mexico ARNG, under the command of Maj. Michael Montoya, deployed to support a brigade task force from the 82d Airborne Division. It was attached to an aviation detachment from the 1st Squadron, 17th Cavalry Regiment, and supported the 67th Combat Support Hospital. Six aircraft and crews were split between Camp Bondsteel and Camp Able Sentry in Macedonia. These crews conducted 60 urgent MEDEVAC missions for U.S. and coalition soldiers, and transfer missions to the large international airport at Thessaloniki, Greece, so that U.S. personnel could be flown to Germany. Crews also provided MEDEVAC for local Albanian and Serbian citizens throughout the KFOR AOR. On 31 December, one of their crews performed a harrowing rescue of a Special Forces team who needed to be recovered from atop a 7,000-foot peak before severe weather overtook them. The crew of Warrant Officers Jason Hyer and Michael Rohrbeck, medic S.Sgt. Robert Parnell, and crew chief Spc. Robert Sage, maneuvered their aircraft onto a narrow ice encrusted ridgeline to safely pick up the fatigued team that was also suffering from altitude sickness. The Guardsmen of the 717th returned home in May 2002, as the American contingent in KFOR dropped to 3,000 troops.[65]

KFOR4A May 2002 – November 2002 and KFOR4B November 2002 – May 2003. The 45th Med Co (AA) from Germany replaced the 717th troops for KFOR4A, and it supported the 67th Combat Support Hospital. The 45th was augmented with personnel and aircraft from both the 236th and 159th Med Cos. On 31 July 2002, their crews MEDEVACed two U.S. soldiers wounded by a mine that detonated as they were conducting clearing operations near the village of Klokot.[66]

As the social and economic landscape slowly stabilized, the UN further reduced

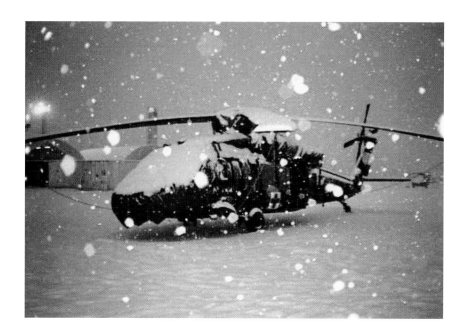

A hard winter in Bosnia.
Source: U.S. Army.

forces in the area. Most incidents included more petty crime like smuggling, drugs, and prostitution, as opposed to ethnic strife or overt challenges to the government or the UN forces. Several national contingents were either reduced or returned to their home nations. Overall, forces had been slowly reduced by 40%.[67]

KFOR5A May 2003 – November 2003 and KFOR5B November 2003 – May 2004. A detachment of helicopters and personnel from the 24th Med Co (AA), Nebraska/Kansas ARNG, supported these deployments. During June 2003, personnel conducted an evacuation exercise with Spanish MEDEVAC helicopters supporting a combined exercise with Spanish Task Force Tizona, and the U.S. Army 2d Battalion, 2d Infantry Regiment. Medics and crews from both units lauded the realism and necessity of the training.[68]

KFOR6A May 2004 – November 2004. The 146th Med Co (AA), Tennessee ARNG, sent a small detachment of helicopters and personnel to support this rotation. The 146th attached to an aviation element from the 1st Battalion, 137th Aviation Regiment, from the Ohio ARNG and worked with the 139th Medical Group, USAR, from Missouri.

In July 2004, 146th crews participated in a mass casualty exercise involving all task forces designed to calibrate operational procedures and communications. Such drills were still necessary because even though the political situation continued to stabilize, the potential for violence to erupt remained.[69]

KFOR6B November 2004 – May 2005 and KFOR7A May 2005 – November 2005. In January 2005, the 717th Med Co (AA), New Mexico ARNG, arrived to support KFOR6B and KFOR7A, as part of an all ARNG aviation task force built around the 1st Battalion, 104th Aviation Regiment, from the Washington, DC ARNG. A detachment from the 332d Medical Brigade (USAR) from Nashville, Tennessee, commanded by Maj. Michael Rieske led the medical task force. The medical task force was also based at Camp Bondsteel. The political situation was relatively stable, and few recovery missions were flown. The medical task force conducted a large mass casualty drill that involved all of the various national units. The 717th also participated in a task force wide celebration of six years of successful peacekeeping operations in the region as dictated by UN Security Council Resolution 1244. Designed to reestablish conditions for a peaceful and normal life for the inhabitants of Kosovo, the KFOR slowly but steadily achieved that goal. The 717th remained part of the KFOR until it deployed home and demobilized in January 2006. Operations in Kosovo remain ongoing, and U.S. Army MEDEVAC units continue to support the deployments.[70]

Nigeria

When the 159th Med Co returned home from Kosovo in late September 2000, the troops expected to have a break. However, as the decade ended, the 159th Med Co (AA) was tasked for another deployment. It sent a team of three helicopters and crews and 23 support personnel as part of a larger task force from the 30th Medical Brigade to support Operation FOCUS RELIEF. This operation directed the Special Operations Command Europe to send a 250-soldier training detachment from the 3d Special Forces Group to train five Nigerian battalions to conduct peacekeeping operations in Sierra Leone. The only aviation asset sent was an aviation intermediate maintenance package of six troops sent specifically to support the 159th. As opposed to the TF Hawk operation, this time the 159th remained under medical control. The task force was in Nigeria mid-October through mid-December 2000. The team flew 59 sorties, mostly operations support and training. No serious injuries or medical problems were encountered. The deployment was uneventful, but it was a classic example of the flexibility of MEDEVAC units to support peacetime operations under medical vice aviation control.[71]

MAST

As the only MEDEVAC unit in Hawaii, the 68th Med Co (AA) at Schofield Barracks in the middle of Oahu was constantly in high demand for MAST calls and had flown an average of 250 missions per year since the beginning of the program. On Thanksgiving Day of 1999, CW3 Tyron Freeman and Capt. Scott Eichel flew the unit's 6,000th MAST mission to transport two teenagers who had been hurt in an automobile accident.

"We didn't make too much of it," said the 68th's commander, Maj. Steve

Bolint, "but we are proud of our record. Any time we can help save someone's life it makes us feel good." Donna Malawa, the state chief of medical emergency services, was more expansive.

"There is no doubt that the 68th has greatly improved survival of patients and made a tremendous contribution to the health and welfare of our citizens," she said.

Freeman was more self-depreciating. "What amazes me is that I get paid for flying around the islands and helping people." Their sentiments represented what MAST had become.[72]

Doctrine

Service Doctrine - Field Manual (FM) 8-10-26, Employment of the Medical Company (Air Ambulance), February 1999

In February 1999, the Army Medical Department Center and School again updated its MEDEVAC doctrine using a different approach. A new document, FM 8-10-26, was written to provide guidance directly for the MEDEVAC companies. The new FM described the tactics needed for implementation of the company's role as a combat service support unit. It was specifically crafted for the company commander and personnel, and individuals on staffs at several levels for the planning for overall combat health support. The aviation community could use it to determine what support it needed to provide to facilitate MEDEVAC operations.[73]

The document reflected the changes in threat environment and possible mission assignments since the end of the cold war. It also expanded the panoply of taskings to include regional instability, ethnic or territorial disputes, proliferation of weapons of mass destruction, and threats to democracy or democratic reform.

The document also reaffirmed the vital role of the CHS system as a force multiplier that protected the health of the soldier in war as well as stability and support operations. Medical evacuation was a part of the CHS system, and the Army was the only U.S. military service with dedicated assets to perform the aeromedical evacuation mission.[74]

The manual continued by explaining that aeromedical evacuation was the execution of this process with the use of aircraft that had the capability to provide en route care. The use of aircraft for patient movement without en route patient care was designated casualty evacuation or CASEVAC.

MEDEVAC or CASEVAC could be accomplished with three different systems:

1. A *dedicated* system is one in which aircraft and crews were solely dedicated to the mission of MEDEVAC. This was the case with the MEDEVAC units.
2. A *designated* system was a system whereby aircraft were identified for use as either a MEDEVAC or CASEVAC platform. During mass casualty situations, other aviation assets, such as CH-47s, could be designated for CASEVAC.
3. A *lift-of-opportunity* system was a system that utilized empty aircraft for backhaul as available.[75]

FM 8-10-26 included a detailed chapter that described the air ambulance company's organization and functions, including a new tasking to conduct combat search and rescue missions for downed aircrews. The company was organized with a company headquarters that provided the unit command and control, and several subordinate platoons. The flight operations platoon provided all flight planning, flight dispatch, aircraft fueling, and operation of the heliport. The aviation unit maintenance platoon provided all unit-level maintenance for the aircraft. The evacuation platoon commanded the three FSMTs of three aircraft and crews that could be deployed forward to directly support maneuver forces. Also assigned was the area support MEDEVAC section consisting of six aircraft and crews that provided general area MEDEVAC support in the vicinity of the company headquarters, performed patient transfers, or reinforced the FSMTs.

The company could be employed in direct support of a division with which it would then establish direct liaison, or in general support of a corps. The company established the necessary communications links with all relevant headquarters.[76]

The rest of the FM was a detailed discussion of the employment of the company in a variety of environments, operations, and contingencies. It included a suggested series of tactical standing operations procedures, team leader's guides, liaison officer's checklists, and commander's checklists for a variety of concerns. Also included was a discussion of relevant portions of the Geneva Conventions pertaining to MEDEVAC operations, a section on risk management, a section on aviation countermeasure techniques and survivability equipment, practical guidelines for the flight medics, and medical support for combat search and rescue operations. It was a doctrinal rewrite for MEDEVAC that was stretched into a useful "how to" guide.

Service Doctrine - FM 8-10-6, Medical Evacuation in a Theater of Operations, Tactics, Techniques, and Procedures, April 2000

Reflecting recent operations in the Balkans, the next doctrinal rewrite was an update of FM 8-10-6. Dated 14 April 2000, it addressed medical evacuation as part of the CHS system and captured the evolving threats and technological trends of the decade since the last iteration of the FM in 1991. Dovetailing nicely with the recent FM 8-10-26, it recognized the new international environment presented to the nation with security challenges unprecedented in ambiguity, diversity, risk, and opportunity, presented by the "new world order," which was neither new nor orderly. The old forces of adventurism, nationalism, and separatism had reappeared with sometimes violent and unpredictable consequences. Challenges to national security now required military forces to participate in peacekeeping operations, nation building, and humanitarian assistance. The U.S. Army had to be prepared to face a variety of threat forces, many with credible military capabilities.

The FM also offered expansive discussion of the evolving medical evacuation system and considerations for specific environments and medical regulating. Several chapters on tactics, techniques, and procedures followed. Lastly, as an ominous harbinger, it included a section on combating terrorism and force projection, and suggested difficult missions ahead for MEDEVAC.[77]

* * * *

The 1990s was a busy period for the U.S. Army. Having developed the concept of AirLand Battle and then reorganizing to wage it, the necessity arrived, but not on the Plains of Europe as had been expected. Instead, the test came in the heat and dust of the Persian Gulf. The MEDEVAC force, busy reorganizing to support the new concept, pushed forth its largest effort ever to serve the needs of the soldiers. It did so, but was stressed in the effort. Yet that experience validated the changes that needed to be made. That process would continue.

The conflict also validated the efforts of Gen. Creighton Abrams, who reorganized the Army after the long war in Vietnam so that it would once again rely heavily on its two Reserve Components as it had historically done. At one point, more than 50% of all MEDEVAC assets were in these two components. They answered the call for DESERT SHIELD/STORM and performed admirably both at home and in the conflict. Necessary force cuts after the war saw the complete elimination of all U.S. Army Reserve MEDEVAC units. In one stroke, the MEDEVAC community lost almost one-third of its capability and an uncounted number of highly experienced and motivated pilots, medics, crew chiefs, and support personnel. There is no pretty way to eliminate forces.

After DESERT STORM, taskings changed for the MEDEVAC units. Nature provided challenges with devastating hurricanes and earthquakes. They required response, as did manmade disasters at places such as Fort Bragg. MAST missions were still being flown, although steadily, and more communities were developing their own capabilities as the program had been designed to stimulate.

With the demise of the Soviet Union and the successful conclusion of the war in the Persian Gulf, the strategic focus changed, because no single adversary dominated the nation's attention. Humanitarian missions and peacekeeping taskings took the Army to places like Northern Iraq, Somalia, Haiti, and Bosnia, and Army doctrine in general—and MEDEVAC doctrine in particular—changed to meet the new challenges. The men and women of MEDEVAC saw duty in all of those locations, doing what they were trained to do. MEDEVAC remained under medical control. However, the increasing sophistication and complexity of aviation operations in DESERT STORM and Albania suggested that MEDEVAC should be more closely aligned with aviation operations.

As the decade approached its end, Gen. Eric K. Shinseki became the 34th Army Chief of Staff. He was commissioned in 1965 and was a Vietnam combat veteran. Throughout the 1990s he served as a commander of mechanized units and held several key posts in Europe, including command of U.S. Army Europe. He was acutely aware of the problems facing the Army as it attempted to address the challenges of the current world political realities with forces optimized for heavy battle. Reflecting on the efforts of former Army Chiefs Gordon Sullivan and Dennis Reimer, he also believed that the Army needed to transform so that it could leverage new and evolving technologies to move faster with a lighter but smarter and more lethal force. He wanted an Army that was highly maneuverable, technologically advanced, and strategically mobile. He was determined to lead that transformation.

That evolution—within just a few short years—would lead to significant change for the Army and MEDEVAC force. Before that process would play out, however, other unforeseen and dramatic events would abruptly intrude.

Part Four

Into the Millennium:
New Challenges, at Home and
Abroad

Chapter Eight
To 9/11, 2000–2001

"Today, our fellow citizens, our way of life, our very freedom came under attack
in a series of deliberate and deadly terrorist acts."
President George W. Bush[1]

Renewed Desire for Change

It was a new millennium, and the Chief of Staff of the Army, Gen. Eric Shinseki, wanted to refocus the Army. The heavy divisions, which stood ready during the cold war and defeated the Army of Iraq in 1991, were too heavy to respond quickly to the panoply of challenges facing the United States. Operations in Somalia, Haiti, Bosnia, and Kosovo had conclusively validated this position. Shinseki concurred that the need for change was inevitable, stating, "If you don't like change, you're going to like irrelevance even less." He wanted a lighter, quicker force designed around brigade-sized packages with the necessary capabilities versus the divisional forces then in existence. His goal was to have brigades that could deploy anywhere in the world within 96 hours and a full division that could move within another five days.

Shinseki established a transformational process that began with the Legacy Force of current units and charted how they would realign as an Objective Force of the Army of the future. It comprised units of action of approximately brigade size that could accomplish distinct mission-essential tasks and units of employment that were higher headquarters designed of nominal division, corps, or army elements structured to accomplish any mission. Units of action were either maneuver or support elements. This process also necessitated changes in doctrine and organization. Subordinate to this effort was a more focused Aviation Restructuring Initiative that addressed reductions to Army aviation forces, possibly including MEDEVAC units.

However, real world exigencies and developments required the Army to continue operations in several parts of the world while responding to attacks on the homeland and the initiation of offensive operations in several more theaters. Shinseki did not see the fruition of transformation on his watch, but his successor, Gen. Peter Schoomaker, continued the process.[2]

Organization

The Army Medical Department (AMEDD)

The winds of change also began to blow across the medical community. Lt. Col. Dave MacDonald became the medical evacuation officer in the Force Development branch on the Office of The Surgeon General staff in Falls Church, Virginia. After completing the Army Command and General Staff College course at Fort Leavenworth, Kansas, he had remained there for two years as an instructor. It became his turn to do a staff tour, but it was a short one. While at Leavenworth, he had been selected for battalion command, and rumor had it that he would get a unit in the summer of 2001.[3]

When he reported to his new position, he was immediately embroiled in an Aviation Restructuring Initiative induced effort to reduce the MEDEVAC fleet. Army aviation accounted for 25% of the overall Army budget, and the Army Staff pushed for efficiencies to reduce that cost, including one proposal that would have reduced the UH-60 MEDEVAC fleet—both active and Army National Guard (ARNG)—by 30%, by reducing all units from 15-ship to 12-ship (and possibly 10- and 8-ship) formations, with the intention of then using the released UH-60s to replace UH-1V aircraft still used by several ARNG MEDEVAC units. MacDonald argued for maintaining the 15-ship Medical Force 2000 companies while developing proposals to reduce the companies as directed. He searched—with little success—for empirical data that he could use to determine the requisite force structure for each package. He discovered that the MEDEVAC community had not been very proactive in maintaining a good database to show its successes and validate the structure of its units. What he found instead was a rather casual attitude that, "We know it works; it's worked in the past; it's working now; we need to keep it." He could not find data showing how many lives had been saved or why the 15-ship company was the best structure to support the needs of the corps or division. A modified Table of Organization and Equipment for the MEDEVAC units requiring 15 aircraft but assigning 12 was developed, but it was not implemented because subsequent events overrode all initiatives to reduce the MEDEVAC fleet. However, the idea for a 12-ship MEDEVAC company was accepted and resurfaced in a few years.[4]

MacDonald stayed engaged in the issues and debates until June 2001, when he was ordered back to Fort Bragg, North Carolina, to command the 56th Medical Battalion (Evacuation), the unit under which he had commanded the 57th Med Co (AA) a few years prior. As he prepared for the move, he recalled those earlier difficult times with the 57th. He resolved that as soon as he arrived at Fort Bragg, he would make office visits to all of his medical *and* aviation counterparts so that he could immediately assume the role of "marriage counselor" between the medicine and aviation units at Fort Bragg.[5]

At Fort Sam Houston, Texas, Maj. John Lamoureux also was involved in these transformation and modernization issues. After his tour with the 421st Medical Battalion in Germany, he served a short tour as an observer/controller at the Hohenfels Training Center and then returned to Fort Sam Houston to serve as an instructor in the Medical Service Corps basic and advanced courses. At Fort Sam Houston he was selected to serve as the executive officer for the AMEDD Center and School Commander, Maj. Gen. Kevin Kiley.

Lamoureux's experiences had clearly shown that on any deployment, MEDEVAC always struggled to establish itself with an aviation element to get the necessary operational and logistical support to operate properly. He and Kiley were impressed with the 101st Airborne Division (Air Assault) model and agreed that it could be the basis for a reorganization of MEDEVAC units as divisional elements rather than corps-assigned companies with their slice of supporting units. However, their analysis also showed that the 101st also always needed to have another MEDEVAC unit in general support for backhaul, so that the Forward Support MEDEVAC teams of the 50th could focus on direct tactical support to the brigades.

At one point, Kiley had his combat developers shape a proposal for MEDEVAC units as divisional assets with the options developed by MacDonald from 15 down to eight aircraft. When the overall proposal was ready, Kiley briefed it to the Surgeon General, Lt. Gen. James Peake. After some detailed and often heated discussions, Peake supported it. He then briefed it to the Training and Doctrine Command commander. Gen. John Abrams listened carefully and responded, "I agree with all of your points. I think you are making all the right arguments, and I really can't counter anything. The problem is, I can't approve it."

Kiley and Peake were taken aback and asked him why. Abrams answered, "We have a troop cap, and if I put a MEDEVAC company in the division, that is so many troop numbers that I have to take out, specifically on the gunfighter side." It was the classic "beans versus bullets" argument. Peake was not finished. "When," he followed up, "would a division ever deploy without MEDEVAC?" Again, Abrams pondered and then said, "No, I cannot do it. We are going to have to make the Corps slice thing work.... I cannot afford to take those slots away from the warfighters."[6]

Another individual keenly watching these initiatives was MacDonald's old Eagle Dustoff compatriot and Lamoureux's early mentor, Col. Scott Heintz, then serving at Fort Rucker, Alabama, as the director of the Medical Evacuation Proponency Directorate. He reported to the AMEDD Center and School at Fort Sam Houston, but also served as the MEDEVAC Consultant to the Surgeon General. This second designation was an unofficial position but afforded him the ability to communicate directly with the Surgeon General on MEDEVAC matters. This was a classic medical phenomenon whereby physicians frequently consulted with specialist experts when dealing with a patient. In this capacity, Heintz advised the Surgeon General on MEDEVAC-related decisions. Scott's varied experience as a MEDEVAC officer and pilot made him the natural choice for this function.[7] He did not want to see the units reduced in size and assigned to the divisions, but understood that Shinseki's drive for transformation would ultimately affect every part of the Army, including MEDEVAC. He was resolved to fight for his units and personnel.[8]

New Aircraft

While working with Kiley, Lamoureux was involved in another long simmering MEDEVAC issue: the procurement of a new helicopter. The MEDEVAC fleet still possessed a large number of UH-1V aircraft, especially in its ARNG units, which were far beyond their best days. Almost all of its UH-60s were "A" models dating back to the early 1980s and some of the oldest helicopters in the overall Army Black Hawk fleet. There were a few UH-60Ls with bigger engines and four UH-60Qs, essentially "A" models but with updated cargo cabins optimized for patients, forward looking infrared systems for better all weather navigation, and improved avionics. All of the new Ls and most of the Qs belonged to ARNG units, thanks to individual senators making specific legislative earmarks. An updated aircraft for the general Army MEDEVAC fleet was needed, but it had to be procured through the overall Army acquisition process and compete with the needs of the aviation community at large.

MEDEVAC Aircraft Variants

Model	Engine	Load	Special Equipment	Range (nautical miles)
UH-60 A	T-700 1,560 HP	6 Litters	Carousel Internal Hoist	319
UH-60L	T-701C 1,880 HP	Same	Carousel Internal Hoist	315
UH-60Q	T-700	Same	Forward looking infrared On board Oxygen Medical Monitoring Litter Lift On board Suction Defibrillation Global Positioning System Glass Cockpit External Hoist	319
HH-60A	T-700	Same	Same	319
HH-60L	T-701C	Same	Same	315[9]

Both Kiley and Peake wanted to replace the older MEDEVAC aircraft with new UH-60Qs, like the four that had been modified postproduction and given to the Tennessee ARNG. However, the UH-60Q aircraft still had the same older engines as the "A" models. Subsequent events would indicate that they just did not have enough power to operate at higher elevations.

Accordingly, the AMEDD modified its request for new aircraft to specify the "Q" model with the better engines of the "L" model. To keep the designations from getting too confusing, the force planners redesignated the new aircraft the HH-60L, using the joint designation for rescue aircraft used by the Air Force. Three had been procured through the acquisition process in the late 1990s and assigned to the 507th at Fort Hood, Texas. Lamoureux attended several conferences as Kiley and Peake met with the Army Staff G-3 and Lt. Gen. Richard Cody to argue for Army procurement of HH-60Ls for MEDEVAC. They forwarded a modernization plan that called for the procurement of 192 HH-60Ls in two force packages at a cost of $883 million, but did not receive any commitment for funding.[10]

Doctrine

Service Doctrine – Field Manual (FM) 3.0, Operations, June 2001

As the new century was beginning, Shinseki directed another rewrite of FM 100-5 *Operations,* the Army's capstone warfighting document, in support of his transformation initiative. Recognizing recent Joint Staff doctrinal literature renumbering guidance, the new manual was republished as FM 3.0 and was fully compatible with joint doctrine. Shinseki knew well that the Army was a doctrine-based institution. Doctrine guided its actions, organization, equipage, and even manning across the range of military operations and spectrum of conflict as part of joint and combined operations in a broad range of events from major wars to peacekeeping to stability and support operations.

As its predecessor FMs had done, this new manual also reaffirmed that the Army forces were the decisive component of land warfare in joint and combined operations. Fighting and winning the nation's wars were the foundation of Army service. The Army was prepared to take action across the full spectrum of conflict, from war to peace. Increasingly in the international security environment, this action included peacetime military engagement like humanitarian, counter-drug, or peacekeeping operations. Additionally, Army forces helped civil authorities — both at home and abroad — prepare for and respond to natural disasters. The document was filled with many vignettes drawn from events that had occurred since the publication of the 1993 edition of FM 100-5, and it graphically showed how the world had changed and the Army had adapted. Shinseki wanted to leverage new and evolving technology to surmount these threats.

Combat service support forces, including medical elements, had to remain prepared to support these operations. Increasingly, the Army was being called upon to mount support operations to assist foreign and domestic civil authorities. In these cases, the real enemy was disease, hunger, or the consequences of natural disasters. The Army, with its mobile and well-organized units of trained specialists equipped with many capabilities, was an obvious asset to meet such potential needs. The Army intended to dominate in both land warfare and in operations other than war. The MEDEVAC units were some of the enabling forces that provided these "soft" capabilities.[11]

Joint Doctrine – Joint Publication 4-02, Doctrine for Health Service Support in Joint Operations, July 2001

Almost concurrently, the Joint Staff published an update to Joint Publication 4-02. It introduced a new term, force health protection (FHP), which rested on three pillars: (1) a healthy and fit force, (2) casualty prevention, and (3) casualty care management. The health service support system facilitated this by conforming to the joint commander's overall plan, being responsive and flexible, being mobile and anticipating the need for rapid movement, providing uninterrupted care, and coordinating for the efficient employment of health service support resources to support the planned operation.

The document reaffirmed that timely patient movement played an important role in FHP and that movement by air was the preferred method. Initial movement to a theater Level III facility was a service component responsibility, but, in any theater, Army MEDEVAC helicopters were used for patient transfer to hospital ships. This publication was released in conjunction with subordinate documents that prescribed joint doctrine and tactics, techniques, and procedures for health services logistics support and patient movement.[12]

This rewrite also included specific functions for assigned joint force surgeons. Under the joint construct or in a coalition environment, combined/joint force commanders and subordinate component commanders (like the combined/joint force land component commander) were assigned a combined/joint forces surgeon as a specialty advisor to report directly to them. The combined/joint forces surgeon was responsible for combined/joint coordination of health service support initiatives and planning, joint coordination of intratheater patient movement that linked into the intertheater movement system, and the reception, staging, onward movement, and integration of assigned and attached medical units.[13]

The update also recognized that in military operations other than war, the health threat had to be evaluated for a patient base much larger than just the U.S. force alone. It stated:

> When preparing for and conducting operations during MOOTW [military operations other than war], elements of the health threat to the indigenous population, allied and coalition forces, U.S. Government employees, DOD [Department of Defense] contractors, and as appropriate, IO [international organizations], and NGOs [non-governmental organizations], must be assessed. The impact of the heath threat as a contributing factor to social, political, and economic stability in both peace and other operational environments must be considered.[14]

This was a significant change because it recognized that the patient base that any deployed MEDEVAC force had to support could be much larger than the traditional military force used to determine its allocation.

Service Doctrine – FM 8-10-26, Employment of the Medical Company (Air Ambulance), May 2002

In May 2002, the Army published Change 1 to FM 8-10-26. Perhaps reflecting lessons learned in several operations—but most prominently in Task Force Hawk—it included several updates designed more closely to integrate the MEDEVAC units into aviation task forces.

These updates specified that units not operating in a theater general support capacity and tied to a medical evacuation battalion should be included in the aviation brigade communications net. Additionally, forward support MEDEVAC teams should have long-range communications capability for battle tracking and situational awareness of ground and air units. They should maintain division A2C2 information and comply with standard use Army aircraft flight routes into and out of the maneuver brigade areas.[15]

The change also included an entire section on combat search and rescue as an additional mission. During the war in Vietnam, MEDEVAC crews made many rescues under fire, but this mission had been absent from subsequent doctrinal manuals. FM 8-10-26 recognized the role that the MEDEVAC helicopter and crew could play in this mission in a general way. It prescribed a mission training plan, standard operating procedures, and event checklists.

The change also pointed out that if a MEDEVAC helicopter was utilized as part of an aviation or larger joint task force to rescue personnel in enemy territory, it could lose its protection under the laws of war and Geneva Convention. Moreover, this use of a MEDEVAC aircraft for combat search and rescue required the removal of the distinctive Red Cross for the mission. However, it did not provide for the arming of the aircraft.[16]

Service Doctrine - FM 4-02, Force Health Protection in a Global Environment, February 2003

FM 8-10 was next to be updated and republished as FM 4-02 in consonance with the Joint Chiefs of Staff joint publications system. The manual was more expansive than the earlier version. The overarching references to AirLand battle and the restructuring of medical support to enable and sustain it were eliminated. The new focus was on FHP enabled by the military health system's capabilities to deliver health care across the continuum of military operations in any environment. These capabilities rested on three pillars, including (1) a healthy and fit force, (2) casualty prevention, and (3) casualty care management, and they supported the joint mission as part of guidance from the Joint Chiefs of Staff under Joint Vision 2020.[17]

A robust capability to evacuate the wounded was a key part of casualty care management. This applied to U.S. soldiers, allied troops, contract personnel under Army employ, or indigenous civilians. Planners needed to be aware of the limits of specific modes of transportation in terms of operational range, speed and lift limitations, and tactical use considerations. The en route teams had to leverage technological advances in communications, computers, and medical equipment to facilitate and enhance medical treatment provided to patients while they were en route between facilities. MEDEVAC was performed as per FMs 8-10-6 and FM 8-10-26.[18]

The new FM also defined medical evacuation and medical regulating as a key functional area for the AMEDD. It formalized the concept of theater evacuation policy and redefined evacuation priorities. Although re-acknowledging that tactical evacuation was still a service component responsibility, it reaffirmed the Army commitment to shore-to-ship evacuation and defined the theater patient movement requirements center as that command and control node responsible for the medical regulation and movement of patients between Level III and IV hospitals.[19]

The manual explained in general terms how FHP was applied in classic offensive and defensive operations, stability operations, and support operations for domestic community assistance (like Military Assistance to Safety and Traffic), domestic preparedness, disaster response, or foreign humanitarian assistance. Such actions were almost invariably joint and/or combined and could be coordinated with other governmental and nongovernmental organizations.[20]

Overall, FM 4-02 was a significant update of medical doctrine. From the perspective of MEDEVAC, it clearly defined the new and more dangerous world environment and the multifold events that could require the dispatch of MEDEVAC units.

From the return of the MEDEVAC forces from Vietnam in 1973 to the tumultuous events of the beginning of the millennium, MEDEVAC doctrine was never static. It was addressed in Army doctrinal manuals at several levels and then in joint doctrine as it evolved. Guided by officers experienced in battle and understanding the intricacies of medicine and aviation, it steadily morphed as the world, nation, and Army changed. Rooted in the past while exploiting evolving technology and anticipating the future, it continues to guide MEDEVAC operations as a key component of the continuum of care.

Operations

Still in the Sinai

Mirroring the ongoing support operations in Balkans and Central America, the country was still honoring its obligation to support the Multinational Force and Observers in the Sinai that had been created to enforce the ceasefire between Israel and Egypt at the Camp David Peace Accords in 1979. The U.S. contingent still consisted of an infantry battalion and an aviation element, which included a MEDEVAC team. Many MEDEVAC pilots and medics from the active and Guard units did tours with the Nomads—the call sign they still used—of the 1st Support Battalion. Beginning in 2002, however, all of the infantry battalions were Guard units.

The Nomads were called for another type of duty in January 2004, when a civilian Boeing 737 crashed shortly after takeoff from the Sharm el-Sheikh Airport.

The alert crew was scrambled from South Camp to recover injured passengers. Unfortunately, all 148 persons on board were killed when the aircraft slammed into the Red Sea. The crew participated in the recovery of human remains. All were decorated for their actions.[21]

In late 2005, UH-60s replaced the UH-1s and were also painted in the distinctive white and orange paint scheme. The Nomads of the 1st Support Battalion continue to provide the same excellent level of support to the soldiers of the Multinational Force and Observers.[22]

11 September 2001

The events of that crisp late summer day are well known and documented. Like the United States and its Army, the MEDEVAC community was shocked by the horrific events. As events unfolded, President George W. Bush said, "No American will ever forget this day." That was certainly true for the men and women of MEDEVAC.[23]

Following his tour as the commander of the 159th Med Co (AA) and then a short tour as the executive officer of the 421st Medical Battalion (Evacuation) in Germany, Maj. Mike Avila was assigned to the Army Staff in the Pentagon. He reported for work in early July, as the aeromedical evacuation support officer for the Director of Military Support Operations. The Army Staff in the Pentagon oversaw military support for civil authorities. Among his many duties, Avila oversaw the Military Assistance to Safety and Traffic program. He also was involved with issues introduced to him from other governmental agencies including the Department of Transportation and the Federal Emergency Management Agency.

Just a few weeks into his job, he was directed to attend Army Staff "new guy" training. The second day of that training occurred on 11 September. Avila was sitting in his classroom located on the "C" Ring, in the newly renovated Army section on the west side of the building with 20 other personnel engaged in some interactive computer training. He had been working away for about an hour when a young sergeant from his office came in and asked him to return to his work area. Avila had almost finished his work and did not want to be interrupted. He asked the young troop why he needed to return. The soldier told him that a plane had just hit one of the towers in the World Trade Center and some air evacuation might need to be worked. As a career aviator, Avila had a bit of trouble trying to understand how an airplane like that could hit a building on a clear day. He told the soldier that he would be right down and quickly tried to finish his work so that he could get credit for the course.

A few minutes later, the building shook noticeably, and the lights flickered. Sound tile fell from the ceiling. Avila had grown up in California and experienced many earthquakes, but the near instantaneous "BOOM" indicated some kind of explosion. Everyone was stunned. The instructor opened the door and smoke rolled in.

"Everybody get out," she shouted. Avila grabbed his backpack and followed the crowd into the hall. There was not a sense of panic, but everybody moved earnestly. As the smoke increased, the rumors started that an aircraft had hit the building. That really unnerved everybody, and they evacuated the building. Then the sirens went off and people started to panic. Avila was not that familiar with the building but made his way back to his new office. He was briefed on what had just happened. He was stunned but called his wife and told her that he was all right, but would be home late.[24]

His office was chaos with phones constantly ringing and people coming and going. Outside, local police, fire departments, and emergency services from the local area responded within just minutes, mirroring the massive response in New York City. Military personnel from within the building and local bases also swarmed to the scene. Wounded persons were immediately treated and dispatched via ground ambulance to local civilian and military hospitals. The ambulances formed in long lines. While waiting for patients, many doctors who had accompanied the ambulances joined the growing medical effort outside the stricken building. Civilian, police, and military helicopters landed in every open area to offer their services. The overall emergency response to both catastrophes was a mix of local, state, and federal jurisdictions that were dealing with combined airplane crashes, fires, and whole or partial building collapses. Since the incipient event in both cases was determined to be terrorist attacks, the United States reacted. When the Secretary of Defense directed that the nation move to Defense Readiness Condition 3, the national airspace was closed and all nonemergency civilian aircraft were ordered to land.[25]

The Department of Justice was the lead agency in charge of the response. Military support for New York was provided under the Joint Forces Command. The Military District of Washington, reporting directly to the Headquarters, Department of the Army, provided the military response to the Pentagon in support of the local authorities.[26]

Operations

MEDEVAC Response

The nearest MEDEVAC unit to the Pentagon was located 12 miles south at Davison Field on Fort Belvoir, Virginia. Detachment 1 of the 148th Med Co (AA), Washington, DC ARNG, received a call from the Military District of Washington requesting launch of MEDEVAC helicopters to the Pentagon. Within an hour, three aircraft had been launched. However, local civilian emergency medical teams, civilian helicopters, and military ground ambulances were handling the casualties. The 148th crews returned to Davison Field, but kept aircraft and crews on alert for the next 72 hours.[27]

Col. Scott Heintz was at the National Guard Bureau Headquarters in Falls Church, Virginia, working with the Army Staff on aviation transformation issues. There was a break in the meeting and everyone was watching TVs positioned in the hallways and the coverage of the breaking news of the planes flying into the Twin Towers. Two Captains ran downstairs and announced to the group that they had just watched—from their window—a commercial airliner fly into the Pentagon, less than 3 miles away. Everyone was stunned. The meeting was cancelled. Heintz immediately drove to the Office of The Surgeon General to offer help. When he subsequently discovered that all civilian aircraft were grounded, he realized that he would not be returning home to Tampa, Florida, for several days and volunteered to work in the operations center in The Surgeon General's office until he could get a flight home.[28]

Col. Pauline Lockard was attending a Command and Staff meeting in the Surgeon General's Office. One of the staff officers came in and reported to Peake (The Surgeon General) that an airplane had just flown into the World Trade Center in New York City. Based on that sparse report, Lockard assumed that it was some kind of pilot error. Then the staff officer interrupted the meeting again with the news of the second aircraft. The Surgeon General suspended the meeting just as they heard the explosion at the Pentagon.

Lockard's husband was a U.S. Marine Corps officer and worked in the Pentagon. She immediately tried to call him on his cell phone but could not make contact. Then she had to subordinate her personal concerns as she and the rest of the Office of The Surgeon General staff were immediately overwhelmed with the momentous events swirling around them and the nation. She recalled that, "Around [2 PM] my husband contacted me and indicated he was ok, so my focus then shifted 100% to what needed to be done to support the situation. …I wanted to be right on the ground to help but knowing the Surgeon General needed his staff to be prepared to shift in any direction, I had lots to do."[29]

Other ARNG units also reacted. In New York, one of its aviation battalions located at Rochester was being converted to what would later become the 249th Med Co (AA). Lt. Col. Chris Holiday, who was the commander, quickly ran a unit recall and locked down the facility. The unit was just beginning its transition, but his troops reported in. Several who lived outside of New York went to some personal expense to report. They were keyed up and prepared for any orders. The unit was not tasked initially to respond, though, and Holiday dismissed them.[30]

Statewide, other armories also filled with Guardsmen reporting for duty. When New York Governor George Pataki declared a state of emergency and signed an order directing 8,000 Guardsmen to report for active duty, they rapidly formed into task forces and departed by convoy to New York City. They maintained security lines, guarded airports, set up medical collection points, constructed emergency shelters for evacuees, and did just about whatever they were asked to do. Other Guardsmen from Maryland and Virginia performed similar tasks around the Pentagon. Fewer were needed because of the large military population in the building, which was composed of many with honed emergency skills.[31]

The nearest MEDEVAC unit to New York City was the 1159th Med Co (AA), New Hampshire ARNG. Within one hour, they had five helicopters and crews at the main facility in Concord. However, they were not called either.[32]

For the next several days the 112th Med Co (AA), Maine ARNG, launched several crews to perform numerous state missions such as pipeline patrols and forest fire surveillance until the Federal Aviation Administration reopened the national airspace to civilian and other nonfederal aircraft.

In Oregon, Matt Brady was driving to work. In his civilian capacity, he was a guard for the Oregon Department of Corrections and had just been transferred to a new correctional facility. He heard the reports on the radio as he drove to the new site. Like most people, he assumed that the first strike was an accident, but when the second aircraft hit, he immediately sensed that the combined event was an act of war. He rushed into the building when he arrived at work, found a television, and stood transfixed as the tragic scenes unfolded. He intuitively knew that he and his unit, the 1042d Med Co, would be directly affected by what he was watching. They had not been home from Bosnia very long and he had not finished unpacking. "Why bother?" it now occurred to him. He knew that he would soon be back in uniform.[33]

Multiple governmental and civilian agencies began mounting steadily growing responses to these devastating events. Avila as the Director of Military Support Operations diligently stayed abreast of the fast-moving developments and expected to get requests to order in MEDEVAC units. The necessary legal instruments under various laws and Army Regulations were in place. However, the Director of Military Support Operations did not receive any requests from the Department of Justice or the Federal Emergency Management Agency for MEDEVAC support.[34]

The troops in the field units were also stunned by the prophetic events. Maj. Bob Mitchell had taken command of the 507th Med Co (AA), at Fort Hood in July 2000, after serving three years as a personnel officer in the U.S. Army Personnel Command and then attending the Army Command and General Staff College at Fort Leavenworth. He was on alert duty that morning and had just done an aircraft engine run when he was called on the radio and told that he might want to come in and see a "weird" television news report about some kind of accident in New York. He was standing in operations watching the news reports when the second airplane hit.

Soldiers were immediately keyed up as they anticipated some "serious butt kicking" to happen soon. The news also solved a bit of a morale problem that Mitchell had with his unit. When he first arrived, he directed a series of readiness drills to ensure that his unit was ready on short notice to deploy. Normally, the 507th was not designated to deploy early in any contingency. Mitchell knew that, but felt that it spawned a bit of a lackadaisical attitude. He had spent a lot of time at Fort Bragg and was used to the "sense of urgency" that was the calling card for the units of the XVIII Airborne Corps. His drills were met with a lot of carping. All of that ended as the news from New York and then the Pentagon spread throughout the unit.[35]

Maj. John Lamoureux was in his office at Fort Sam Houston with the television on in the background when the first reports appeared. Listening to the initial comments that a small plane had hit one of the Twin Towers, he immediately noticed that the weather was clear. Then he saw a close-up shot of the impact hole in the building and realized that the tower had been hit by something larger than a small plane. As a career pilot, none of this made sense. He was watching when the second plane hit and knew immediately that this was a premeditated attack on the United States.

Kiley was at a conference in Florida. His senior staff was having a routine meeting led by the Chief of Staff, Col. Frank Blakely. Lamoureux entered the meeting and briefly announced what had transpired. Then he had the news coverage piped in on the video teleconferencing screen. The staff discussion switched to the ongoing events. A short time later, Fort Sam Houston, like all military installations, received a FLASH message from the Pentagon announcing the crash of the aircraft there and directing all bases to immediately go to Force Protection Condition Delta, which meant that the entire base had to be secured. The staff meeting then became a planning session to determine how to do this at Fort Sam Houston. They also had to keep Kiley briefed on developments via cell phone as he and his aide drove the 11 hours back to the base in a rental car because of the cancellation of all air traffic.

Fort Sam Houston, in existence since 1845, had grown up side-by-side with San Antonio and their road structures were completely integrated. Fort Sam Houston was a completely open post and had never been totally secured. Over the next several hours, approximately 26 vehicle and pedestrian access points were either locked down or secured with military police, members of the command band, and soldiers attending various courses at the medical schools there.[36]

At Fort Polk, Louisiana, Capt. John Fishburn, a MEDEVAC pilot with the 717th Med Co (AA), New Mexico ARNG, was on a training flight and preparing with a detachment from his unit for deployment to Kosovo as part of KFOR 3B. The situation in Kosovo had been steadily improving, and he and his fellow Guardsmen anticipated a relatively smooth deployment and tour. His flight was abruptly terminated, though, when the tower controller called him and ordered him to return to base. When he queried the controller, he was informed of the developments in New York and Virginia, and the closure of all U.S. airspace. He and the members of his unit were subsequently confined to Fort Polk. When the airspace restriction was lifted, they finished their predeployment training, and then shipped out for their tour with KFOR. As they left, they could not help but wonder if this was just the beginning of a much longer and larger effort.[37]

Maj. Mike Pouncey was serving with the 498th Med Co (AA) on deployment in Bosnia with Task Force Eagle under SFOR 10. He remembered these events clearly:

> I remember that day like it was yesterday. I was walking back to the Task Force Med Eagle area of the compound and remember seeing about 15 people in a horseshoe formation around someone's door. I could tell by the look on everyone's face that something wasn't right, so I walked up right after the first plane hit the first tower and I remember seeing the smoke coming from that tower and the report of a plane crashing into the building.... We knew...we knew the easy, relatively stable deployment environment we were enjoying 10 minutes prior, was over. Prior to 9-11, we flew up to New York ...in order to put our aircraft on the ship for deployment [to Bosnia]. The port was right there in New Jersey - just a mile or so south of the Statue of Liberty. I couldn't help but think to myself as I watched all those people jump to their death... If we could have been there, we might have been able to save a few from the roof. It only took a matter of minutes before the call went out to take off our soft caps and go to full battle-rattle (meaning, put on all your gear). At that time, we didn't know if we were about to be attacked either.[38]

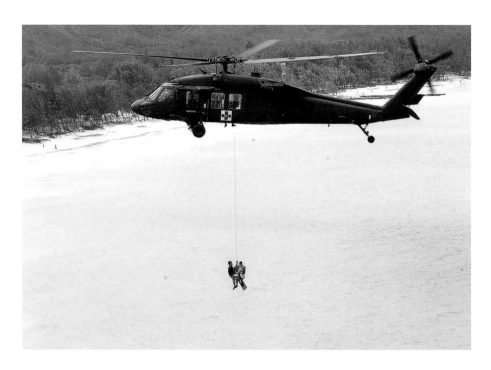

MAST. A 68th Med Co performing a beach rescue on Oahu in 2003.
Source: U.S. Army.

A Path to War

That evening, President George W. Bush addressed the nation regarding those horrible events, by stating:

> Today, our fellow citizens, our way of life, our very freedom came under attack in a series of deliberate and deadly terrorist acts. …Thousands of lives were suddenly ended by evil, despicable acts of terror…The pictures of airplanes flying into buildings, fires burning, huge structures collapsing, have filled us with disbelief, terrible sadness, and a quiet, unyielding anger. These acts of mass murder were intended to frighten our nation into chaos and retreat. But they have failed; our country is strong…A great people has been moved to defend a great nation. Terrorist attacks can shake the foundations of our biggest buildings, but they cannot touch the foundation of America…America and our friends and allies join with all those who want peace and security in the world, and we stand together to win the war against terrorism.[39]

Nine days later, President Bush addressed a joint session of Congress. He said:

> On September the 11th, enemies of freedom committed an act of war against our country…All of this was brought upon us in a single day – and night fell on a different world, a world where freedom itself is under attack.

Americans have many questions tonight. Americans are asking: Who attacked our country? The evidence we have gathered all points to a collection of loosely affiliated terrorist organizations known as al Qaeda…Our war on terror begins with al Qaeda, but it does not end there. It will not end until every terrorist group of global reach has been found, stopped, and defeated… These terrorists kill not merely to end lives, but to disrupt and end a way of life. With every atrocity, they hope that America grows fearful, retreating from the world and forsaking our friends. They stand against us, because we stand in their way.

Americans are asking: How will we fight and win this war? We will direct every resource at our command – every means of diplomacy, every tool of intelligence, every instrument of law enforcement, every financial influence, and every necessary weapon of war – to the disruption and to the defeat of the global terror network…This war will not be like the war against Iraq a decade ago, with a decisive liberation of territory and a swift conclusion. It will not look like the air war above Kosovo two years ago, where no ground troops were used and not a single American was lost in combat. Our response involves far more than instant retaliation and isolated strikes. Americans should not expect one battle, but a lengthy campaign, unlike any other we have ever seen. It may include dramatic strikes, visible on TV, and covert operations, secret even in success. We will starve terrorists of funding, turn them one against another, drive them from place to place, until there is no refuge or no rest. And we will pursue nations that provide aid or safe haven to terrorism. Every nation, in every region, now has a decision to make. Either you are with us, or you are with the terrorists. From this day forward, any nation that continues to harbor or support terrorism will be regarded by the United States as a hostile regime.[40]

The President's declarations quickly came to be labeled the "Bush Doctrine." They were incorporated into the next iteration of the National Military Strategy and fundamentally changed the way the United States would ensure its national security. Preemptive action became a strategic cornerstone of security and required a fully expeditionary force capable of rapidly imposing America's will on hostile foreign soil and then maintaining a robust presence to ensure lasting change.

The men and women of MEDEVAC joined their fellow soldiers as the nation initiated sustained combat operations in what would soon be called the war on terror. It would be a clash between two cultures: Western democratic ideals and Eastern Islamic fundamentalism. The first valued freedom, equal rights, and religious tolerance. The second was based in prejudiced hostility—especially for the United States and Israel—and the suppression of women, demonization of any religion other than Islam, and a strict adherence to radicalism that embraced terrorism and viewed death in holy war as glorious martyrdom.[41]

Chapter Nine

Again, Into Battle, 2001–2003

I want beans. I am not going to tell you how I want them cooked. I just want beans.

Lt. Col. Bryant Harp,
36th Medical Battalion[1]

Afghanistan

Intelligence reports quickly linked the 9/11 attacks to elements of an extremist organization called al Qaeda (meaning literally "the base") led by a shadowy Saudi named Osama bin Laden. As calls mounted for retaliation, intense diplomatic efforts began to isolate his influence, pinpoint him and his organization, and hold them accountable. Anticipating the President's actions, on 14 September the U.S. Congress passed a joint resolution that authorized "the use of United States armed forces against those responsible for the recent attacks launched against the United States." The Secretary of Defense, Donald Rumsfeld, immediately signed orders calling thousands of Guardsmen and Reservists to active duty. Bin Laden and a subordinate bevy of his group leaders were reported to be in Afghanistan as "guests" of its brutal Taliban regime. All signs indicated a winter combat campaign in the high terrain of that distant and little-understood nation. After reviewing options, President Bush directed the United States Central Command, commanded by Gen. Tommy Franks, to initiate a joint and combined air-ground effort that relied primarily on airpower, and—initially at least—special forces elements.[2]

Operations

Operation ENDURING FREEDOM (OEF)

Initial Engagements. Air and missile strikes began on the evening of 7 October, destroying key Taliban facilities and locations. Concurrently, Air Force C-17 heavy transports began air dropping tons of rations, signaling that the war was against the Taliban and those they harbored, not the Afghani people or nation. Twelve days later, Army Special Forces Operational Detachment Alpha teams were inserted into the northern mountains of the country, and in conjunction with teams from other U.S. governmental agencies, linked up with forces allied against the Taliban regime.[3]

The teams were an immediate conduit for the flow of direct logistical support for the allied forces. They were also authorized to direct airstrikes for the Afghanis. Equipped with sophisticated communications gear, Global Positioning System receivers and LASER (light amplification by stimulated emission of radiation) precision designators, they immediately linked with B-1s, B-52s, and a steady flow of fighter aircraft overhead systematically to demolish enemy forces. In use since the Vietnam War, these precision weapons became a staple of the American way of war. Mass production made them extremely cheap, and an almost endless supply ensued. What could be seen could be hit—and destroyed.[4]

Although the actual number of Americans fighting in Afghanistan was very small, American presence in the theater grew. A task force of about 2,000 soldiers from the 10th Mountain Division deployed to the large Karshi-Khanabad Air Base in southern Uzbekistan to provide base support and security. This task force was the first significant conventional ground force into the area.[5]

The indigenous forces in conjunction with their American advisors consistently destroyed or defeated the Taliban units that either surrendered or slipped into the high mountains along the Pakistan border. As the main cities were recaptured, more special and conventional U.S. forces moved in. United States Special Forces elements began operating also in southern Afghanistan. They were joined by a Marine Corps task force that seized a remote forward base and then the airfield near Kandahar, which they immediately began building into a main base. A company of infantry from the 10th Mountain Division task force in Uzbekistan secured a prison at Quali Jangi when prisoners there revolted. As the large former Soviet airfield at Bagram was captured, another task force of military police and engineers occupied the base, secured it, and began preparing it for follow-on operations. Effectively, the Taliban collapsed and the capital, Kabul, was captured, allowing for the formation of a new government. The enemy remnants fled to the Tora Bora region of southeast Afghanistan. Apparently, Osama bin Laden was with them.[6]

On 11 December, exactly three months after the horrible events in the United States, Hamid Karzai was sworn in as the president of the interim government of Afghanistan. Within weeks a United Nations International Security Assistance Force, ultimately consisting of 5,000 soldiers from 18 nations, began to fan out from Kabul to stabilize the nation.

MEDEVAC Units

In early 2002, the 3d Brigade, 101st Airborne Division was deployed to Kandahar to replace the Marine task force there. Its support package included one of the air assault battalions and the attached 50th Med Co (AA) Forward Support MEDEVAC Team (FSMT) consisting of 18 soldiers and three UH-60s, under the command of Capt. James Stanley. Arriving in Kandahar, the team was the first and only MEDEVAC asset in country, and it garnered high-level attention. For higher risk missions launch authority had to be obtained from a general officer, which significantly slowed down launch times. Due to limited assets, the team also performed traditional lift missions. The long-distance missions in Afghanistan caused the team to operate with long-range tanks on all flights and generally with a support UH-60 and AH-64 Apache.

The accompanying medical support slice package consisted of Task Force 261, a 40-soldier detachment from the 44th Medical Command (MEDCOM) based at Fort Bragg, North Carolina. It had attached to it several smaller medical detachments from subordinate units. The FSMT from the 50th Med Co (AA) worked directly with Task Force 261.[7]

In March 2002, a strong force consisting of indigenous and special forces and troops from the 3d Brigade, 101st Airborne Division, and recently arrived elements from the 10th Mountain Division mounted Operation ANACONDA. This effort was designed to capture or destroy enemy elements in the high terrain near the Pakistan border between the small towns of Gardez and Khowst. From 2 through 19 March the operation cleared 129 caves and 40 buildings, killed an unknown number of Taliban, and destroyed or captured vast amounts of enemy equipment and supplies.[8]

The FSMT from the 50th Med Co participated in Operation ANACONDA, the highest fight—in terms of terrain elevation—in U.S. Army history. Two aircraft from the team initially repositioned to Bagram Air Base and then moved forward to forward arming sand refueling point (FARP) Texaco to conduct MEDEVAC missions. They also occasionally flew as an aerial retransmission platform for the widely dispersed ground elements.

On 9 April, the detachment at Bagram received a nine-line MEDEVAC request to recover five patients wounded in a grenade blast suffered by a team in contact with enemy forces. Arriving at the site 40 minutes later, the medic, Sgt. George Hildebrandt, dismounted and assessed the wounded while the crew chief provided extra security. Within five minutes the three most critically wounded were loaded aboard while the two less seriously wounded waited for another inbound aircraft. Once airborne, Hildebrandt had to constantly work on all three to keep them alive. Frequently, he called on the crew chief to assist. Arriving at Bagram, Hildebrandt then directed the quick movement of all three into immediate intensive care at the forward surgical team facility. Due in large part to his quick and decisive actions, all three patients survived.[9]

After Anaconda, the team reconsolidated at Kandahar and provided general area support. On 17 April 2002, the 50th launched a crew to support Canadian

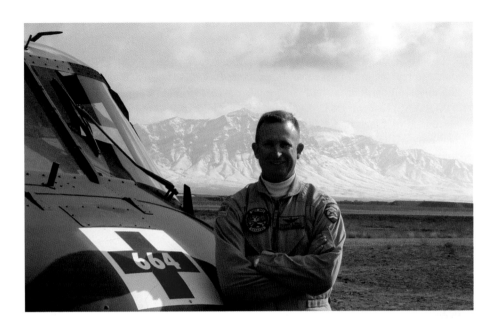

Maj. Matt Brady, 1042d Med Co (AA) Oregon ARNG in Afghanistan 2002.
Source: Matt Brady

forces when an Illinois Air National Guard F-16 dropped a bomb on 15 Canadian soldiers conducting night live-fire anti-tank exercises at Taramac Farms outside Kandahar. Four soldiers were killed and several were wounded.

Also in April, the 57th Med Co (AA) at Fort Bragg deployed an FSMT with three aircraft and 20 personnel to Bagram, and effectively split the theater effort with the 50th. It directly supported several task forces of U.S. and allied units. On 27 July a crew of pilot in command Capt. Michael Stone, co-pilot CW2 Ezekial Coffman, Medic Sgt. Frank Caudill, and crew chief Spc. Jose Peru recovered several U.S. Special Forces soldiers wounded while searching a village for weapons and enemy forces. When the MEDEVAC arrived at the incident site, the friendly forces were engaged with the Taliban. Both helicopter and fighter airstrikes were called in to suppress the enemy fire so that the pickup could be made. The entire event was a well-choreographed exercise of cool professionalism under fire that successfully recovered several wounded soldiers.[10]

After six months in the country, the soldiers of the 3d Brigade, 101st Airborne Division redeployed to Fort Campbell, Kentucky. A brigade from the 82d Airborne Division replaced them. The element from the 50th remained for another two months to support the new troops, earning the team combat patches from both divisions. When he arrived back at Fort Campbell, Stanley of the 50th wrote a detailed after-action report. In it he cited several issues:

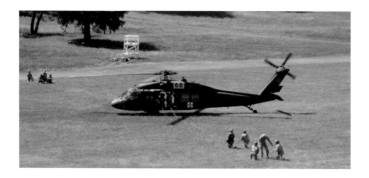

A 1042d Med Co (AA) UH-60 of the Oregon ARNG supports weekend training at Camp Rilea, Oregon. The number 68 on the side is used for identification while performing firefighting support missions, a classical state mission.
Source: Author

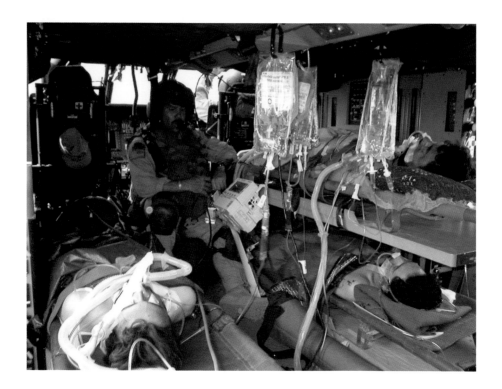

Flight medic S.Sgt. Gene Teves of the 126th Med Co (AA), California ARNG, on active duty in Afghanistan in 2003. In civilian life, Teves was a paramedic with the Sacramento Fire–Rescue Department. Many guardsmen have civilian careers that directly complement their military duties, especially in the medical units.
Source: Lt. Col. Pete Smart

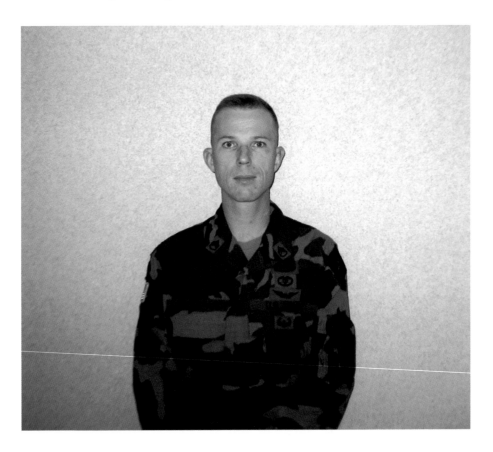

Medic S.Sgt. George Hildebrandt of the 50th Med Co in Operation Enduring Freedom.
Source: Author

1. MEDEVAC launches were delayed because of launch approval issues. At one point, approval was maintained by a Major General who was occasionally hard to contact. Launch authority should rest with the aviation brigade or battalion commander.

2. Army MEDEVAC needed to move away from its unarmed approach when functioning in combat operations. On many occasions U.S. Air Force HH-60s were used for recoveries because of the enemy threat.

3. Medics needed increased medical training to the paramedic level.

4. The medical equipment set and aid bag for MEDEVAC needed to be reassessed. The high elevations decreased the lift ability. Weight had to be reduced as much as possible, to include pulling out the carousels.

5. "A" model UH-60s did not have the power available to operate at the same level as other Army aviation aircraft.

6. FSMTs needed to be attached to the aviation battalion or brigade during combat operations.
7. MEDEVAC aircraft should be deployed to forward operating locations for better responsiveness.[11]

Col. Scott Heintz reviewed these lessons learned and recommended that an Army National Guard (ARNG) unit with UH-60L aircraft be mobilized and deployed to Afghanistan. He also recommended that because of the austere conditions in Afghanistan, MEDEVAC teams deployed there should be attached to the aviation task forces less operational control (OPCON) that would be given to the medical task force, with a 67J assigned to the medical task force operations center.[12]

In response, two FSMTs from the 1042d Med Co (AA), Oregon ARNG, replaced the teams from the 50th and 57th. Under the command of Maj. Mathew Brady, the 1042d was ordered into federal service and activated as Operation ANACONDA concluded. Initially three aircraft, crews, and support personnel were sent to Fort Bragg, where they were assigned to the 56th Medical Battalion (Evacuation) commanded by Lt. Col. Dave MacDonald.

The rest of the company joined them a month later. They assumed some base taskings and covered Army Ranger training at Dahlonega, Georgia. However, training exercises for overseas deployment consumed the majority of their time. The unit deployed the two FSMTs with six aircraft, crews, and support personnel in late July 2002 to Afghanistan. The UH-60L aircraft had the more powerful engines and were better suited to the demands of mountain flying. Replacing the 50th, the 1042d FSMTs assumed responsibility for operations at Kandahar, moved two aircraft and crews forward to Bagram, and positioned another two helicopters and crews to forward Operating Base Salerno near the Pakistan border. The crews subsequently flew more than 90 missions recovering 130 patients and logged more than 900 flight hours, 300 of which were flown with night vision goggles (NVGs). An estimated two-thirds of their patients were local children, who had been hurt by land mines or improvised explosive devices. In another incident, 1042d crews responded to the crash of a German CH-53 that was an International Security Assistance Force MEDEVAC asset and had gone down with a medical team on board. With its demise, the 1042d picked up coverage for the International Security Assistance Force, too.[13]

Brady deployed with the Afghanistan contingent and located his headquarters at Bagram where he developed an excellent working relationship with the 82d Aviation Brigade that supported his unit. The brigade commander retained launch authority over all sorties, but most often relented when Brady asked for a waiver. Although Brady appreciated the additional logistical, intelligence, and gunship support provided by the linkup with the brigade, he still wanted the unique status of a medical unit versus an aviation unit. On several occasions, his crews had to delay launching on a recovery because it took several more minutes for the AH-64s to prepare for takeoff.

A detachment of three aircraft and crews also remained at their home station in Salem, Oregon, for state taskings and firefighting duties. On 30 May 2002, the unit supported rescue operations for nine hikers involved in a terrible accident on Mt. Hood. An Air Force Reserve rescue helicopter from the 304th Rescue Squadron at Portland, Oregon, crashed trying to recover the hikers. The 1042d crews subsequently rescued the downed 304th crew, the surviving hikers, and the bodies of the three who had died in the original accident.[14]

Brady was also ordered to deploy four aircraft, crews, and support personnel to Kuwait. After activation, that contingent departed directly from Oregon to the theater. Two aircraft and crews provided general MEDEVAC support out of Camp Doha, Kuwait, for American forces in that area, and the other two were sent to the Prince Sultan Air Base in Saudi Arabia. The unit was put under Air Force control and directed to remove its crosses so that they could be used for base security surveillance missions. Both teams remained in their assignments as U.S. forces were built up in the area for action against Iraq. At one point, Brady had aircraft and crews at five different locations around the world. They all finally returned home in July 2003. As the 1042d contingent in Afghanistan departed, teams from the 45th Med Co (AA) from Germany and the 126th Med Co (AA) California ARNG, also equipped with the more powerful UH-60L aircraft, replaced it. As of this writing, operations are still ongoing in that theater.[15]

The Second Persian Gulf War

Operation IRAQI FREEDOM (OIF)

Background

When the United States led the great coalition that freed Kuwait in 1991, numerous pundits and governmental leaders felt that it was just a matter of time before Saddam Hussein would be overthrown by disparate, disaffected elements within Iraq. Almost immediately, primarily Shia groups revolted in the southern portions of the country. Very quickly after their victory, however, U.S. and coalition forces pulled back into Kuwait and could only watch as Hussein unleashed his remaining forces on the rebels and brutally suppressed them. These actions and similar ones taken in the north led to the death of tens of thousands of Shiites and Kurds, and resolidified Hussein's grip over the nation.

Encouraged by the rapid departure of the allied forces from his country and the success of his suppression of the rebels, Hussein reassumed a defiant pose toward the western powers. Once again, he began subtle but aggressive actions against Kuwait and was allegedly involved in an assassination plot against President George H.W. Bush when Bush visited the Gulf region. Hussein ordered his Air Force to fly in violation of a United Nations–imposed no-fly edict, triggering continuous patrolling of two formalized no-fly zones in northern and southern

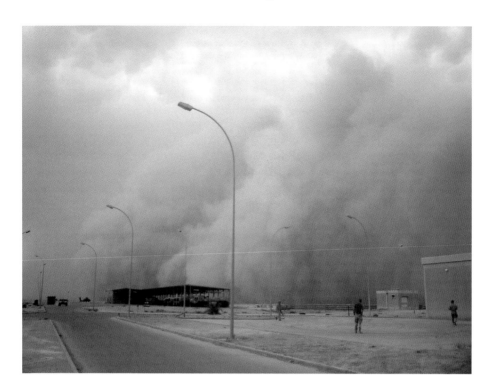

A fast moving Iraq dust storm.
Source: Lt. Col. Brad Pecor

Iraq. He also challenged these no-fly zones by ordering his anti-aircraft gunners to fire on allied aircraft patrolling the sectors.[16]

When he took office in January 2001, President George W. Bush directed his administration to review these actions. His administration determined that Hussein's hostile actions and intent and stated determination to develop and use more weapons of mass destruction or pass them to international terrorists presented a serious danger to the United States and its interests in the Gulf region. Bush addressed this threat in a speech at the United States Military Academy on 1 June 2002. To the gathered cadets, their families, faculty, and friends, he said:

> The gravest danger to freedom lies at the perilous crossroads of radicalism and technology. When the spread of chemical and biological and nuclear weapons, along with ballistic missile technology—when that occurs, even weak states and small groups could attain a catastrophic power to strike great nations. Our enemies have declared this very intention, and have been caught seeking these terrible weapons. They want the capability to blackmail us, or to harm us, or to harm our friends—and we will oppose them with all our power...

> For much of the last century, America's defense relied on the cold war doctrines of deterrence and containment. In some cases, those strategies still apply. But new threats also require

new thinking. Deterrence — the promise of massive retaliation against nations — means nothing against shadowy terrorist networks with no nation or citizens to defend. Containment is not possible when unbalanced dictators with weapons of mass destruction can deliver those weapons on missiles or secretly provide them to terrorist allies.

We cannot defend America and our friends by hoping for the best. We cannot put our faith in the word of tyrants, who solemnly sign nonproliferation treaties, and then systemically break them. If we wait for threats to fully materialize, we will have waited too long.[17]

Laid out in such stark terms, Bush's speech was immediately labeled a doctrine of preventive or preemptive war. The Army Chief of Staff, Gen. Eric Shinseki, realized that it most probably meant renewed hostilities with Iraq in addition to Afghanistan, and he accelerated preparations, although he had already ordered the Army to a wartime footing right after the attacks of 11 September.

Weighing Iraq's belligerence, its interest in producing and using weapons of mass destruction, and potential connections to international terrorist groups, Bush decided to remove Hussein and his Baathist Regime from power. He was heartened in that decision by the realization that the American people also saw Hussein and his regime as a threat, and in the face of the dramatic events of 9/11, they had lost their aversion to war casualties.[18]

While Bush made his case for war and Secretary of State Colin Powell appealed to the United Nations for diplomatic support, the commander of U.S. Central Command, Gen. Tommy Franks, directed his staff to develop the detailed plans necessary to execute the attack. As opposed to its unlimited support in DESERT STORM, Saudi Arabia put strict limits on its backing for the proposed campaign. Although Air Force and some ground units could be based in Saudi Arabia, the ground campaign would have to be mounted from Kuwait. This main attack would be mounted with three plus divisions and numerous supporting elements. Task Force Horse consisting of the 4th Infantry Division and associated support units including the 62d Medical Brigade would mount a secondary attack south out of Turkey. Additionally, the insertion of significant special operations forces into western Iraq would tie down Iraqi units there and prevent the launching of surface-to-surface rockets from the region against Israel and Saudi Arabia, as had been done in DESERT STORM. The timing of the campaign was not yet set. However, Franks wanted to initiate it as soon as possible, preferably in the cool weather of the winter months instead of the blinding heat of late spring and summer. February or March of 2003 seemed to be the most propitious time.

Combat Units. As the preparations to attack Iraq proceeded, Franks organized his forces for the operation. The Third Army, based at Fort McPherson, Georgia, and commanded by Lt. Gen. David McKiernan since September 2002, would wage the ground campaign. With the initiation of combat operations in Afghanistan, it had been task organized as the Combined Forces Land Component Command (CFLCC), as authorized under the Goldwater-Nichols Legislation passed in 1986. This was the first time that land forces were so organized. For operations against Iraq, the CFLCC commander, McKiernan, controlled two powerful units:

1. The U.S. Army V Corps, commanded by Lt. Gen. William S. Wallace, and consisting of the 3d Infantry Division (Mechanized), the 101st Airborne Division (Air Assault), two brigades of the 82d Airborne Division, the 12th Aviation Brigade, the 11th Attack Helicopter Regiment (AHR), the 31st Air Defense Artillery Brigade, and many support units.
2. The U.S. Marine Corps I Marine Expeditionary Force (MEF), commanded by Lt. Gen. James T. Conway, and consisting of the 1st Marine Division, the 3d Marine Aircraft Wing (MAW), the 2d Marine Expeditionary Brigade the 15th Marine Expeditionary Unit, the 24th Marine Expeditionary Unit, the 108th Air Defense Artillery Brigade, U.S. Army, the 1st United Kingdom Armored Division, and numerous support units.[19]

For combat operations in Iraq, the CFLCC staff was expanded with soldiers, marines, airmen, and allied officers and troops. Shortly after assuming command, McKiernan welcomed Brig. Gen. George Weightman, MC, aboard as his (first ever) CFLCC Command Surgeon. Almost immediately, Weightman deployed forward to Kuwait to serve in that capacity and also as the commander of the 3d MEDCOM (Forward). Per Joint Publication 4-02, he was responsible for the planning and execution of the medical support for the operation for that much larger patient base that Joint Publication 4-02 defined. He discovered that the initial plan, Operations Plan 1003V, needed substantial updating and modification as actual combat operations were considered.[20]

Weightman noticed that the I MEF did not have any MEDEVAC capability and requested augmentation for that purpose. As the CFLCC Surgeon, he had to find the capability for that force. Initial planning called for five MEDEVAC units to deploy to support the operation. He resolved to assign one to directly support the I MEF when the units arrived (it was one of more than 40 U.S. Army units of varying sizes that augmented the I MEF). As he requested necessary medical support units to deploy to the theater, he noticed that the Secretary of Defense was delaying his requests. This was a deliberate action because Secretary Donald Rumsfeld wanted to push combat units into the theater first, assuming that a campaign quickly initiated and conducted yielded fewer casualties and required less support. However, Weightman continuously pushed to bring his medical units forward.[21]

Medical Units. The following medical evacuation elements eventually deployed to support the operation:

- 3d MEDCOM (Forward – CFLCC)
  - 86th Combat Support Hospital (CSH)
  - 3d Medical Battalion (Provisional)
  - 804th Medical Brigade
    - 47th CSH
    - 865th CSH
    - 115th Field Hospital
    - 110th Medical Battalion (Evacuation)

- ▷ 498th Med Co (AA) (OPCON to I MEF)
- ▷ 1042d Med Co (AA) (-)
- ▷ 112th Med Co (AA)
- ▷ 159th Med Co (AA) (-)
- ▷ 437th Med Co (GA)

- 30th Medical Brigade
  - ○ 36th Medical Battalion (Evacuation)
    - ► 82d Med Co (AA)
    - ► 159th Med Co (AA) (-)
    - ► 507th Med Co (AA) (DS to 3d Infantry Division)
  - ○ 28th CSH
  - ○ 61st Medical Battalion
  - ○ 93d Medical Battalion
  - ○ 212th Mobile Army Surgical Hospital (MASH)

- 1st Medical Brigade
  - ○ 56th Medical Battalion (Evacuation)
    - ► 57th Med Co (AA)
    - ► 571st Med Co (AA) (DS to 4th Infantry Division)
  - ○ 21st CSH
  - ○ 111th Medical Battalion

- 62d Medical Brigade
  - ○ 421st Medical Battalion (Evacuation)
    - ► 54th Med Co (AA)
  - ○ 109th Medical Battalion
  - ○ 172d Medical Battalion[22]

The 101st Air Assault Division had its own 50th Med CO (AA).[23]

However, many of these units were not in place when combat operations were initiated on 20 March 2003. Only four U.S. Army hospitals were completely fielded and operating, and they only provided 500 beds for patients.[24]

As forces continued to build in Kuwait for the southern portion of the attack, the government of Turkey voted not to allow the passage of Task Force Horse through its territory to mount the northern attack. Some of the soldiers and most of the equipment of the 4th Division and support units were aboard ships in the eastern Mediterranean Sea, and Franks ordered that they be diverted to ports in Kuwait and Saudi Arabia. They were fed into the campaign as they arrived.[25]

The southern scheme of maneuver called for both the V Corps and I MEF to attack generally northwest to destroy Iraqi forces, clear the main roads and adjoining towns and cites, and capture Baghdad. Subsequent operations would send forces farther north to seize Tikrit and Mosul. Coalition special forces units would conduct supporting operations in western Iraq and another supporting operation in conjunction with the 173d Airborne Brigade and Kurdish forces in northern Iraq.

Springing forth from Kuwait, the V Corps would attack on an axis generally through the cities of Jalibah, As Samawah, An Najaf, Karbala, and then surround Baghdad. To V Corps' right, the I MEF would use the British forces to clear the city of Al Basrah and also sweep generally northwest to surround Baghdad from the east, and then be prepared to continue operations to the north as needed.

More than 1,800 U.S. and allied fighter, bomber, and support aircraft were standing by to support the offensive unit. Arrayed at airfields across the region and aboard aircraft carriers in the Gulf region, a portion of these forces had actually been in action against Iraq almost continuously since the imposition of the no-fly-zones over Iraq after DESERT STORM.

Intelligence sources indicated that Hussein believed an extensive air campaign would precede any allied ground attack, as had occurred in DESERT STORM. Sensing an opportunity to achieve at least operational surprise, Franks decided to initiate the ground campaign with the forces in Kuwait before the initiation of an air campaign. He would do it in March, before the heat had significantly built up.[26]

Conflict

On 17 March, President Bush addressed the nation. He gave Hussein and his sons, Uday and Qusay, 48 hours to leave Iraq, explaining that, "Their refusal to do so will result in military conflict, commenced at a time of our choosing." Hussein immediately responded with his own appearance on television saying, "This will be Iraq's last great battle with the malicious tyrant in our time, and America's last great war of aggression, too."[27]

Actual combat operations began on 19 March, when special forces elements entered Iraq at several locations. However, the actual initiation of the larger campaign was triggered not only by precise planning, but also a perceived fortuitous combination of events. In the early morning hours of 20 March 2003, the Central Intelligence Agency indicated that Hussein and his two sons were gathered with possibly other key national leaders at a compound southwest of Baghdad called Dora Farms. Franks was prepared for such an opportunity to decapitate the regime in one bold action, and he ordered the launch of 39 Tomahawk Cruise Missiles into the site, followed by two F-117s, each dropping two 2,000-pound bombs. Unfortunately, Hussein and his compatriots were not present. Franks then ordered the offensive to begin. Within hours, V Corps and I MEF task forces crossed into Iraq and allied fighters and bombers were striking targets all over the country. In response, Iraqi forces launched cruise missiles at the locations of the headquarters for both the CFLCC and the I MEF. Little damage was sustained at either location, but all troops had to quickly don their chemical suits.[28]

Within 24 hours, the 3d Infantry Division moved into Iraq and had lead elements operating near Al Najaf. The 5th Regimental Combat Team from the 1st Marine Division seized the vital Rumaylah Oil Fields near Safwan, while its 7th Regimental Combat Team destroyed several Iraqi units, secured three oil pumping stations, and seized the Al Basrah Airport. The I MEF then passed control of that area to British forces and turned northwest. Almost simultaneously, British forces captured the key port of Umm Qasr and cleared the Al Faw peninsula as the Marine Division's 1st Regimental Combat Team attacked northwest to Jalibah.[29]

For the most part, regular Iraqi Army units either surrendered or ran away. As the U.S. units moved into the country, however, Fedayeen irregular units and Republican National Guard units began to present a spirited defense. Some of the attacks mounted against the lead elements of the 3d Division were almost suicidal in nature as enemy fighters in pickup trucks tried to swarm in among the armored convoys. The heavy M1 tanks were not affected, but lighter M2 Bradley fighting vehicles and trucks suffered losses and casualties mounted.

In the rapid movement forward, many towns and cities had been by-passed. More Fedayeen forces sprang forth from them to intercept and attack the large and ill-defended supply and logistics convoys now moving forward to support the rapidly advancing heavy forces. In one particularly bloody encounter near An Nasiriyah, these forces isolated and captured a convoy of soldiers from the 507th Maintenance Company, killing several and taking six others prisoner. Their pictures were shown on television. Marines who then rushed in to try and free the prisoners were embroiled in a particularly nasty fight with more Fedayeen who dressed as civilians, who pretended to surrender and then opened fire. They used the local populace as shields and attacked out of schools, hospitals, and mosques. They quickly learned and exploited the American rules of engagement and mounted suicide attacks against security checkpoints.

After an intense engagement near Samawah, Capt. Clay Lyle, a cavalry officer with the 3d Division, reported that, "Several hundred Hussein loyalists had recently arrived in Samawah and had taken over the town … and the fighters had moved into the schools and occupied the mosques. Iraqi soldiers who failed to demonstrate sufficient determination were being executed. Townspeople were being pressed into service against the U.S. troops."[30]

The marines of the I MEF continued to fight northwest along Routes 1 and 7, fighting sharp battles at An Nasiriyah, Ash Shatrah, Ar Rifa, and Ad Diwaniyah. These marines faced still resistance as they fought and eventually crossed the Tigris River at An Numaniyah and Al Kut on 2 and 3 April, respectively. From there, Baghdad was 90 miles northwest.[31]

On the night of 23–24 March, the 11th AHR launched a two-battalion attack against the Republican Guard Medina Division located a few miles northeast of Karbala. The enemy used cell phones and flashing lights to signal the advance of the helicopters and alerted the considerable enemy air defenses located in the villages and towns in the region. Every aircraft in the attack was damaged. One AH-64 was forced down and the crew was captured. Task Force Gabriel, the personnel recovery task force including MEDEVAC helicopters, was with the 11th AHR but did not respond to the downed aircraft because the recovery aircraft had not been refueled at an intermediate Forward Operating Base (FOB) set up for the operation.

Reviewing the debacle, Wallace said, "Deep operations with the Apaches, unless there's a very, very, very clear need to do it, are probably not a good idea."[32]

For the next two days, the battle area was encased in the "Mother of all Sandstorms" (MOASS, as the troops quickly dubbed it), with winds routinely as high as 50 knots. Aviation units were grounded, and even ground vehicles had a hard time traveling. The storm was interspersed with rain showers, which made it worse.

Said one soldier as he tried to dig out a stuck vehicle, "It's raining mud!"[33]

The Aviation Brigade of the 101st Division did a detailed review of the attack of the 11th AHR and mounted a second and more successful raid against enemy formations just north of Karbala, destroying 47 enemy vehicles and crewed weapons and suffering only one damaged AH-64.[34]

The enemy forces adjusted their tactics, too. They used the cover of the severe sandstorms to mount close-in individual attacks. More troubling, the enemy began to detonate bombs placed along roads or in derelict vehicles. These hellish creations were quickly named "improvised explosive devices," or more simply, IEDs. Commanders also noticed that the populace was not rallying to the allied forces as had been predicted.

Reviewing the first two weeks of operations, the V Corps commander, Lt. Gen. William Wallace, commented that the Iraqis were "not the enemy we war-gamed against."[35]

Wallace realized that changes in tactics were necessary. He resisted the temptation to pull back his armored units to provide convoy escort. Instead, he brought forward strong task forces from the 101st and 82d Divisions to clean out the Fedayeen pockets in the cities and towns and provide overall rear-area and main-supply-route security forces.

The efforts allowed supplies and sustenance to flow forward to the lead task forces of the 3d Division as they steadily destroyed the Iraqi elements being pushed back toward Baghdad. Heavy battles were fought to secure Samawah, Najaf, Karbala, and Al Hillah.

In western Iraq, special forces units worked closely with U.S. Air Force, Navy, Marine, and allied airpower steadily to decimate Iraq units and prevent the area from being used to launch missile strikes against other nations in the region. Concurrently, Turkey allowed U.S. and allied aircraft to transit its airspace, and a task force consisting of the Italy-based 173d Airborne Brigade and strong special forces units parachuted into northern Iraq. Reinforced with a company-plus of M1 Abrams tanks and supported by thousands of air strikes using precision weapons, this strong force linked up with Kurdish Peshmerga fighters to tie down significant enemy units along the "Green Line," thus preventing their movement south to reinforce their countrymen in the looming climactic battle for Baghdad.[36]

By early April, the 3d Infantry Division had fought through the Karbala—Al Hillah Gap and approached Baghdad. On 4 April, its lead brigade seized the Baghdad International Airport (BIAP) on the southwest edge of the metropolitan area. To the east, the lead elements of the I MEF crossed the Tigris River and closed in on Baghdad from that side, before engaging and destroying a Republican Guard Division dispersed in the suburbs of the capital. The 173d Airborne Brigade and attached elements in the north broke through the "Green Line" and prepared to seize Mosul and Tikrit. All forces closed in on the remnants of Hussein's regime now squeezed within its last bastion in Baghdad.

On 5 April, a reinforced armor battalion from the 3rd Infantry Division attacked into the heart of the capital and then withdrew. Two days later, a 3d Division heavy brigade conducted a "Thunder Run" into the western sector of the city and then formed into defensive laagers. The enemy response was ferocious. Mayhem broke out as Iraqi soldiers and—apparently—civilians assaulted the American units with every conceivable weapon that they could bring to bear, including suicide bombers who rushed up to the tanks and personnel carriers in vain attempts to destroy them and their soldiers inside. Firing was continuous as the Americans held their ground, expending vast amounts of ammunition and calling in continuous airstrikes from ever-present allied fighter aircraft and attack helicopters. Despite the enemy response, the soldiers of the 3d Division steadily crept forward into the center of the city, and the lead elements of the I MEF entered from the east. Both came into full view of the international media recording the event. On 9 April, a small team of U.S. Marines and Iraqi civilians pulled down the Saddam Monument in the center of Baghdad. Almost instantaneously broadcast to the world by the now ever-present press, it seemed to signal the final end of the Saddam regime and a successful conclusion to the war.[37]

Task Forces Tarawa and Tripoli from the I MEF continued north and attacked enemy units in Baqubah, Samarra, and Tikrit, freeing seven American soldiers: five who had been taken prisoner in the ambush in An Nasiriyah, and two who were aboard the AH-64 shot down in the 11th AHR raid near Karbala.[38]

On 14 April, the press office of the Secretary of Defense in the Pentagon released a terse message that all major combat operations had ended. The campaign's casualties had been relatively light. The CFLCC declared that the U.S. Army reported 42 killed and 133 wounded, the Marines reported 41 killed and 1,521 wounded, and the British reported 19 killed and 36 wounded. As symbolic as the fall of Saddam's Monument was, however, there was no precise end to Hussein's regime, no formal surrender or treaty, cease-fire, or capitulation. For the most part, the soldiers of the various parts of the Iraqi Army and Fedayeen just deserted and went home. Many kept their weapons or stashed their armaments in weapons caches. The Iraqi national identity and infrastructure had been fragmented by the war, both physically and emotionally.

Postcombat planning attempted to address this with mop-up and reconstruction efforts. Campaign planning had assumed that the majority of the Iraqi people would welcome the invading forces as liberators and willingly support them as they removed Hussein and his supports. Experience gained in the recent combat indicated that this was not a valid assumption. Hostility was already being noticed throughout the country, and as the Iraqi military forces and even local police elements melted away, the locals massively vandalized government offices, commercial centers, and even their neighbors' homes. Only the Kurds in the north fully excised the Baathist party, maintained order, and welcomed the Americans. On 24 April, a task force from the 82d Airborne Division occupied Fallujah, a lawless Sunni city 25 miles west of Baghdad. The local populace demonstrated against the troops. Somebody fired shots that triggered a street battle. Seventeen Iraqis were killed and 60 were wounded. The demonstrations continued. Protesters hung out a sign that said, "U.S. killers, we'll kick you out." These were troubling harbingers and indications that perhaps the war was not over.[39]

Postconflict plans for U.S. forces called for a reduction to 30,000 residual troops by September. However, efforts to engage other nations to send troops for occupation duty were not very successful. Several nations agreed to small contingents, many with significant caveats as to how their forces could be used. Most notably, though, Arab countries and even India declined to participate. As the "Phase IV" reconstruction efforts began in earnest to address the drastic needs of the people and nation, crimes of violence, and then attacks on American and allied troops, contract personnel, and governmental employees steadily increased. Those who still opposed the liberation seemed to rejuvenate and reappear Phoenix-like to precipitate a guerilla war of indeterminate scope and eventually allied with the larger antiwestern elements active throughout the world. It appeared to those who understood events that perhaps this would not be a short war, but a long and involved one, with more troops, including MEDEVAC units, needed ultimately to pacify and stabilize the country.[40]

MEDEVAC Units

1042d Med Co (-) (In place in Kuwait). Capt. Brian Houston commanded the detachment of two aircraft from the 1042d Med Co (AA), Oregon ARNG. He and his troops sat alert for MEDEVAC duties as the allied forces built up in Kuwait. As the war approached and the other MEDEVAC units arrived, Houston and his troops stood down and packed up their gear and helicopters to go home. When Weightman interceded and had their orders changed, they unpacked and went back on alert. As the battle unfolded, they remained in general support under the 3d MEDCOM and flew backhaul missions in support of the other units that provided direct support to the combat units. They returned to Oregon in July 2003 for demobilization.[41]

Weightman also tried to take control of the 1042d detachment that was supporting the Air Force at the Prince Sultan Air Base in Saudi Arabia, but could not get them released from that assignment.[42]

159th Med Co (-) (In place in Kuwait). An FSMT from the 159th Med Co led by Capt. Dustin Elder had also been pre-positioned. However, it was attached to the 2d Squadron, 6th Cavalry Regiment, as part of the personnel recovery task force, Task Force Gabriel, and located at the huge Ali Al Saleem Air Base in Kuwait. Elder and his troops had trained with aviation units for this mission in Germany and on deployments into eastern European nations. They used the three-ship package first tried in Albania. The command UH-60 lead followed by the security aircraft with a small infantry team onboard and special heavy crash equipment for extricating trapped crewmembers. The MEDEVAC aircraft was number three. In December, Elder was transferred to the 421st Medical Battalion (Evacuation), and his second in command, 1st. Lt. Anthony Borowski, took over the FSMT.[43]

Evacuation Battalions. At Fort Hood, Texas, the 36th Medical Battalion (Evacuation), commanded by Lt. Col. Bryant Harp, received a warning order for deployment to the Gulf region on 15 January 2003. Harp had initially enlisted in the Army and trained as a crew chief before entering the warrant officer program and attending pilot training. While serving a tour with the 498th Med Co (AA), he received a direct commission into the Medical Service Corps (MSC) in 1984. He subsequently served a ground tour with a medical company of the 2d Armored Division in DESERT STORM and then commanded the 571st Med Co (AA) at Fort Carson, Colorado. Next he served a tour as a medical planner with the Army component of Central Command, which gave him a very good knowledge of contingency plans for operations in the Gulf region. He took command of the 36th in July 2002.[44]

At home station, the 36th commanded three air ambulance units: (1) the 507th also at Fort Hood, (2) the 82d at Fort Riley, Kansas, and (3) the 571st, still at Fort Carson. The warning order specified that the 36th would deploy with the 507th Med Co (AA). Separately, the 82d would also deploy. The 571st was on a completely different order and would deploy to Turkey as part of Task Force Horse under the 62d Medical Brigade. That order was subsequently cancelled, when the government of Turkey refused to allow the deployment. The 571st eventually was diverted to Kuwait to join the southern campaign.

By early February, all 36th vehicles, equipment, and shipping containers full of Class VIII medical supplies had been shipped by rail to the port of debarkation. On 12 February, the troops of the 36th departed Fort Hood by commercial charter aircraft for the long flight to Kuwait. Arriving 26 hours later, Harp and his troops were met by representatives from the 3rd MEDCOM who helped with their initial in-processing and then moved them to Camp Udairi. The 36th was placed under the 30th Medical Brigade, with the mission of commanding and controlling the evacuation assets for V Corps. It was physically located with the 12th Combat Aviation Brigade from Germany, which provided operational and logistical support.

The 421st Medical Battalion (Evacuation) also deployed from Germany. Like the 571st, it was initially designated to support Task Force Horse, but was diverted to Kuwait with all the other units. Upon arriving, however, it was not assigned a mission and returned to Germany two months later.[45]

The 110th Medical Battalion (Evacuation) from the Nebraska ARNG was activated in February and deployed to Kuwait in April. It served under the 3d MEDCOM and eventually provided military command and control for the MEDEVAC detachment from the 1042d and the 159th Med Co (AA) and 112th Med Co (AA) when they arrived in theater. The unit returned home in August 2003.[46]

The 36th Battalion moved to Camp Doha as the 507th and 82d arrived. They were both also slated to be under the 30th Medical Brigade, but their roles had not yet been determined. All commanders assumed that air evacuation was the primary mode of movement for all casualties. The 507th was placed at Doha, and the 82nd went to Camp Arifjan. Harp got involved in the discussion about possibly putting an air ambulance company in direct support of the 3d Infantry Division. He recommended that the 507th was the best unit to do so, and the 507th received the mission.

As combat approached, Harp moved his headquarters and headquarters detachment to collocate with the 12th Aviation Brigade. This move gave him the ability to directly monitor the Army Airspace Command and Control arrangements under which his crews would operate. Harp also appreciated that the aviation brigade commander was responsible for airspace management, and he (Harp) wanted to make sure that the commander knew what the MEDEVAC helicopters and units were doing. All other Army helicopters were equipped with a new tracking device called "Blue Force Tracker." These devices were specifically designed to provide for constant real time flight tracking, and they gave the brigade the ability to quickly determine the overall aviation picture. However, the MEDEVAC helicopters had not been equipped with these devices, and their movements had to be coordinated manually, which required close coordination with the aviation units. Harp resolved that he would make a special effort to get his aircraft equipped with these devices when they returned to their home stations.

To facilitate the necessary flight coordination procedures, Harp made arrangements to have liaison personnel in the various command centers, which enabled the expeditious handling of MEDEVAC requests. His planners helped develop a plan to handle mass casualty (MASCAL) events, and they were promised the use of CH-47s configured to haul casualties if needed. The planners also developed tactics, techniques, and procedures with the aviation battle captains so that when a MEDEVAC aircraft was dispatched into an area with a significant enemy threat, an AH-64 would be concurrently dispatched without any launch delay to provide en route and on-site security.

The 82d Med Co also joined the 12th Aviation Brigade at Udairi. They were actually in a compound that belonged to the 35th Armored Brigade of the Kuwaiti Army. Working with planners at the 30th Med Brigade, Harp and his operations officer, Capt. Corey Beaudreau, developed the overall evacuation plan for the V Corps. The 507th directly supported the 3d Division. The 101st Division had its 50th Med Co (AA), but, by design, needed general support from the 36th and its companies for backhaul. The 36th maintained control of the 82d and a possible additional air ambulance unit and provided overall area general support as the campaign developed. The 3d MEDCOM remained in Kuwait and provided theater support with the 110th Medical Battalion, the detachment from the 1042d, and the FSMT from the 159th that was released from its assignment to the 2d Squadron, 6th Cavalry Regiment, for personnel recovery operations with Task Force Gabriel. That tasking went to another unit.[47]

As combat operations commenced, the 36th moved up to Tallil with the 82d Med Co. It established an ambulance transfer point called AXP Beaudreau, named after the 36th operations officer because he set it up.

As soon as Harp's crews started hauling patients, he realized that they had a communications problem. Their assigned high frequency long-range radios were not working. The FM radios were adequate, but only had a short range at the lower altitudes at which the helicopters were flying. The issued TACSAT radios worked adequately, but not all command centers nor the MEDEVAC helicopters were equipped with them. The only system that worked reliably was Iridium cell phones. Harp procured several and distributed them to his commanders, liaison officers, and as many crews as possible. Then the 86th CSH moved a hospital detachment up to Tallil and began accepting patients. As the battle developed, this became the location for all enemy wounded prisoners. To make room for them, Harp used the 82d to move the wounded U.S. soldiers back to Udairi.

All battalion-assigned helicopters monitored common "MEDEVAC" frequencies while in flight and generally diverted if they received a call from somebody hurt along the heavily used main supply routes. The battalion also routinely received requests to provide support to special forces elements operating in support of the campaign all the way from Kuwait to Baghdad.

Urgent MEDEVAC requests were answered without delay. As the operations tempo increased, Harp and his planners tried—as much as possible—to delay noncritical patient pickups so that the wounded could be gathered into larger loads and handled during the day. He also closely monitored crew usage at his units to ensure that flight safety was not compromised because of flight personnel fatigue. He was very concerned about his crewmembers flying while wearing chemical warfare suits, body armor, and survival vests. He assigned either a flight surgeon or physician's assistant to each unit with the authority to remove from the flight schedule any person that they thought was either over-tired or over-stressed. The company commander could override this decision, but only for clear operational reasons. On many occasions, too, the flight surgeon or physician's assistant provided direct psychological counseling to soldiers who were overwhelmed with what they were seeing in their work.

As the V Corps gathered its combat power near Karbala for the fight into Baghdad, the 212th MASH moved forward and set up at FOB Rams. It was a Level III medical facility with beds for 36 patients. The 82d Med Co located several aircraft, crews, and even a small maintenance team there, and picked up a direct support tasking from the 82d Airborne Division when it committed a brigade to clean out enemy elements in the key city of Samawah. Harp then took control of the 159th Med Co and moved it up to Tallil, also in the general support role. Once the 159th was established at Tallil, Harp gave it the general support mission all the way from FOB Rams back to Kuwait, while the 507th and 82d moved forward with the battle as it closed on Baghdad.[48]

When the BIAP was seized, the 507th with the 3d Infantry Division was one of the first units to move in. Harp took a small detachment from the 36th and moved it forward to co-locate with them to provide for the best possible responsiveness in the Baghdad area. A few days later, he decided to leave a liaison officer with the 12th Aviation Brigade at Tallil and move his entire headquarters to BIAP. His unit and its attached MEDEVAC companies were responsible for evacuation operations for a swath of southern Iraq spanning more than 400 miles.

498th Med Co

Maj. Greg Gentry was still in command of the *498th Med Co* (AA) at Fort Benning, Georgia, when he received a call on 24 December 2002 to alert him that his unit would deploy to Kuwait to support future operations. The official order arrived two days later. At home station, the 498th was assigned to the XVIII Airborne Corps, but the Corps was not deploying. Initially at least, the 498th was the only Corps unit slated to go to Kuwait.

Serving with Gentry as the 498th Operations Officer was Capt. Casey Clyde. He had been with the unit about nine months and was preparing them for a required deployment of four aircraft and crews to the Gulf region to support Operation DESERT SPRING, when Maj. Sean Bailey, the 3rd MEDCOM MEDEVAC officer working for the G-3 Air, called him and suggested that he go to the Gulf region for a deployment conference. When Clyde arrived, he was informed that the planned four-ship deployment was being cancelled, and the entire unit was deploying over for a larger operation. Bailey also told him that the 498th would be directly supporting a Marine Division. When Clyde returned home, he briefed Gentry, who found this information perplexing because the unit had an almost habitual relationship with the 3d Infantry Division that was already in the Gulf region.[49]

The 498th deployed in late January 2003. Clyde led the advance team with three aircraft and 42 troops aboard C-5s. The rest of the unit shipped their other aircraft by sea and then departed Fort Benning on chartered commercial air. Clyde's C-5 broke down and he and his troops arrived after the rest of the company. When the 498th arrived in Kuwait, they settled at Camp Arifjan. Initially, they were assigned to the 3rd MEDCOM pending the arrival of a medical evacuation battalion. The first three aircraft were quickly assembled so Gentry could start training his crews for desert flying and, especially, maintain their currency with NVGs. The rest of the aircraft arrived by sea two weeks later and flight training began in earnest, especially night flying. The pilots needed to become comfortable using their NVGs while flying over terrain much different than home.[50]

As the 498th crews trained, Bailey visited the unit and confirmed for Gentry that his unit was aligning under the operational control of the I MEF for the upcoming operations. Additionally, the 498th would provide general support on an area basis for all units in Kuwait as they arrived. Gentry received a set of formal orders directing the unit's assignment OPCON to the I MEF. He immediately contacted the I MEF staff to begin the necessary coordination and was directed to contact the staff of the 3d Marine Air Wing. He was informed that he would be further assigned to the Marine Air Group 39 (MAG 39) commanded by Col. Richard Spender. This unit already had six helicopter units assigned to it. It was the Marine equivalent of an Army combat aviation brigade. Gentry immediately began to establish the necessary connections to operate with them and draw upon them for general support such as security, lodging, meals, etc. The Marines did not have UH-60 helicopters, so Gentry quickly established a relationship with an

Army helicopter maintenance unit at Camp Doha for necessary Aviation Intermediate Maintenance support.[51]

At first, the Marines did not know what to do with the MEDEVAC guys. Their attitude was, "You've got to stay out of our way and not hurt yourselves." The Marines' evacuation procedure was CASEVAC and they were very proficient at bringing out their wounded on backhaul cargo helicopters. However, CASEVAC was one of many missions accomplished by the Marine lift units including the movement of KIAs. As combat operations approached, the 3d MAW commander, Maj. Gen. James Amos, developed an overall evacuation plan. He would use his CH-46s to pick up casualties at the forward aid stations and deliver them back to medical companies that were Level III facilities. The crews from the 498th would then move them to theater hospitals or to hospital ships at anchor in the Gulf region.

Gentry tried to convince the planners to use his helicopters forward. He was unsuccessful until the 3d MAW held a "rock drill" walk-through of how they would logistically support the movement of the I MEF forward into Iraq. Gentry made his case, and once Amos and his planners saw how the 498th operated, they realized that Gentry's troops were a true force multiplier and completely supported the 498th and its concept of operations. Gentry then moved his unit from Arifjan over to the Ali al Salem Air Base where MAG 39 was located. He set up his operations center right next to the MAG 39 operations center, which gave him excellent access to intelligence, operational updates, and overall battle space command and control.

As the unit commander, Gentry retained launch authority for his aircraft. Only he or Clyde would dispatch their crews. Spender did not put any restrictions on them. As the crews would report for duty, Gentry or Clyde would brief them on the weather and operational conditions under which they could launch. The pilots in command were then free to fly within those parameters. If conditions changed, either Gentry or Clyde would be immediately available for a more detailed analysis and decision. If necessary, they could then go to the MAG 39 commander for operational support or their medical commander, Weightman, the CFLCC Surgeon General, for medical support.[52]

MAG 39 and the 498th were both linked to the direct air support center (DASC) for integration into the overall operations of the I MEF. All nine-line requests for MEDEVAC would come in through the DASC. They would then be immediately passed to the 498th and shared with the Navy patient evacuation team for overall medical regulation of the patient and determination of the optimum medical facility to which the patient should be evacuated. All of the I MEF medical companies were assigned to the 1st Force Services Support Group. Clyde maintained direct contact with the patient evacuation team so that the 498th's MEDEVAC efforts were closely integrated with the CASEVAC missions being flown by the Marine lift units.[53]

Gentry then task organized his unit to support the upcoming operation. He designated his 2d and 3d FSMTs to support the 1st Marine Division. Capt. Adrian Salvetti was the overall leader for that element. Capt. John Hartman led the third

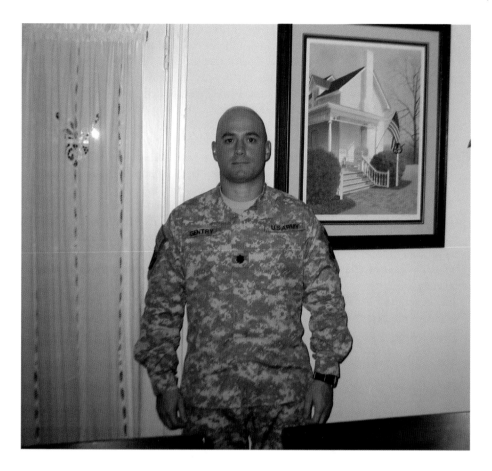

Lt. Col. Greg Gentry commanded the 498th Med Co in Operation Iraqi Freedom.
Source: Author

FSMT that supported Task Force Tarawa and the United Kingdom forces operating with the marines. The other five aircraft of the area support medical team remained behind for general support and provided spare aircraft for the FSMTs. Gentry maintained contact with his crews through the Secret Internet Protocol Router Network (SIPRNET) system.[54]

The crews would fly single-ship or obtain armed escort (if available) from the other units in MAG 39 or even fixed-wing fighters if it was necessary. The FSMTs would move forward with the combat task forces and deliver their casualties to the Level III medical facilities. The CH-46s would then be used to move them in larger numbers back to the larger theater hospitals, just the opposite of what Amos had first proposed. Subsequent movement of patients to the off-shore hospital ships would be done—as necessary—by the crews from the 1042d.[55]

Many casualties could also be carried to Fleet Hospital 3, a Level III facility that had been forward deployed to Iraq. It had 116 beds and 21 distinct surgical specialties, and was the most advanced Navy medical facility ever deployed so far forward into a combat zone.[56]

At 0600 local time on 21 March, the I MEF initiated combat operations and crossed the border into Iraq. Almost immediately, the 498th was called into action and its crews carried casualties. It was also directed to send its large tanker trucks forward to carry fuel to a temporary refueling site being set up by the Marines on Safwan Hill, a small rocky edifice located just three miles north of the border. They refueled helicopters and AV-8 Harriers in direct support of ongoing operations as the Marine task forces surged forward. Although the site only existed for a few days, the fuelers of the 498th pumped more than 100,000 gallons of aviation gas into the thirsty machines before operations moved farther north. For the next two weeks, the 498th fuelers stayed with the support units and gassed up both Army and Marine aircraft at the FARPs.[57]

As the campaign progressed, Gentry's crews displaced forward 23 times with the advancing marines, even at night. They had never trained to do this and literally developed the procedures on-the-fly and even slept in their helicopters when a lull in the action occurred. Most crews flew at 50 feet or lower, so in-flight communications were a problem. When they could, the crews talked to the Marine DASC. Gentry procured several satellite cell phones and issued them to the teams. They provided the best and most reliable way to maintain contact with the Company Tactical Operations Center (TOC).

Salvetti and his two-FSMT element collocated their six-ship team with either the "Main" or "Forward" Division Headquarters at all times to receive missions and maintain situational awareness. They worked diligently with the Marine Corps and Navy operations personnel at the division headquarters to familiarize them with the Army concept of MEDEVAC. Despite these efforts, there were attempts early on to assign classic lift missions to the Army MEDEVAC crews, including one to transport a Navy Sea, Air, and Land team. The FSMT aircrews had to be diplomatic but resolute in handling these requests. They found that if reminded, the Marine Corps and Navy Operations personnel understood that any MEDEVAC helicopter dispatched on a nonmedical or nonpriority mission was not available to evacuate critically wounded marines. This simple logic slowly permeated the thought process of the DASC and patient evacuation team personnel as the value of MEDEVAC on the battlefield was demonstrated in the large number of successful evacuations performed by the 498th. Yet among the marines on the ground, the Army MEDEVAC mission was not always understood. On one occasion, a small Marine Corps element pinned down by enemy gunfire along a main support route flagged down a MEDEVAC crew. The crew made a hasty approach to their position—thinking injured may be on the ground—despite possible enemy gunfire. At the bottom of the approach, it became clear through the marines' hand and arm signals given to the crew that they simply wanted the aircraft to make a gun run on the suspected enemy position, which was an impossibility.

Clearly the unarmed status of the Army MEDEVAC aircraft with the red crosses was not communicated to all.[58]

Even though he stayed very busy as the operations officer, Clyde flew his share of missions, including some night low visibility runs where he and his crew operated with their NVGs. On several occasions, he carried marines who were in terrible pain or near death. He remembered:

> My rule is ...try not to look back. Don't focus on what is going on in the back of the aircraft. You've got a job to do and that is to get that patient somewhere as quickly as you can.
>
> There are a few missions that really stick in my head with guys who were dying or very close to death or did die in the back of the aircraft. It sticks with you because you know that if you stop and think about it that that's the same guy who . . . He's got a family, he's got a mom, he's got a dad.
>
> If you let yourself think about it, you jeopardize the crew and the airframe.... But sometimes you've got to look back because you hear the medic in your [intercom] system. You'd hear the medic telling the crew chief, "Put pressure here! Hold this!" Sometimes the crew chief is not into it . . . He's scared. He's a nineteen, twenty, twenty-one-year-old guy who never thought he was going to be doing that. Now he is applying pressure to an amputated leg or he is bagging a patient while the medic is working on the other patient... When they chose their MOS [military occupational specialties], I don't think a lot of them figured they would be seeing things like that.
>
> Yes, there are a few missions that stick in my head. Guys dying. And even afterwards, cleaning out the back of the aircraft. ...A lot of blood ... a lot of biological matter. We brought out the pressure washer and it failed on us, so we were using 5-gallon water jugs to clean out the back of the aircraft.[59]

Salvetti and his teams received nearly all of their missions and situational awareness through the 1st Marine Division DASC. Unfortunately, the speed of the advance of American forces into Iraq made it difficult for the MEDEVAC crews to procure accurate intelligence on enemy forces. Salvetti worried about the safety and accountability of his crews as they departed on their single-ship missions because there was little he could do to mitigate the inherent risks in their mission.

The 2d and 3d FSMTs jumped between the Main and Forward Division Head-quarters locations 17 times during the 30-day Marine Corps advance to Baghdad. The intensity of this constant movement was a test of endurance for the aircrews. Everybody flew; Gentry himself flew 34 MEDEVAC missions. The two division headquarters were not designed to support or sustain aviation operations. The DASC was simply an air support coordination group, and logistical support had to be procured to facilitate the six Army MEDEVAC UH-60As frequently at their location.[60]

In a disheartening turn of events some weeks into the operation, Salvetti's team was criticized by a Fox News reporter, retired U.S. Marine Corps Lt. Col. Oliver North, for not carrying out the body of a deceased U.S. Navy medical corpsman. North later wrote a book that contains his version of the incident in an inaccurate and perhaps sensationalized account.

The 2d and 3d FSMTs crossed paths with North while stuck at an FARP during the murky aftermath of the MOASS [Mother of all Sandstorms]. No aircraft could fly that day because of the extremely poor visibility. Luckily all six of the team's aircraft assembled at the FARP that morning to wait out the weather with several other Marine Corps helicopters. As soon as the weather lifted, the team planned to jump to the DASC to receive any missions that were waiting.

At one point during the day, Salvetti was informed that one of the pilots in command on his team had just had a discussion with a Marine aviation crew regarding a KIA held by a Marine Corps CH-46 also stuck at the FARP. The MEDEVAC crew had not taken possession of the KIA. Salvetti understood that one of the missions of the CH-46s in the area was to transport remains. As Salvetti discussed the situation with another pilot, CW3 Barnett, North approached their position.

North explained that he was flying with a CH-46 crew that had a very important mission and had to leave and had no time to transport the KIA and that it would be "a shame if they had to leave him on the side of the road." Salvetti listened but did not offer to take the KIA because it was clear no aircraft were going anywhere that day and did not feel it necessary to debate mission priority with a reporter.

In North's written account of the exchange he claims the FSMTs' aircraft were full of supplies and food headed for the rear. However, this was false. One of six aircraft carried the team's supplies that were meant to sustain the team as it advanced forward with the division headquarters. All other aircraft were mission ready. North also suggested a dramatic exchange between Salvetti and himself. However, according to Salvetti, it never occurred.[61]

The next day the CH-46 crew flew forward and dropped off the KIA at another FARP. Once the MEDEVAC team flew forward and established contact with the DASC, one crew went back to the FARP and transported the KIA rearward. During the conflict the 498th moved KIAs as directed.

The day after the sandstorm turned out to be the busiest flying day of the war for the 2d and 3d FSMTs because many casualties had accumulated while the helicopters could not fly.

Unfortunately, the "encounter" with North spawned criticism of the 498th. In reality, the 498th provided the best medical evacuation possible for the Marines. The 498th FSMTs stayed forward without replacement throughout the conflict, and at the conclusion of the mission, there was little doubt that Army MEDEVAC was valued a great deal by the Marine Corps.[62]

However, difficulties such as this incident were minor and few in number. As the operation proceeded, the relationship between the 498th and the 1st MEF steadily strengthened. The rapid 300-mile advance tested the tentative plan for MEDEVAC support that Gentry and his staff had created. The flexibility of the company structure and the dedication of the crews showed the 498th fully capable of the mission.

Some of the 498th flight medics initially had trouble dealing with the severity of wounds that they encountered. All had been well trained for their work. But little actual combat had occurred in the past 10 years, so most of the younger troops had

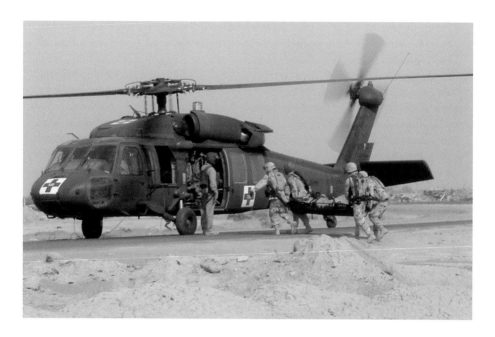

Roadside MEDEVAC in Iraq 2003.
Source: U.S. Army.

no real experience dealing with severe trauma. S.Sgt. Greg Givings was forward with Salvetti's team. With 13 years of Army service as an Army medic and his share of Military Assistance to Safety and Traffic (MAST) missions, he felt that he knew what to expect. He later remembered:

> I was very well prepared with my medical skills, but as far as being mentally prepared to see so many severely wounded patients, I don't think I was ready for that…Most of my missions consisted of marines that had either been shot, or that had been in vehicle rollover accidents. Also, I provided aid for a few enemy prisoners of war, … and maybe five or six civilians and three children. Dealing with civilians that were hit—most were females who had stepped on land mines.[63]

All of the medics learned quickly. As a team sergeant, Givings also had to watch over his younger troops as they instinctively recoiled from the shock and horror of war. After several missions, he assembled his soldiers and provoked them to express their feelings that they frequently suppressed to get their missions done.

Givings was on one mission that diverted from a flight forward when the crew spotted a fuel truck that had turned over and was hanging on the edge of a ravine. One of the drivers was waving frantically and pointing to the truck cab. As the pilot hovered the aircraft, Givings jumped off and ran to the marine. He was okay, but told Givings that the other driver was pinned in. The two of them extricated the second driver from the cab just before the truck fell into the ravine. During his time in Iraq, Givings cared for many wounded marines and civilians. This was the one time that he actually believed his actions directly saved someone's life.[64]

Some of the crew chiefs also had difficulty adjusting to the realities of MEDE-VAC work. Trained as helicopter mechanics and responsible for maintaining the aircraft, all learned very quickly that they had duties beyond caring for the machine. First, they were also crewmembers with designated duties such as providing an additional set of eyes to scan for external threats: towers, power lines, other aircraft, enemy fire, etc. They had to stay on the intercom system at all times and monitor the communications flow between all crewmembers and, sometimes, external agencies. Second, they had to acquire a basic set of medical skills so that they could effectively serve as the backup medic in case the primary was wounded or was just overwhelmed with critically wounded patients.

Spc. Robert Dahlen was a 22-year-old crew chief and also forward with Salvetti's team. He remembered his initial exposure to MEDEVAC:

> This was my first dealing with MEDEVAC, and I had no clue…I had no idea what my job was, what I was supposed to do if I was supposed to help out with the medical part, with the medic and the patient. It wasn't until I got over there and sat down with some of the medics and we had little classes, they walked me through the crew brief on how to load patients into the carousel…We had a kind of crash course on combat life saving, stick an IV, just basic stuff.

> The first time I was helping somebody, we picked up seven guys that walked into a minefield, a bunch of Navy guys. Two of them had lost their legs and three or four had a bunch of shrapnel, just miserable guys…We only had room for four litter patients in the litter pans and two ambulatory patients able to sit down in our seats. So one of my pilots said, "Well, let's run half of them down to Kuwait and we'll come back up and get the other guys." I told him, "I don't think that it is a good idea, sir…If I was in their shoes I wouldn't want to be split up right now, I'd want to stay with my guys. Get them in and we will work something out."

> Me and the medic gave up our seats, and I took a cargo strap and strapped one guy sitting down with his back against the wall…I just didn't feel comfortable splitting these guys up. It was just a good feeling …I am doing something that is important and that helps.[65]

On 4 April, the bulk of the 498th moved 250 miles forward with MAG 39 and its squadrons to a temporary air base called "Three Rivers" near Al Kut. That dramatically cut their reaction time for MEDEVAC missions in the Baghdad area. The 498th directly supported the I MEF until the company was relieved and shipped home on 10 June. They did not have any personnel killed or wounded, or aircraft shot down, although several did take hits from small arms fire.

There were aircraft maintenance challenges. The maintenance officer, Capt. Tom Mallory, later stated that the biggest single problem was broken windscreens—caused by the blowing rocks thrown up by rotor blast of helicopters taking off and landing. Also, the blowing sand played havoc with the engines, rotor blades, infrared jamming devices, and electrical wiring and components. Overall, the maintenance platoon did an outstanding job of keeping the aircraft flyable. For the previous three years, the 498th had won the Army Master Readiness, Operational Readiness Award. The unit's performance in the desert reinforced these honors.[66]

The 498th evacuated 740 patients, including 126 enemy prisoners and 118 Iraqi civilians. Most were delivered to Marine medical companies or the Fleet Hospital 3. Throughout the operation Clyde maintained contact with the 3d MEDCOM operations section and tracked the location of U.S. Army Level III facilities. On a few occasions, his crews crossed command boundaries to deliver critically wounded marines to Army hospitals so that their wounds could be more expeditiously treated.[67]

The 498th crews flew 1,600 flight hours, the majority in combat. The maintenance teams performed superbly, in many cases dispatching on short notice to forward locations to fix aircraft and return them to duty. The unit was well recognized for its outstanding work and received the Navy Presidential Unit Citation for the tour. All soldiers of the 498th proudly wear the 1st Marine Division patch on their right shoulders.[68]

For the soldiers of the 498th, the deployment was a powerful and bonding experience. Salvetti later recorded:

> I will always remember the folks I was with, especially the 30 days when the major portion of the fighting was actually going on. The crew I flew with, us four individuals, that's always going to be a real crisp, clear memory. And...the first time we ever went into Iraq, ...I remember looking at those guys and going, "Okay, this is the real thing."[69]

112th Med Co

Another MEDEVAC unit sent to the Gulf region was the ***112th Med Co*** (AA) from the Maine ARNG. Commanded by Maj. Mark Sullivan, the unit was activated in February 2003 and processed for deployment at Fort Drum, New York. The unit then flew to Kuwait, arriving on 28 March, as the V Corps and the I MEF were engaged in heavy combat on the road to Baghdad. Arriving at Camp Arifjan, the unit was assigned to the 110th Medical Battalion (Evacuation) under the 3d MEDCOM and provided general support in Kuwait, including the transfer of patients out to hospital ships.

With the termination of combat operations in early May, the 112th moved forward into Iraq and assumed area responsibility for the area south of Baghdad down to Kuwait. The 112th maintained detachments at different times at Camp Doha and the Ali Al Salem Air Base in Kuwait, and Tallil, Ad Diwaniyah, and Al Kut in Iraq. This included some direct support to the I MEF elements as they disengaged and withdrew. The unit flew 761 MEDEVAC missions and carried 1,170 patients. While deployed, the unit was awarded the Master Readiness Award for maintaining the highest operational readiness of any aviation unit in the theater. The soldiers of the 112th returned to the United States in March 2004.[70]

82d Med Co

The ***82d Med Co*** (AA) based at Fort Riley was also alerted for deployment. It was commanded by Maj. James Schwartz, who had commissioned into the MSC in 1989 after graduating from Wofford College in Spartanburg, South Carolina. He initially served with a divisional medical company before attending flight school at Fort Rucker, Alabama. His initial posting as a MEDEVAC pilot was to the 498th at Fort Benning. Subsequently, he served with the 377th in Korea and had the requisite staff and school assignments before taking command of the 82d in June 2002.

In October 2002, Schwartz began to hear rumors that his unit would deploy to the Gulf region. This caused a bit of a morale problem because the unit had just returned from a one-year tour in Kuwait as part of Operation DESERT SPRING. However, many of the personnel who deployed—like his executive officer, Capt. Ricky Ortiz—were still with the unit, and knew how they needed to prepare the unit to return to the Gulf region. The rumors were confirmed when Schwartz received a warning order on 8 January and a deployment order four days later. The unit kicked into high gear to prepare and delivered 14 of their assigned 15 UH-60A aircraft to Beaumont, Texas, for surface shipment to the Gulf region. One aircraft was left behind because of structural damage discovered just before the deployment. Another deploying aircraft was undergoing a required phase inspection and had to complete it in theater before it could fly. Schwartz anticipated austere operations and packed lots of extra Class VIII medical supplies for his crews. The unit personnel traveled by commercial contract air from Topeka, Kansas.[71]

The troops of the 82d arrived in Kuwait on 16 February. Their equipment pulled into port a week later. Schwartz and his soldiers used the time to acclimatize and accomplish myriad tasks necessary to prepare for operations. Frustrations abounded when they hunted for individual support units to provide them with specific types of equipment or personal gear. One of the biggest difficulties was getting their Heavy Expanded Mobility Tactical Truck tankers certified to carry fuel. The unit had been required to purge them with water before shipping. Before they could be used in Kuwait to carry aviation fuel, they had to be inspected by a special laboratory, which took three weeks before all of their Heavy Expanded Mobility Tactical Trucks were released. Since the tankers were at a premium in the area, Schwartz worked around this limitation to get his helicopters and crews flying to prepare for the upcoming missions. His training requirements were not that heavy because his unit had experience in the area on the earlier DESERT SPRING deployment. Most of his pilots knew the hazards of night desert flying and brown-out landings. He did get three crews qualified to land aboard Navy hospital ships, if that was necessary. However, he could not procure the maintenance help necessary to complete the phase inspection on his 14th aircraft, which meant that it was not available for combat operations.

Once all in-processing was complete, the unit moved to Camp Doha and co-located with the 36th Medical Battalion (Evacuation) and the 12th Aviation Brigade with an associated Aviation Intermediate Maintenance battalion. The brigade provided them with intelligence, weather, and flight operations support. The 36th also supported the unit during in-processing. It also provided the unit with some cell phones that were indispensable because the troop buildup overwhelmed the base phone system.[72]

The 82d would provide general support to backhaul casualties for the 507th and the 50th as they covered their divisions, and possibly the 498th Med Co (AA), which was providing direct support to the I MEF.

The 82d Med Co effectively lost two more aircraft and crews when it was ordered to assign them to the 5th Battalion, 158th Aviation Regiment, to serve as recovery vehicles for personnel recovery missions with Task Force Gabriel. That battalion had taken over the personnel recovery tasking from the 2d Squadron, 6th Cavalry Regiment, and the 82d crews replaced the crews from the 159th so that they could join their unit, which was arriving in Kuwait. Capt. Justin Avery led the 82d detachment.[73]

Schwartz and Ortiz were very concerned about the personnel recovery tasking because their crews had never received any training on the mission. However, the aircraft and crews went to Task Force Gabriel, and the 82d went into combat, not as a 15-ship company but as an 11-ship company.

With the initiation of combat operations, the 82d operated out of Camp Doha until 24 March, when Schwartz deployed a three-aircraft package to Camp Udairi to support the 86th CSH. He also ordered a four-aircraft package with a small maintenance team and two Heavy Expanded Mobility Tactical Truck tankers and refueling personnel to the newly seized Tallil Air Base near Nasiriyah. They located next to a detachment of the 86th Combat Surgical Hospital, which was a Level III facility with 40 beds.[74]

The next day, Schwartz dispatched another five aircraft, crews, and maintenance team up to FOB Rams near Najaf. They launched just at sunset and adjusted to the almost zero illumination and the obscurant mix of dust and smoke as they flew over the barren desert. When they stopped at Tallil for fuel, they also loaded up with medical supplies and fresh blood for the flight north. Arriving at Rams, they found the landing on the crusty soil that rapidly converted to fine dust when dislodged by the helicopter downwash to be very challenging. The spotlight mounted on the nose of the helicopter helped the pilots with the landings and immediately became a priority item for night flights.

The 82d crews located with the 212th MASH, another Level III facility. When not flying, the 82d medics worked in MASH helping take care of the massive number of Iraqi civilians—some with severe trauma—who were seeking care. The Iraqi Army had shut down many of the local hospitals and told their people to go to the American units and ask for help. When the 82d medics arrived, the hospital was full. S.Sgt. Dan Ledbetter and his fellow medics helped clear out many patients to make room for anticipated casualties from the upcoming battles.[75]

The crews and helicopters of Task Force Gabriel, the personnel recovery team, were also at Rams. They saw little action except for the evacuation of one AH-64 pilot wounded on the ill-fated attack mounted by the 11th AHR. Most of their flying consisted of logistical runs to support the task force or transport VIPs. On one occasion, one of the 82d crews assigned to Gabriel spotted two soldiers left behind to guard and repair a maintenance vehicle belonging to one of the aviation units. The 82d crew contacted the aviation unit to inform it of the status of the soldiers and stayed with them until a detachment from their unit came back and picked them up. Their actions possibly precluded a repeat of the horrific events of the ambush and capture of the soldiers of the 507th Maintenance Company.[76]

Avery did launch one aircraft on 2 April to look for the pilot of a U.S. Navy F-18 that had been shot down by a Patriot Missile over Lake Razzaza, northwest of Karbala. The crew joined a large armada of U.S. Navy and Air Force air and ground units looking for the pilot. Eventually, the aircraft wreckage and pilot's body were located and recovered. In comparison, though, the troops of Avery's team posted to Task Force Gabriel were doing very little while their fellow 82d crews were constantly flying MEDEVAC missions.[77]

The 82d Med Co crew chiefs had their hands full keeping the aircraft mission ready. Routine duties were difficult enough in the austere conditions. Additionally, the wind and talcum-like sand played havoc with the windshield, wiring bundles, engines, and sophisticated electronic elements such as radios, transponders, and jamming systems. Fortunately, Schwartz included in the package sent to FOB Rams a small maintenance team to assist with the upkeep of the aircraft and give the crew chiefs a break so that they could rest when they were not flying.[78]

In addition to their maintenance duties, the crew chiefs were also crewmembers and had to perform those functions inherent in that capacity. Many had served as crew chiefs on non-MEDEVAC helicopters and were familiar with their job description. One of the critical functions was to control the approach of any personnel to the aircraft when they were on the ground. Often the aircraft settled into the soft dirt, and the whirling blades drooped down to head height. The crew chiefs had to dismount and physically block and then lead anybody approaching the aircraft.

On MEDEVAC they had to also become proficient at providing medical assistance to the medic. The reason was simple: First of all, the medic could be wounded or killed at any point, and the crew chief would have to take over. More commonly, the medic was overwhelmed with several wounded on board, or one seriously wounded patient who needed his or her immediate and continuous attention to the exclusion of the other wounded. The crew chief was medical plan B. Most crew chiefs and medics developed into a smoothly running team and anticipated each other's needs to accomplish the mission.[79]

As the 3d Infantry Division fought past Najaf, the 212th MASH began to receive casualties delivered by crews from the 507th. Once the patients were stabilized, the 82d helicopters either moved them to Tallil for more care, or tail-to-tail transferred them for further transport to the 86th CSH at Udairi, or other medical facilities as necessary. More often than not, coming out of Udairi, the 82d helicopters were loaded with class VIII medical supplies for delivery to Tallil or Rams.[80]

For communications, Schwartz tried to use the aircraft HF radios, but they would not work. This was a problem because many missions took the crews out of range for the other tactical radios that they were issued. Schwartz noticed that battalions and higher had satellite radios that worked. He requested some for his unit but was not issued any. He found that the only thing that worked with any consistency were the satellite cell phones that he had received from the 36th. They were also used with secure voice mode and became his most reliable link to his teams for everything to include passing MEDEVAC requests.

Communications were a problem throughout the operation. Many times, the crews arrived at a medical facility for a pickup only to find that the patients were not ready to go or subsequently land for a dropoff only to discover that the receiving facility had not been notified that they were coming or were expecting a different number of patients than they were carrying. Schwartz had to work through this because the long flight distance back to Kuwait meant that fewer flights could be flown. Each flight carried more patients, which required more communication properly to coordinate for proper individualized medical care. Challenges abounded.[81]

There was another problem. As his crews moved forward to more austere and remote locations, they did not have access to secure communications for intelligence updates and Army Airspace Command and Control or weather information. They had to scrounge it from whatever TOC or headquarters that they could find.[82]

Schwartz brought six sets of long-range fuel tanks for his aircraft. Because of the long distances involved, he made sure that all of the aircraft sent to Rams were equipped with the tanks so that they had the range necessary to fly back to Tallil or Udairi. As the temperatures increased, however, he had to restrict the external tank fuel load to 100 gallons each versus the full 230 gallons because of thrust limitations dictated by the heat.

On 29 March, the 2d Brigade, 82d Airborne Division, began operations to secure Samawah. At Tallil, Schwartz received a request from the 82d Division Medical Operations Center to provide MEDEVAC support for its operation. Schwartz relayed the necessary radio frequencies to use for requesting MEDEVAC and then detailed one aircraft and crew to move forward and locate with the forward support battalion medical company in direct support of the brigade. Simultaneously, he also directed the main body of the 82d Med Co to move forward to Tallil and again to collocate with the 12th Aviation Brigade, which had moved into the airfield.

As the rest of the company arrived at Tallil on 3 April, Schwartz brought forward his FSMT from Udairi and also moved his entire company up to Rams on 4 April. Then he dispatched four helicopters and crews to backhaul for the 507th now located at FOB Chickenhawk and another helicopter to support the 2d Brigade of the 82d Division at Samawah. This gave him aircraft at three locations. Additionally, three aircraft and crews from the 159th Med Co (AA) that had arrived from Germany moved up to Tallil.

For the next several days, Schwartz's crews picked up patients from the 507th in tail-to-tail transfers and either brought them to the 212th at Rams or down to Tallil, where the 86th CSH detachment cared for them, or the 159th crews further backhauled them to medical facilities in Kuwait. They also made a few point-of-injury recoveries to pick up wounded for the 82d Airborne Division. The 82d Med Co crews also responded to numerous vehicle accidents along the main supply routes used by the endless supply convoys moving back and forth. Many of these resembled the MAST missions that many had flown in the United States.

When the 3d Infantry Division seized the BIAP, the 36th Medical Battalion (Evacuation) and the 507th Med Co moved to the airport. Schwartz gave the mission to support the 2d Brigade of the 82d Airborne Division to the 159th Med Co and consolidated his entire unit at Logistics Support Area (LSA) Dogwood, 60 miles south of Baghdad, co-located with the 28th CSH. For the next several weeks, he shuttled teams of aircraft and crews to support the I MEF as it pushed Task Force Tripoli up to Tikrit. Schwartz also dispatched aircraft and crews to again support the 2d Brigade, 82d Airborne Division as it moved into western Baghdad, and even a team back down to Tallil when the 159th redeployed north.

The team sent to support the Marine Task Force going to Tikrit was Avery's detachment, recently relieved of its assignment to Task Force Gabriel. Lashing up with the task force, Avery discovered some residual ill will among the marines about the Salvetti–Ollie North incident. He assured the task force commander that his crews would provide the best support possible. Relations improved rapidly as he and his soldiers provided the task force with the MEDEVAC it needed for the drive to Tikrit. Avery and his crews were then dispatched to Al Taqaddum Air Base to support a brigade from the 82d Airborne Division as it swept through that area.[83]

On 13 May, the 82d Med Co moved six aircraft and crews to BIAP to provide general support to forces around Baghdad. However, all of the 82d Med Co elements were relieved a few days later by aircraft and crews from the 159th and then returned to Camp Arifjan in Kuwait. Simultaneously, Schwartz's aircraft and crews that were working with Task Force Tripoli were replaced by CASEVAC assets from the 3d MAW, and they also flew back to Arifjan. The soldiers of the 82d Med Co spent the next week cleaning their aircraft, vehicles, and equipment, and packed up so that they could go home in late May. During the combat portion of the operation, they had logged 1,023 flight hours and carried more than 500 patients.

However, the 30th Medical Brigade planners decided that one FSMT from the 82d Med Co needed to remain in Iraq longer to augment the MEDEVAC units in place. Avery and three full crews volunteered to stay. They were dispatched back to Tikrit where they were then parceled out piecemeal to different MEDEVAC units. Avery and his crew joined the 159th—now at BIAP—and flew with them until August, when they were finally allowed to go home.[84]

Like the other units, the troops of the 82d discovered that the harsh desert conditions were very hard on the aircraft. They only had to change out two engines, but they also had trouble with damage to the auxiliary power units, electrical systems, and windscreens. Overall, Ortiz noted that they never cancelled a mission because of nonavailability of aircraft.[85]

Schwartz was extremely proud of his 141 troops and their unselfish accomplishments. The general support mission was very challenging. They had to fly long flights to support a multitude of units. Most of their patients were backhauls, but some crews did work directly with units in enemy contact and had to do point-of-injury recoveries. Frequently, they were out of contact with anybody, especially medical units. Ortiz had difficulty on several occasions as they moved forward with getting current intelligence updates for his dispersed troops. He felt that at several points his troops' integration with aviation units was poor. However, the troops made the best of the situation and were very proud that none of their crews had a patient die while under their care.[86]

159th Med Co

As OIF approached, Maj. Art Jackson commanded the ***159th Med Co*** (AA). He had entered the Army in 1988 as a distinguished military graduate from the University of Guam. His first choice for branch was aviation, but he was given the MSC. After graduating from the basic course, he was assigned as a medical platoon leader for the 2d Battalion, 18th Infantry Regiment, 197th Brigade at Fort Benning. He was there when Hussein invaded Kuwait in 1990. Shortly thereafter, the 197th was ordered to deploy to the Gulf region as part of the 24th Infantry Division. Unfortunately, Jackson had broken his ankle and the necessary surgery to repair the damage kept him from deploying. He stayed behind as a rear detachment commander.

In the summer of 1991, Jackson learned that he was supposed to be in flight school. For some unexplained reason, he had been selected to attend right after the MSC basic course, but instead had received the orders to Fort Benning. He headed off to Fort Rucker and flight school. After graduation, he served with the Flatiron Detachment at Fort Rucker where he flew many MAST missions, and then he did a tour with the 229th Med Det (RA) at Fort Drum that included duty with a medical detachment under a United Nations tasking in Haiti in 1996. After a subsequent tour working with reserve forces in Atlanta, Georgia, he was posted to Germany and the 421st Medical Battalion (Evacuation) in 2000 as the executive officer. At this post he was selected to command the 159th.[87]

The 159th actually deployed to OIF in pieces. In October 2002, the unit was participating in a major V Corps exercise in Poland when it was ordered to deploy an FSMT to Kuwait. This was Capt. Dustin Elder and his team. Arriving in Kuwait, they located with the 2d Squadron, 6th Cavalry Regiment, and prepared for their personnel recovery tasking. Additionally, they shared MEDEVAC duties with the crews from the 1042d Med Co as the massive ground combat units arrived in Kuwait.[88]

Four months later, Jackson was working with the 421st Medical Battalion as it was preparing to be part of the northern task force when he received orders to deploy the rest of his unit to Kuwait. Within two weeks, the unit flew its 12 remaining aircraft to Antwerp, Belgium, for shipment to the Gulf region, and then the 102 unit personnel were flown to Kuwait. Assembling at Camp Doha on 13 March, the rest of the unit quickly became combat ready and was assigned to the 36th Medical Battalion. Jackson then learned that Weightman wanted his initial FSMT to stay under 3d MEDCOM control for intra-theater transfer or movement of casualties to the hospital ship off shore. Effectively, Jackson commanded a 12-aircraft company.

When the V Corps crossed the border on 21 March, the 159th started receiving

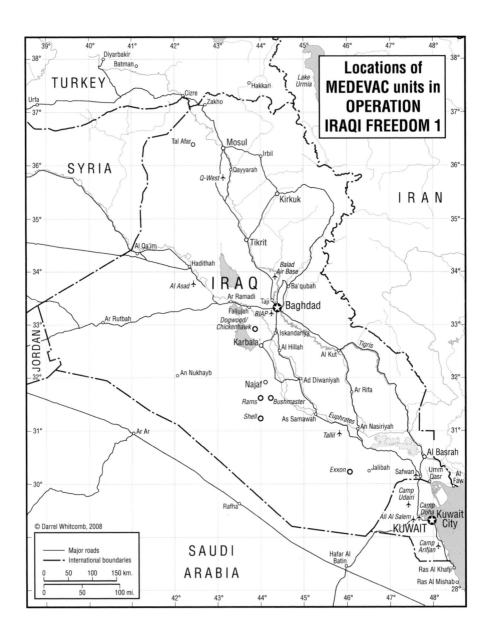

Locations of MEDEVAC units in OPERATION IRAQI FREEDOM 1

missions. They moved forward to Tallil Air Base near Nasiriyah on 27 March. They were in general support of the V Corps. When Jackson asked Harp what the 159th's mission was, Harp responded, "I want beans. I am not going to tell you how I want them cooked. I just want beans." Jackson got the message. They were the MEDEVAC swing force. They had to be ready for anything. Jackson told his troops, "Guys, this is it. We're just going to have to be ready to do whatever it is he [Harp] needs us to do and there's not going to be any excuses. I want the aircraft flying. I want the vehicles out. I want the fuelers ready. I want people ready to go."[89]

To Jackson, this general tasking made sense because he knew that the ebb and flow of the battles to come would dictate a very irregular flow of casualties. Every injured soldier was important, so they had to be ready 24 hours a day. When they started operating out of Tallil and then LSA Dogwood, north of Karbala, they received even more immediate taskings.

When the MEDEVAC helicopters flew, the crews monitored common radio frequencies. These frequencies were passed to the ground units. As more convoys were ambushed along the main supply routes, they spontaneously called for MEDEVAC on the common frequencies. Additionally, teams from the 82d and 101st Divisions operated in many dispersed locations trying to destroy the scattered Fedayeen elements. They took casualties and followed the same procedure. Therefore, Jackson and his crews received taskings through the 36th and also immediate point-of-injury requests directly from soldiers in combat. The crews of the 159th were very busy.[90]

Jackson generally maintained launch authority for his aircraft, although he did designate it to some of his more senior and experienced officers. His vast medical experience in several capacities helped him develop a sharp mental matrix for determining mission execution. He explained:

> If the medic on the ground said that this guy needed to be air-lifted well then I was not going to question that. Because I'm not there…seeing how bad this person is injured. And as long as we …had good weather, we had cleared the C2 [military command and control] — I had an aviation [liaison officer] and we would call and make sure that the skies were basically clear from anything…So as long as we cleared those two or three nodes I would go ahead and brief the mission was okay to fly. And then on some occasions depending on the risk category my Captains would have the ability to make that decision on whether or not we flew a mission. I'm talking my pretty senior Captains… I had some great Captains, guys that had been flying MEDEVAC and they'd been med platoon leaders… guys that I just had trust and confidence in based on their performance throughout their career and were totally capable of making those decisions…I mean it's the last thing you want is to see your guys get shot up or shot down. But, having been a med platoon leader in an infantry battalion and seeing guys get hurt and working in the environment and being trained on what it is that a MEDEVAC pilot does, and working with mentors that have been doing MEDEVAC for years…and then having done it in MAST missions in the past and you look back and you know what your medics are doing. Clearly that lends an enormous amount of weight to a decision on whether or not you're going to launch an aircraft to pick somebody up. The thing is, is you don't have much time. You've got to make the decision otherwise soldiers die.[91]

On rare occasions, if there was a significant risk to a mission because of weather or enemy threat, Jackson passed the launch decision to Harp. It all worked, and Jackson prided himself on getting his MEDEVAC flight airborne in seven minutes

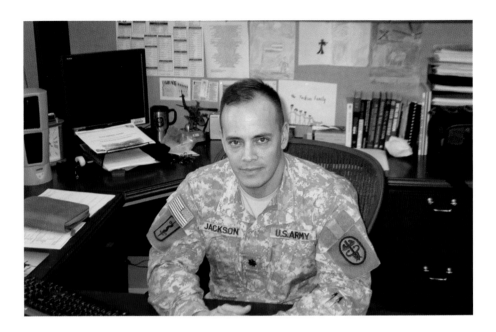

Lt. Col. Art Jackson commanded the 159th Med Co during Operation Iraqi Freedom.
Source: Author

or less. The 159th also received mission requests from the 212th MASH, and all of those also had to be cleared through the 36th.[92]

One of the youngest pilots in the 159th was 2d Lt. Tom Powell. He had just reported to the unit when they received their deployment notice and was not able to do any qualification training before leaving for Kuwait. When he arrived in Kuwait, he was initially assigned duty as a liaison officer in the S-2 section of the 12th Aviation Brigade. Before being commissioned, Powell had been an enlisted soldier and served in the intelligence field. He used that background to prepare the daily intelligence briefings and updates sent to all of the flying units on the SIPRNET.

When the 159th deployed forward into Iraq, he led the ground convoy of the unit support elements up to Tallil Air Base and then worked in the unit TOC. When the operations tempo slowed down, he started his mission qualification and was paired with CW3 Mike Hackworth, one of the unit instructor pilots, who gave him his initial aircraft and combat checkout.

One evening, Powell and another pilot, CW3 Clint Miller, were scrambled to pick up a soldier who had been shot in the face in Baghdad. Landing in the city using NVGs, they successfully picked up the soldier and headed for the nearest hospital. While the medic, S.Sgt. Eric Hartmann, worked desperately to keep him alive, the soldier died en route. Three hours later, the crew received another call to return to the same location. This time they picked up the enemy who had shot the soldier. He had been injured and captured. Without hesitation, Hartmann gave him the same level of care, and he was delivered alive for necessary medical care. On two occasions, the crew also recovered injured military working dogs.[93]

The flight medics and crew chiefs greatly impressed Powell. He remembered:

> I don't know how they do it. I swear, sometimes I'd look back and . . . [S.Sgt.] Eric Hartmann was the medic I flew with most. And I have more respect for that guy than almost anybody else I know in the military. There were several times I'd looked back and he was back there working on a patient. I mean his elbows all the way into this guy...

> I have seen him back there doing CPR on a guy who didn't have a face. The crew chief is back there trying to hold somebody's head together, trying to save his life.

He also remembered another somber detail from his deployment, the unforgettable smell of MEDEVAC. He recalled:

> [It was like] metallic blood. Mixed with—I don't know—it's like a body stench. I can't even describe it. For me, the smells are all mixed up. We would fly . . . I can still smell burning flesh. I can still smell stinky body odor. I can smell . . . there were a lot of patients back there that defecated all over the place. The fire department [would] come out and spray down our helicopters, but the smell still stuck there. The blood and guts kind of seeped under the boards, the floorboards. I don't know how else to describe the smell.[94]

After initial hostilities ended, the 159th was ordered to move to BIAP, then to Balad Air Base near Baqubah, and eventually to Mosul. In all instances, it was located with an aviation element that provided all necessary intelligence, and operational and logistical support necessary to operate. When Jackson had teams at remote sites, he made arrangements to pass all necessary data to them via the classified SIPRNET. Before returning home in April 2004, the 159th crews flew over almost every part of Iraq, logging more than 5,000 combat hours on almost 2,500 hundred missions and carrying more than 5,200 patients.[95]

507th Med Co

Maj. Scott Drennon commanded the ***507th Med Co*** (AA). He had taken over the unit from Maj. Bob Mitchell in May 2002. Drennon had entered the Army in 1988 after attending Georgia Southern University. He initially asked for military police, but there were no openings. So he selected the MSC with hopes that he would fly. At the completion of the basic course, there were no flight school slots. Instead he was assigned as a medical platoon commander with the 1st Battalion, 64th Armor Regiment, 24th Infantry Division at Fort Stewart, Georgia. Subsequently, he deployed with the division to DESERT STORM and experienced Army medicine at the ground combat level. Afterward, he completed flight training with Art Jackson, and then served with the 507th, where he flew his share of MAST missions. He attended the aviation advanced course and then did a tour as an observer/controller at the Joint Readiness Training Center at Fort Polk, Louisiana.

His next posting was in Korea where he commanded a ground ambulance company assigned to the 52d Medical Battalion (Evacuation), led by Lt. Col. Scott Heintz. He was sent to Panama to command the 214th Med Det and inactivated the unit. He also attended the Command and General Staff College at Fort Leavenworth, Kansas, and graduated in June 2000 with Mitchell. Then he moved to Fort Hood to be the executive officer of the 36th Medical Battalion (Evacuation). He held that job until February 2002, when he took command of the 507th.[96]

Later that year, the unit was notified that it would deploy a six-aircraft package to Kosovo in the spring of 2003 for a six-month rotation. In preparation, Drennon took his aircraft and crews to the High Altitude Army Aviation Training Center near Eagle, Colorado, for mountain training. When that was complete, he deployed them to Fort Irwin, California, for a training cycle at the National Training Center with the 1st Cavalry Division. Extended-range fuel systems were used there to practice long-range missions. On both deployments, he sent the three HH-60L aircraft assigned to the 507th, the newest and most advanced MEDEVAC aircraft in the fleet. These training cycles allowed the unit to get these aircraft fully certified and released for combat operations.[97]

All of that changed in February 2003 when he was notified that the deployment to Kosovo was cancelled and that within 72 hours his unit would deploy to Kuwait. Drennon and his soldiers frantically scrambled to meet the movement schedule that also required them to fly their aircraft to Galveston, Texas, to be loaded aboard cargo ships for the passage. They took the three HH-60Ls, 14 UH-60As, and their long-range fuel kits. The unit deployed with 132 soldiers plus several augmentees from the base and three highly experienced ARNG MEDEVAC pilots. All the personnel flew over on contract airliners that were now being called upon for the massive personnel movement to the Gulf region. They arrived in Kuwait in mid-month.

Theater in-processing and environmental training began immediately as they awaited the arrival of their aircraft, maintenance package, and other gear. As the aircraft arrived, the 507th troops picked them up, reassembled them, and got them flying so that the crews could accomplish their area orientations and practice desert dust landings. Drennon and his crews also discovered that the Forward Looking Infrareds (FLIR) on two of the HH-60Ls of the 507th had all been broken in the shipment. They would not be easy to fix.[98]

Weightman informed Drennon and Harp that he was going to attach the 507th to the 3d Infantry Division so that it could provide direct support to that unit. Drennon visited the commander of the 3d Division Aviation Brigade, Col. Curtis Potts, and made arrangements to attach to it. The 507th located and integrated with the 3d's battalions. This provided the 507th with all of the aviation support that it needed to operate. Very shortly thereafter, his troops were directly working with the aviation brigade planners and attending their "rock drills," as they reviewed in detail the projected flow of the campaign. Drennon also coordinated with their planners and the 36th Battalion for medical resupply, medical regulation, and patient movement.

In analyzing the projected operation from both a medical and aviation perspec-

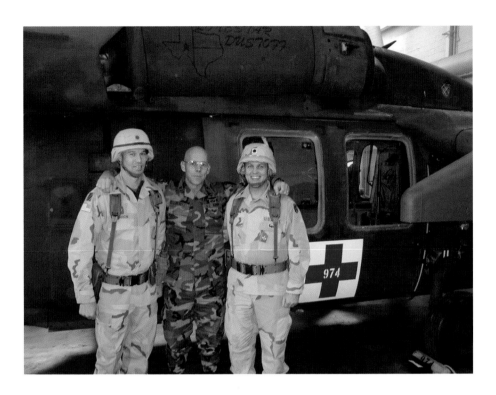

Change of command of the 507th Med Co (AA), 2002. Left to right: Maj. Scott Drennon, new commander, Col. Scott Heintz, Lt. Col. Bryant Harp, commander of the 36th Medical Battalion (Evacuation). Source: Scott Heintz.

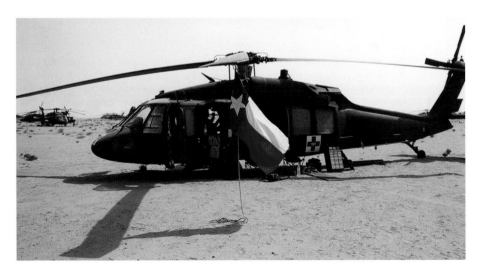

"Lonestar Dustoff," UH-60 of the 507th Med Co in Operation Iraqi Freedom 1. Source: Scott Drennon.

tive, Potts and Drennon decided not to disburse the unit as FSMTs but to keep it together. Then he could use his aircrews and maintenance teams more efficiently to provide constant coverage for anticipated significant night combat operations. His plan was simple—he put his strongest and most experienced crews on nights and his younger troops on days.[99]

Anticipating communications challenges, he coordinated with the medical companies assigned to the division combat brigades so that they could contact the 507th TOC via cell phone with their nine-line requests.

Few missions were flown by single MEDEVAC aircraft. Potts and Drennon were concerned about the enemy threat. Accordingly, Potts decided to provide escort for all MEDEVAC missions with up to two AH-64s if the threat warranted it. Drennon knew that the Apaches needed more time to prepare for takeoff, but felt that the potential threat to his crews justified the minimum delay.

To make his system work, Drennon worked through liaison officers in the division, aviation, and combat brigade TOCs. He explained:

> Because we were all together at the same location…launch authority was extremely easy. I had two LNOs [liaisons] that I kept in the aviation brigade TOC. The missions came through Iridium telephone to me or the aviation TOC and every one of the Charlie company commanders [in the forward support battalions] was given an Iridium telephone—that is how we did better in OIF than we did in DESERT STORM for comm[unications].

> I would say, for the first three weeks, I got about 70% of my MEDEVAC missions called directly to me or my ops officer over those Iridium phones because the other [communications systems] were either too busy… So I would relay those missions to the brigade TOC where my [liaison officer] was; he would tell the battle captain in the TOC "MEDEVAC mission, this is a request." They would plot it on the map, they would look at the threat, see what the threat was, and determine the best route. The Apache [pilots] were also in the TOC so my MEDEVAC PIC [pilot in command], the escort Apache [pilots] took the brief at the same time from the brigade S2, the battle captain, and the S3…[and then] they would go out to the aircraft and launch.

> Launch authority was delegated within the TOC to the S3, the battle captain, and my MEDEVAC LNO [liaison]. All had launch authority, particularly during the day. At night, the aviation brigade commander a lot of times, particularly when we had zero illum[ination] nights in the desert—he would direct serious mission analysis. The division commander delegated to him to make sure that the aviation operations were conducted safely and timely. He did, and he gave us a lot of room to do things when we needed to…Col. Potts was a great combat commander who fully supported MEDEVAC and ensured that we had the tools to accomplish the mission. It worked very well.[100]

With the other aviation elements, the 507th moved into Iraq on 21 March. It flew constant missions in support of the divisional units and relocated to Jalibah, FOB Rams near Najaf, FOB Chickenhawk north of Karbala, and finally settled at BIAP on 4 April. 2d Lt. Mark Knight led the first 507th team of two aircraft and crews into BIAP. The pilots in command were CW3 Craig Richardson and CW2 C.D. Foster. During combat, the unit flew 206 missions of which 170 were urgent. The unit carried 401 patients including 236 U.S. military personnel and 121 enemy prisoners.

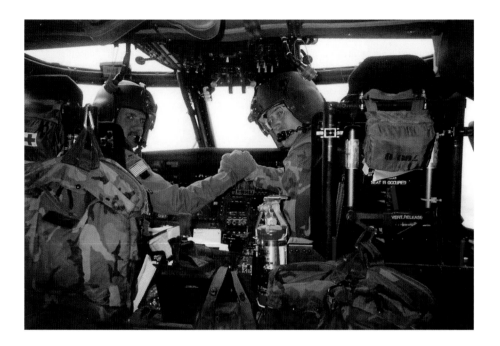

CW3 Dave McCurry and Maj. Scott Drennon of the 507th Med Co in Operation Iraqi Freedom 1.
Source: Scott Drennon

The 507th experienced the same tough maintenance challenges as the 498th. The big problems were wind and sand damage that necessitated the continuous taping of blades, seven engine changes, and the replacement of 16 infrared jamming devices, 10 windshields, and three auxiliary power units. The HH-60Ls were mission ready 95% of the time, and the UH-60As were mission ready about 86% of the time.[101]

As the campaign ensued, the evacuation distances continuously increased. Working with Harp and his soldiers at the 36th Medical Battalion, the crews from the 507th rendezvoused with helicopters from the 82nd Med Co (AA) and transferred patients to that company for transport to medical facilities in the rear areas, which maximized the presence of the 507th crews with the 3d Infantry Division as it closed in on Baghdad.

On 24–25 March, the 507th, like all other aviation units, was grounded because of the Mother of all Sandstorms. Ground ambulances had to perform all medical evacuation. Doctrinally, air ambulances are ideal, but there are still times when they cannot fly.[102]

Drennon's command and control system worked very well, but he had to draw upon his own manning to provide the TOC liaison officers. Fortunately, he had received the extra manning before deployment. In his after-action report Drennon noted:

Issue: **Location of MEDEVAC, AVN BDE vs. BCT(s)** (Sustain)

Discussion: Due to the nature of OIF combat operations during the initial combat operation (fast moving offense over great distances) it was advantageous for the 507th to co-locate and maneuver the entire company with 4th AVN BDE. This enabled us to stay within supporting distance of the BCT(s), increased our survivability, ensured reliable communications, and provided access to essential aviation products (weather, intelligence, maintenance, aviation fuel, ATO Routes, SPINS [Special Instructions], Mode 4 [IFF], etc.). Most importantly, it allowed for the integration of AH-64 escort and CASEVAC. The 4th BDE CDR was an advocate for MEDEVAC and fully supported the 507th, making us part of his team.

Recommendation: Continue to train MEDEVAC units with AVN TF during FTX(s) and at the CTC(s).[103]

Potts effusively praised the MEDEVAC effort. In an interview after the war, he stated, "I will tell you that I was very impressed with the heroism of the 507th.... Those MEDEVAC pilots were the bravest guys. ... Those were really the heroes of the battlefield."[104]

The 507th returned to Kuwait on 9 May, packaged up all of its equipment and then departed for home on 3 June. After some well-earned leave time, Drennon directed the unit to recover its equipment and address training deficiencies caused by the long deployment. Numerous personnel left for new assignments and new troops arrived. He sent several more crews to Colorado for mountain training and worked closely with his maintenance crews to repair the hard wear and tear suffered by the helicopters and other unit equipment in the harsh desert conditions. There was a certain urgency to their work because ongoing events in Iraq indicated that the 507th might have to do another tour in the theater. Drennon commanded the unit until January 2004, when he passed it to Maj. Jack Leach, and moved to Alexandria, Virginia, where he served as the MEDEVAC assignments officer at the Army Human Resources Command.[105]

50th Med Co

The **50th Med Co** (AA) deployed with its parent unit, the 101st Airborne Division (Air Assault). Maj. John Lamoureux was in command, having taken over on 26 June 2002. At that time, the unit had an FSMT with three aircraft and crews in Afghanistan as part of an aviation package to support the 101st's brigade fighting. Within days of assuming command he heard rumors of some kind of larger deployment to the Gulf region. The Afghanistan team came home in August. The 50th was still busy with MAST commitments and range coverage for Fort Campbell and Fort Knox, Kentucky. Lamoureux stepped up the unit training program—especially for his pilots—and accomplished the myriad details necessary to take his unit to combat.[106]

In November and December, the entire division conducted an exercise to prepare all units to pack and deploy on short notice. Lamoureux had to push his maintenance crews to ensure that the three aircraft that had just returned from Afghanistan were ready to go again. He also had his troops pack the shipping containers with extra carpentry tools and plywood so that they could build showers and latrines for their soldiers when they were in the field.[107]

Lamoureux was finally notified that his unit would deploy to Kuwait in February for a projected four-month tour. He was also told that the 812th Med Co (AA), a UH-1V unit from the Louisiana ARNG, would activate and a detachment from that unit would deploy to Fort Campbell to provide MAST and range support for the post and Fort Knox. Lamoureux was directed to plan and execute the swap-out. In communicating with the 812th, he discovered that their activation orders would not have them in place before the 50th deployed. He had to plan to keep some of his aircraft on alert at Fort Campbell and Fort Knox until the day before his aircraft were due at Jacksonville, Florida, for shipment by sea to the Gulf region. Working with the two bases, he crafted a plan to have civilian helicopter ambulance companies provide coverage on a contract basis for both installations between his departure and the arrival of the 812th.[108]

Once the unit was packed up and relieved of its base duties, Lamoureux had his pilots fly their UH-60A aircraft (some of the oldest UH-60s in the entire Army fleet) to Jacksonville, Florida, in two flights of six aircraft each. They made one stop near Atlanta for fuel and delivered all 12 aircraft with no en route break-downs. They were the last of the 275 aircraft from the division to arrive for the journey to the Gulf region. The pilots then returned to Fort Campbell by chartered bus. For the next several days, they finished packing the unit and put all of their ground vehicles and CONEX storage boxes aboard the chartered train. They welcomed in the arriving 812th and gave them orientation briefings and rides. On 1 March, they boarded a charter airliner for Kuwait.[109]

When they arrived in Kuwait, the troops of the 50th were transported to Camp Victory. The 159th Aviation Brigade of the 101st Division, commanded by Col. Bill Forrester, was located there, and upon arrival, Lamoureux was advised that the 50th would be attached to the 159th for the war. Additionally, each of his FSMTs would align with the aviation assault battalions supporting each of the brigades. Forrester made it very clear to his staff that the 50th would be treated as one of their own, and it would be fully integrated into their operations. This arrangement guaranteed that the 50th had the maintenance, logistical, and operational support necessary to do its job. Lamoureux was pleased and said, "It couldn't have worked better. We were always considered for all of the things we need[ed] to make our mission successful aviation wise."

Falling back on his experiences as a ground medical company commander, Lamoureux designed a simple medical support plan. He would locate his FSMTs with the medical "Charlie" companies of the forward support battalions. However, he did not do that until the Charlie company commander assured Lamoureux that he had a plan for supporting the FSMT with a place to sleep and eat and a way to get fuel for their helicopters. He also realized that—most probably—his biggest challenge would be to effectively integrate into the theater medical plan.[110]

A few days later, the 50th's first shipment of equipment arrived and it included only three helicopters. Lamoureux pushed his troops to get the helicopters flyable so that all crews could get their theater indoctrination flights. In anticipating when

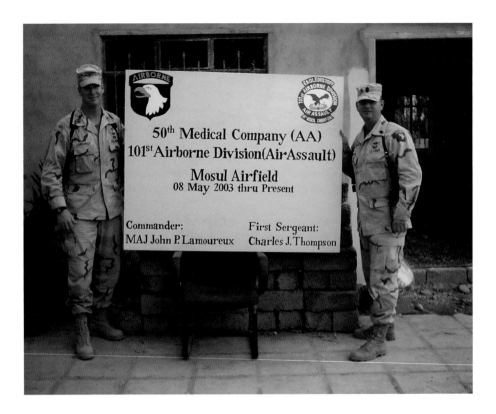

Maj. John Lamoureux and 1st Sgt. Charles Thompson of the 50th Med Co.
Source: John Lamoureux

the attack would begin, Lamoureux worked with the 36th Medical Battalion to use an FSMT from the 82d Med Co for the initial push. However, the other nine aircraft arrived before hostilities started, and the plan was scrapped. Just before the operation started, one of the aircraft had a total transmission failure and was not usable. The 50th had to go to war with 11 aircraft.

The attack on Hussein at Dora Farms signaled the initiation of the campaign. The 50th moved its TOC to Camp Udairi near the border with two FSMTs ready to fly forward. Almost immediately, Lamoureux assessed that communications would be problematic. The high frequency radios did not work. Cell phones were issued, but his unit did not receive any. His unit also did not have any of the satellite radios or the blue force trackers. Out of necessity, he located the 50th TOC with the 159th Aviation Brigade TOC and placed ground assets at the FARPs being established by the 159th Brigade as the division moved forward. This methodology was also used to procure the unit daily intelligence updates and SPINs (special instructions) updates.

The first FARP, which was called Exxon, was 155 kilometers into Iraq. The

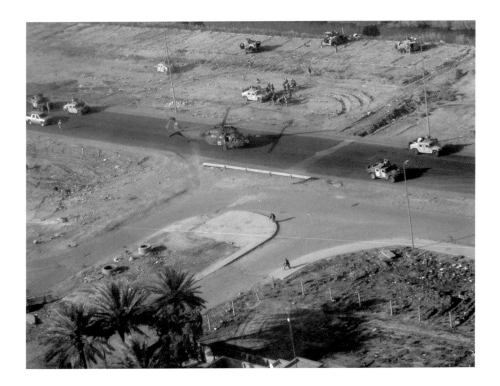

50th Med Co (AA) roadside recovery in Iraq 2003.
Source: Maj. Bill Howard

50th dispatched its first FSMT to that location to provide cover for the massive convoys moving northwest. The next day, the 159th established FARP Shell 220 kilometers farther northwest. It was not far from Objective Rams, just south of Najaf. The second 50th FSMT flew there and assumed alert. The medical company from the 626th Forward Support Battalion and a forward surgical team accompanied the second 50th FSMT. However, when the 212th MASH, a Level III facility, moved to Rams on 24 March, the 50th started taking its patients there. One week later, the 21st CSH set up another Level III facility at LSA Dogwood. Throughout the campaign, the 50th elements repositioned 14 times. The aircraft held up well, although Lamoureux noted that the maintenance trends that he saw replicated the problems of the other units, which were caused mostly by the high operations tempo, the intemperate wind, and the fine sand.

As the battle closed in on Baghdad, the 159th Aviation Brigade and the 50th headquarters moved to a small airfield near the city of Iskandariyah, 20 miles south of the capital. The 626th Forward Support Battalion and the 2d Brigade, 101st Airborne Division joined them. As the Iraqi defenses steadily crumbled and their forces capitulated, the emphasis shifted to Phase IV stabilization operations.

The 3d Brigade was ordered to Tal Afar, 250 miles to the north, to guard the Syrian border. The 1st Brigade was ordered to move to Qayyarah, 40 miles south of Mosul. Both brigades took their forward support battalions and FSMTs with them. In support, the 159th Brigade set up FARPs so that the lift helicopters and MEDEVAC aircraft could overfly the movement of all of their ground vehicles. The elements of the 50th settled into their dispersed locations with their brigades. A few months later, the 2d Brigade and support package moved to Mosul, and the division was assigned responsibility for the northern half of Iraq. It became apparent to the soldiers of the 50th that their projected four-month tour in Iraq would last longer.[111]

571st Med Co

Maj. Bill LaChance commanded the ***571st Med Co***. After he left his reserve advisor job in Salt Lake City, Utah, in 1996, he was the comptroller and then hospital company commander for two years at Landstuhl, Germany, before reporting to Falls Church, Virginia, where he was the aide-de-camp to the Surgeon General, Lt. Gen. Ron Blanck. When Blanck retired in 2000, LaChance attended the Command and General Staff College at Fort Leavenworth. After graduating in 2001, he then reported to the 10th CSH at Fort Carson until he took command of the 571st in the summer of 2002.

He had been commander of the Fort Carson-based unit for about six months when he was informed that some III Corps units were going to be deployed to the Gulf region. The 571st belonged to the 36th Medical Battalion (Evacuation), which was one of the Corps medical units, so LaChance lobbied the medical planners at the Corps. He was rebuffed in his effort. Instead, he was ordered to deploy detachments to Forts Riley, Hood, Sill (Oklahoma), and Bliss (Texas) to cover units from those bases that were deploying. In an abrupt about-face, four days later, 20 January, his unit received a warning order. The 571st would deploy as part of Task Force Horse into northern Iraq. As he prepared the unit, he received the actual deployment order one day later. His unit was ready to deploy within five days. As his troops at home station scrambled to prepare, he had the crews just dispatched to the assigned bases fly directly to Corpus Christi, Texas, for shipment.[112]

Almost immediately, the commander of the 4th Aviation Brigade of the 4th Division contacted LaChance and informed him that the 571st would locate with the brigade's 2d Battalion, the General Support Aviation Battalion (GSAB). He also found out that he would be working with the 421st Medical Battalion (Evacuation) from Germany and the 62d Medical Brigade from Fort Lewis, Washington, that would be the overall medical command in direct support of Task Force Horse.

The troops of the 571st loaded their 15 UH-60A aircraft and equipment aboard the ships. When the ships arrived in the eastern Mediterranean Sea, their helicopters sat out on the decks in shrink wrap as the Turkish government debated and then rejected access for Task Force Horse. As the troops waited back at Fort

Carson, LaChance and his crews had no aircraft to fly and all went non-current for required flight operations. LaChance had to scramble to develop training programs to keep his troops occupied and focused.

In late March, as the campaign began, the ships carrying the vehicles and equipment of Task Force Horse were ordered to steam to Kuwait and unload. LaChance and his troops departed snowy Colorado Springs in charter airlines on 30 March and arrived the next day in the 90 degree heat of Kuwait.[113]

Allied forces were heavily involved in combat operations, and their reception was at best chaotic. There was no prearranged billeting for his soldiers. LaChance claimed his vehicles from the ships, and on the first night he formed them in a circle in an empty field and had his troops sleep in the middle for protection from randomly driving convoys. The next day, LaChance checked in with the 30th Medical Brigade. He discovered that the 62d Medical Brigade, with the 421st Medical Battalion, and the 1st Medical Brigade were also arriving. Instead of lashing up with them, he was given orders *attaching* the 571st to the 4th Infantry Division. He would not work with the 421st or the 36th that was closing in on Baghdad. He would travel with the 4th Division. The 4th Infantry Division Aviation Brigade commander contacted him again and sub-attached him to the GSAB.

Subsequently, the operations officer for the 30th Medical Brigade contacted LaChance to determine his location and status. LaChance reported that the 571st was with the Aviation Brigade of the 4th Division and preparing to move out together. The operations officer told LaChance that he needed 30th Medical Brigade approval to do that. LaChance explained to the operations officer what *attached* meant and quickly obtained from him the designations and locations of all Level III medical facilities. LaChance then fully integrated with the battalion and brigade, which provided all of the maintenance, logistical, and operational support necessary to perform the mission. It was specified, though, that LaChance would maintain launch authority for his aircraft.[114]

When the 571st departed Fort Carson, it was reinforced with additional personnel from the collocated 3d Armored Cavalry Regiment, its home base parent unit. The 571st was assigned 154 troops, but left with 168 that included additional maintenance personnel and aviation officers. The unit suffered misfortune as it prepared for operations in Kuwait. As its aircraft were unloaded and reassembled, one of the crews taxied an aircraft into a light pole. All four blades and the transmission were destroyed. The aircraft was lost for combat operations pending a complete rebuild.

The 571st pressed on and departed with the Aviation Brigade on 17 April as they all flew to BIAP. The next day, the unit was scheduled to fly to Tikrit, with an intermediate stop at the Balad Air Base, 45 miles northeast of Baghdad. Before the war, Balad had been a premier Iraqi Air Base, and the 4th Division had dispatched its cavalry unit to seize it. That operation was delayed, but the crews from the 571st were not so notified. When the MEDEVAC crews landed at Balad, they only saw Iraqis, none of whom were hostile. The 571st crews remained until the cavalry troops arrived, wondering if they would get credit for "seizing" the air base. Then the crews flew the last leg to Tikrit, where the 571st set up with the 4th

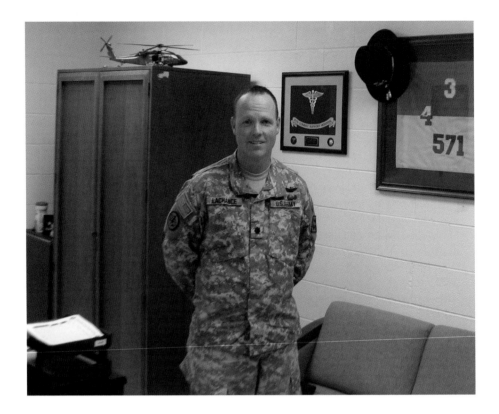

Lt. Col. Bill LaChance commanded the 571st Med Co during Operation Iraqi Freedom.
Source: Author

Infantry Division Aviation Brigade. LaChance dispatched FSMTs to each of the 4th Division maneuver brigades. The crews literally flew "top cover" as the brigades moved into Iraq and assumed their assigned sectors. The aviation brigade commander directed that all units would fly all missions as two-ship elements because of the lack of reliable communications and radar control or tracking facilities in Iraq. LaChance felt that it was not the optimum way to use MEDEVAC but did as he was told, although as the units settled in, the GSAB could occasionally supply the second aircraft.[115]

A few weeks later the 3d Armored Cavalry Regiment arrived in Iraq and was sent to the Al Anbar Province in western Iraq. Its commander, Col. David Teeples, requested that the 571st be reassigned to him. Subsequently, the unit was moved west to Al Asad Air Base to be attached to the 3d. It stayed in action until March 2004, when it was finally returned to Fort Carson.[116]

57th Med Co. As OIF began, Maj. Brad Pecor commanded the 57th Med Co (AA). Initially entering the Army in 1984 as an aviation warrant officer, he had been commissioned in 1988 and served MEDEVAC tours with the 571st Med Det, the Flatiron Detachment at Fort Rucker, the 159th Med Co, and 421st Med Battalion in Germany, including deployments to Bosnia and Kosovo. He took command of the 57th in June 2002.

The company was notified in February 2003 of deployment to Kuwait for combat duty. The unit rapidly prepared for the move. It was hectic at times as its soldiers competed with other Fort Bragg deploying units for supplies and equipment issue.

The unit deployed with the 56th Medical Battalion, still commanded by Lt. Col. Dave MacDonald, and arrived in Kuwait on 13 April. Like the 56th, the unit initially did not have an assignment. MacDonald pushed Pecor to get the unit's helicopters flight ready. When he had the first one in commission, he and MacDonald flew into Iraq and visited hospitals and medical units at several sites before MacDonald decided to move both units to Tikrit. When the rest of Pecor's helicopters were all flight ready, he and MacDonald dispatched the aircraft and a 70-vehicle convoy to move all of the equipment and personnel for the two units to that northern city.[117]

Upon arrival, the 57th crews assumed alert for area support to any units in the vicinity. A few weeks later, MacDonald changed the 57th's orders and directed it to move to the Al Asad Air Base to support the 3d Armored Cavalry Regiment as it arrived in Iraq. However, when its commander requested that the 3d be assigned the 571st Med Co because of their home base relationship, MacDonald complied

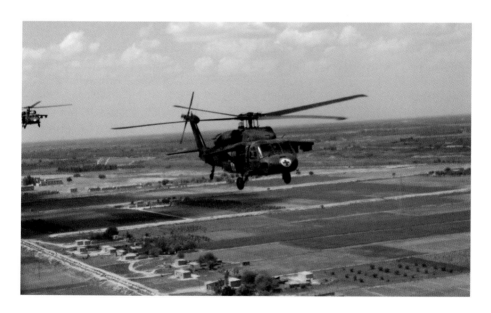

Two 57th Med Co (AA) UH-60s in flight over Iraq in 2003.
Source: Lt. Col. Brad Pecor

and redirected the 57th Med Co to return to Tikrit to be attached to the 4th Infantry Division. When the unit arrived back at Tikrit, Pecor set up his area support section and dispatched FSMTs to airfields at Tikrit south, Baqubah, and Balad. Pecor aligned his unit under the GSAB. He was satisfied with this arrangement because he was given all the help he needed and allowed to run MEDEVAC with little supervision. However, Pecor was directed to fly all missions dual-ship, with the second aircraft occasionally coming from the GSAB or Brigade. Pecor put a liaison officer in the aviation brigade TOC, which expedited the passage of nine-line requests, and then operated well with the 4th Division until ordered home in February 2004.

With redeployment orders, Pecor moved the unit back to Kuwait where the crews cleaned, packed, and shipped their equipment. Just 48 hours before scheduled departure, the unit was informed that it would stay longer. Unit morale immediately began to collapse, and Pecor convinced his troops that they had no choice but to follow orders. His next concern was to reclaim his aircraft and return them to flight status. Most of his aircraft had been badly worn down by a year of desert flying and needed significant maintenance. Fortunately, a contract maintenance team was in Kuwait and was able to answer many of their maintenance needs.

Once the aircraft were ready, the unit was placed under the control of the 429th Medical Battalion (Evacuation), a U.S. Army Reserve unit from Savannah, Georgia. Under that unit, the 57th did not need most of its support troops, and Pecor sent many of his enlisted troops home. The unit then sent detachments to Al Kut, Tal Afar, and Diwanyah, and operated under the 429th until June 2004, when they were finally shipped back to the United States.[118]

54th Med Co

The **54th Med Co** (AA) was the last MEDEVAC company to join the initial units. Commanded by Maj. Martin Kerkenbush, the unit deployed its 13 UH-60A aircraft and equipment from Fort Lewis with the 62d Medical Brigade starting in early February. Both were slated to support Task Force Horse with the 421st Medical Battalion (Evacuation), as part of the operation through Turkey. Initially slated to ship out its equipment through the port at Beaumont, Texas, with the 4th Infantry Division, the 54th Med Co was subsequently ordered to load aboard transports at the huge port at Tacoma, Washington.

When the attack through Turkey was cancelled, the 54th's equipment was also diverted into Kuwait, and the troops joined it there after flying over by commercial contract airlift in mid-April. Several members of the 54th accompanied their equipment aboard the transports and spent 72 days at sea awaiting the Turkish government's decision. When the main body of 54th Med Co troops arrived in Kuwait, the unit moved to Camp Udairi and was aligned under the 56th Medical Battalion (Evacuation).

As the V Corps and the I MEF closed in on Baghdad, the 54th deployed an FSMT that joined the 62d Medical Brigade at Mosul to provide general support to the 101st Division. The entire 54th then deployed to Balad Air Base/LSA Anaconda to provide general area support for northern Iraq. At times, the 54th Med

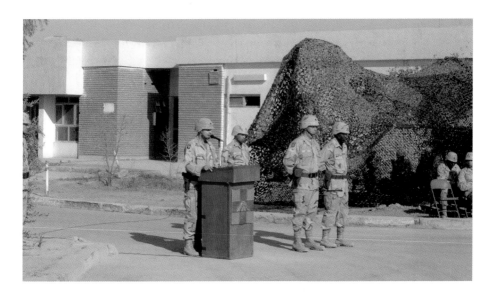

Change of command for the 56th Med Battalion, June 2003. Left to right: Lt. Col. Dave MacDonald (departing), Cmd. Sgt. Maj. George Sosa, Lt. Col. James Rice (incoming), and Col. Charles Hightower, 1st Med Brigade commander.
Source: Dave MacDonald

Co also provided specific direct support to brigades of the 101st and 4th Divisions, and special operations forces operating in northern Iraq. At Balad, the 54th Med Co set up its operations at the southern end of the air base. Some of the more enterprising unit soldiers there set up the Tiki Bar and Coffee Shop, which quickly became a popular gathering spot for the troops at LSA Anaconda.

Before returning home to Fort Lewis in March 2004, the 54th flew more than 3,700 hours, conducted 660 life-saving missions for U.S. and allied personnel, and logged 631 medical re-supply missions in support of area medical units. The men and women of the unit were justifiably proud of the great work that they had done during their long tour in Iraq.[119]

Rotation of Units

Harp traveled to the 30th Medical Brigade on 8 May 2003 for a planning update conference. Col. Donald Gagliano, the 30th commander, notified Harp that the 36th had completed its mission and the just arrived 56th Medical Battalion (Evacuation) commanded by Lt. Col. Dave MacDonald would replace it. The 36th, the 507th, and the 82d were going home. Harp saluted smartly and then ordered the 159th to move its entire unit to BIAP. When the unit assumed the mission, he directed the 507th and 82d to return to Kuwait for redeployment.

The 56th Medical Battalion (Evacuation) had arrived in Kuwait on 12 April with the 57th Med Co. It was assigned to the 1st Medical Brigade and located with the Aviation Brigade, 4th Infantry Division located at Tikrit. As the 36th Battalion, 507th Med Co (AA) and the 82d Med Co (AA) were released and sent home, the 56th assumed control of the 159th Med Co (AA), the 57th, and two ground ambulance units. The 50th was still with the 101st Division, the 571st was still at Tikrit attached to the 4th Infantry Division, the 54th was at Mosul working with the 62d Medical Brigade providing general support to several units, and the 112th remained in Kuwait and southern Iraq.

As he settled in, MacDonald met with Harp at the 36th for a theater briefing. He discovered that there was—in fact—no overall theater evacuation plan.

"I was making it up as we went," Harp explained, as the evacuation units tried their best to adjust to the movements and placements of the combat units and hospitals, which provided for the movement of soldier casualties. However, it made no allowance for humanitarian needs or the evacuation of Department of Defense civilians or contractors, members of nongovernmental or international organizations, displaced civilians, or enemy prisoners of war. MacDonald could not find an overall combat health service support plan. One subsequent lessons learned noted that:

> MED[ical] planners at all levels failed to plan as a team. The maneuver elements recognized this and began to make the medical plan on their own. We saw air ambulance teams being moved and reorganized by the maneuver elements they supported. Those moves placed duplicate efforts within minutes of each other, while other maneuver elements were left uncovered.[120]

Consequently, he and Harp developed a theater evacuation plan. MacDonald explained:

> He [Harp] and I sat down and looked at the map and he, understanding how the operational forces work, gave me that knowledge and we drew the boundaries for the areas…that are currently being used in Iraq. We briefed that, or I briefed that with Brian sitting in the audience. Col. Gagliano, [30th Medical Brigade] he checked the box and gave that to V Corps.[121]

MacDonald also had to deal with the somewhat onerous issue of the assignment of the 571st Med Co to work directly with the 3d Armored Cavalry Regiment. In May that unit arrived from Fort Carson and was assigned to the Al Anbar Province, a very dangerous sector west of Baghdad. Initially, MacDonald directed the 57th to support the 3d with nine aircraft and crews, although a regiment-sized unit was normally assigned one FSMT with three aircraft and crews. Nine more MEDEVAC aircraft from other units were available in the same area in general support. Pecor, the 57th commander, complied and moved his aircraft and crews to Al Asad Air Base. However, Col. David Teeples, the 3d Armored Cavalry Regiment commander, was not happy with that assignment. At Fort Carson, he and his unit had developed a strong habitual relationship with the Fort Carson co-located 571st Med Co, and he sent a request to the V Corps commander, Lt. Gen. Wallace, asking that the 571st be taken from the 4th Division and exchanged with the 57th. MacDonald heard about this and strongly objected. He saw no value in swapping out the two units that were settled in their very different areas of responsibility and established with their supported units. He briefed the commander of the 1st Medical Brigade, Col. Charles Hightower, and his executive officer, Lt. Col. Bob Mitchell, who concurred with his position. Hightower also tried to intercede. MacDonald followed up with a detailed background paper explaining that doctrinally, the 3d Armored Cavalry Regiment rated the support of an FSMT. The 57th supported it with the equivalent of three FSMTs. The assignment of an entire company of 14 aircraft provided an over-abundance of evacuation assets to the 3d Armored Cavalry Regiment, which meant that some other area or unit had fewer than it was authorized. He also explained that the necessary communications and administrative links were established and fully functioning, and that the 4th Infantry Division was satisfied with its present arrangement and did not support the unit swap. MacDonald also pointed out that it was also doctrinally incorrect to attach any MEDEVAC unit to a combat maneuver unit.

When briefed on the issue, Wallace concurred with the 3d Armored Cavalry Regiment request and ordered that the unit change be carried out. MacDonald saluted smartly and directed the changes. Both units had to be ready to respond to evacuation requests during the switch. Consequently, the move had to be phased out over five days and required support from the 159th and 54th Medical Companies. The units completed the move with only minor challenges. MacDonald was disheartened that the maneuver unit commanders ordered the realignment of medical units without any concern for the medical consequences of the move.[122]

Three months later, MacDonald passed command of the 56th to Lt. Col. Jim Rice, another career MEDEVAC officer, and departed for the Army War College. He was determined to return to the MEDEVAC community to resolve some of the disconnects that he saw in Iraq. While he was in Iraq, his unit oversaw the evacuation of 1,086 patients by air in 571 missions and 2,155 patients by ground ambulance. The MEDEVAC units then settled in for the long haul of stability and support operations that are still ongoing.[123]

ARNG MEDEVAC Units Activated for Continental United States Backfill

The 641st Medical Battalion (Evacuation), Oregon ARNG, was called to active duty in April 2003 and deployed to Fort Bragg to backfill the recently departed 56th Battalion. The 641st was activated for a year, and it provided military command and control to MEDEVAC teams from the 146th Med Co, Tennessee ARNG, the 1022d Med Co, Wyoming ARNG, at Fort Benning, and the 812th Med Co, Louisiana ARNG, and later, the 249th Med Co, New York ARNG, at Fort Bragg. The 641st was released from federal duty in April 2004.[124]

In actuality, several units from the base generation force were activated under Operation NOBLE EAGLE for backfill duties. The 812th Med Co (AA) was mobilized in January 2003 for a year and located at Fort Bragg, with detachments at any one time at Forts Stewart, Benning, Campbell, and Knox. At the same time, the 832d Med Co (AA), Wisconsin ARNG, was activated and subsequently deployed with 60 personnel to Fort Lewis to replace the 54th Med Co (AA). Just a month prior, the unit deployed a detachment of three aircraft and 20 personnel to Hohenfels, Germany, to support a larger training exercise, and it had to scramble to support the second tasking. Arriving at Fort Lewis, the unit assumed responsibility for base support and MAST tasking. It also dispatched three aircraft and crews to assume alert at the Yakima Firing Center in central Washington. In December, the original 60 personnel were replaced. The second crew served until May 2005, when the unit was released from active duty after 840 days of continuous service. During that time, the unit conducted 245 MEDEVAC missions, of which 48 were hoist missions. About 25% of the sorties were in support of military operations, and the rest were civilian support missions. The unit flew 3,738 accident-free hours.[125]

Also in January, the 148th Med Co (AA), Georgia ARNG, with its Detachment 1 from Washington, DC, was activated for federal service. The unit was ordered to Fort Hood to backfill for the 507th Med Co (AA) as it deployed to Iraq. The 148th was split into detachments that also eventually covered Forts Bliss, Carson, Sill, and Riley, as the MEDEVAC units and detachments at those bases also deployed.

Like so many of the ARNG units, several of the crewmembers were more senior in rank and were veterans of combat operations as far back as Vietnam. CW4 Jim Brennan was a classic example. He had flown 1,100 hours in Vietnam as a UH-1 pilot with a lift company in 1969, earning 42 Air Medals. After a break in service, he joined the Georgia ARNG in 1977, just as it was forming a MEDEVAC unit. He had served with the unit ever since, doing state activations for disaster response and federal active duty tours to support operations. His unit was not activated for Operation DESERT SHIELD/STORM. But the unit was tagged to fly hospital transfer missions for severely wounded soldiers returning to the United States for care. However, the casualties in that conflict were minimal, and the unit was not needed. The unit did provide on-call MEDEVAC and general support for the Olympics in 1996.[126]

The troops of the 148th remained at their assigned locations until February 2004, when they were released and demobilized. The unit then picked up a commitment to keep two aircraft and crews at Camp Shelby, Mississippi, on volunteer federal active duty to support Reserve Component troops receiving training there for overseas duty.[127]

In November 2003, the 249th Med Co (AA), New York and Rhode Island ARNG, was activated into federal service under the command of Maj. Marc Boies. Previously, the New York unit had been an attack battalion equipped with AH-1 Cobra aircraft. It worked through an intense transition period to meet its MEDEVAC tasking, and then the unit deployed en masse to Fort Bragg, where it was assigned to the 641st Medical Battalion (Evacuation), and eventually replaced the 812th. The unit served there and sat alert for soldier support and MAST tasking at Forts Benning and Stewart and two remote Ranger training sites until May 2005 when the unit was released from active duty. The unit flew 4,100 hours directly supporting the soldiers of the base and XVIII Airborne Corps, and it accomplished 138 MEDEVAC missions.[128]

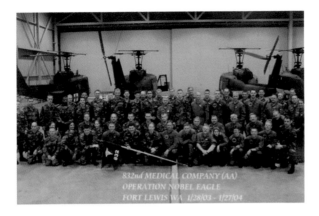

The 832d Med Co (AA), Wisconsin ARNG, mobilized and deployed to Fort Lewis in 2003.
Source: Maj. Matt Strub

* * * *

As U.S. military forces entered combat in Afghanistan and Iraq, active and ARNG MEDEVAC forces were dispatched with them. Reflecting the current joint and Army doctrine, they lined up with their medical evacuation battalions and supported the joint and combined force, evacuating whomever they were called to medically evacuate. Additionally, several more ARNG MEDEVAC units were activated for varying lengths to support various continental United States operations. These operations in both theaters and at home are ongoing.

Chapter Ten

Aviation Transformation and Domestic Operations, 2002–2005

"What does assigning Dustoff to the aviation battalion do for the patient's needs?"

Maj. Gen. (ret) Patrick Brady, U.S. Army[1]

The Aviation Transformation Initiative

Background

In the spring of 2002, Lt. Col. Pauline Lockard was serving on the Office of The Surgeon General (OTSG) staff as the assistant executive officer when she was notified of her selection for promotion to colonel. As part of that selection, she was queried as to whether she wanted to be considered for colonel-level command. She decided against it so she could do one more tour in the Army and then retire. Subsequently, the Army Medical Department (AMEDD) executive officer, Col. Bill Thresher, asked her to assume the dual positions of the MEDEVAC proponent, replacing Lt. Col. Gino Montagno who was leaving for battalion command, and the MEDEVAC consultant to The Surgeon General.

Lockard discussed this with Lt. Col. Scott Heintz, the current consultant, Montagno, and his Proponency deputy, Lt. Col. Van Joy. Heintz was already reassigned to U.S. Special Operations Command (USSOCOM) headquarters in Tampa, Florida, but asked to remain as the consultant to the Surgeon General for MEDEVAC matters. Lockard and Heintz agreed that they could work together with her as the proponent and him as the consultant, and Thresher concurred.

The Medical Evacuation Proponency Directorate (MEPD) was still at Fort Rucker, Alabama, and still reported to the AMEDD Center and School at Fort Sam Houston. Thresher and Heintz were concerned that MEDEVAC needed more visibility in the Washington area, and they told Lockard that she could set up her office in the OTSG complex in Falls Church, Virginia. Her MEPD staff would remain at Fort Rucker with its day-to-day functions directed by the deputy, Joy.

After his tour at the Joint Readiness Training Center at Fort Chaffee, Arkansas, ended in the summer of 1993, Joy had served in medical units in Panama, as an advisor to Reserve Component units at Fort Leonard Wood, Missouri, and at Fort Bragg, North Carolina, with the 56th Medical Battalion (Evacuation) and the 44th Medical Brigade. At Fort Rucker, Joy established strong relationships with his counterparts on the Aviation Center staff and handled affairs there as the MEPD deputy.

This all sounded reasonable to Lockard, and she accepted the job and arrangement. She believed that she could continue to work effectively on the OTSG staff while maintaining control over the MEPD Office and affairs at Fort Rucker through teleconferences, occasional visits, and her working relationship with Joy.[2]

She threw herself into her new job and became engaged in a plethora of medical and MEDEVAC issues including the ongoing Aviation Transformation Initiative (ATI), which included the proposals to reduce MEDEVAC companies from 15 to 12, 10, or even eight aircraft to help reduce the overall Army aviation budget. Wholesale inactivations of units—both continental United States (CONUS) and overseas—were being considered, and the AMEDD Center and School commander, Maj. Gen. Kevin C. Kiley, proposed to align MEDEVAC companies with the divisions similar to the 50th Med Co (AA) with the 101st Airborne Division.[3]

Larger efforts developed. Gen. Eric Shinseki retired from the Army in June 2003 and his successor was Gen. Peter Schoomaker, a career Special Forces soldier who had already retired from the Army and last served as the commander of USSOCOM. However, the Secretary of Defense, Donald Rumsfeld, had not been satisfied with the pace of change being set by Shinseki. With a desire to transform the Army, he had asked Schoomaker to return to duty as the Army Chief of Staff. Assuming office that summer, Schoomaker was very aware of Shinseki's initiatives and almost immediately instructed the Army Staff to convert to a modular brigade-sized force. He and a transition team developed a set of focus areas highlighting aspects of the Army that needed immediate attention to facilitate the change. Several key items emerged:

- The Army needed a better public relations program;
- Commanders had to be better prepared for the "long war"; and
- The post–Vietnam policy of putting most support elements into the Reserve Components had to be reversed.

However, the most prominent need was to reorganize the fighting forces under the modularity concept. Each of these key items became a focus area. Schoomaker directed the Training and Doctrine Command to develop a set of essential tasks for each area.[4]

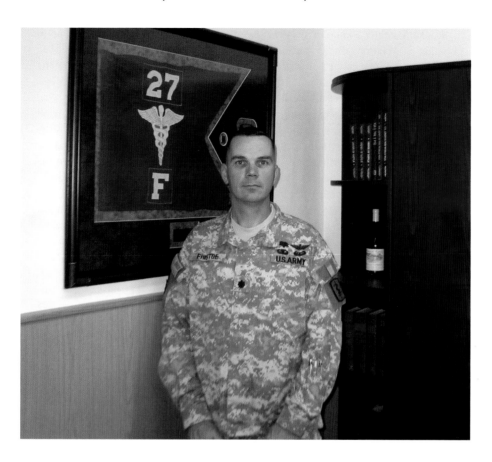

Lt. Col. Jon Fristoe as the commander of the 421st Multifunctional Medical Battalion in 2007. While assigned to the OTSG Staff, he played a key role in the Aviation Transformation Initiative.
Source: Author

Process

Responding to the chief's tasking, the commander of Training and Doctrine Command, Gen. Kevin Byrnes, organized Task Force Modularity, under the direction of Maj. Gen. Robert Mixon. The team of 50, with another 35 analytical support personnel, was drawn from across the Army to address all viewpoints. It also had representation from the regional combatant commanders and the other services. Task Force Modularity had several parallel task forces with specific areas of interest. One was Task Force Aviation, which had the lead for developing concepts and designs for aviation in the modular force. Its autonomous nature reflected the complexity of designing aviation units and concepts of use. The earlier ATI was ongoing and eventually absorbed by this effort. Its report was due by early November 2003.[5]

Lockard heard about Task Force Aviation. She called the action officer in charge, an aviation officer, and discovered that the actual task force leader was Brig. Gen. (P) James D. Thurman, an armor officer who had flown AH-64s. His assigned deputy was Brig. Gen. Edward J. Sinclair, a career Army aviation officer. They were charged to do a "holistic review of Army aviation."[6]

Before this temporary assignment, Sinclair had served as the assistant division commander for support with the 101st Airborne Division and had been with the unit during the initial phases of Operation IRAQI FREEDOM. His next assignment was as the commander of the U.S. Army Aviation Center and chief of the Aviation Branch at Fort Rucker. Sinclair maintained a close liaison with the senior aviator in the Army, Lt. Gen. Dick Cody, and had recommended Thurman to Cody as the head of the ATI project. Sinclair and Cody spoke directly several times a week, and Cody shared with Sinclair his thoughts on transforming Army aviation, especially the configuration of aviation brigades and maintenance structure.

Cody was also concerned about the integration of MEDEVAC into aviation and the fact that the MEDEVAC aircraft fleet was older than the overall Army fleet. He would act as a behind-the-scenes sounding board as the ATI progressed. Sinclair had Col. Ellis Golson working with them as the head action officer.[7]

Lockard attended the initial meeting at Fort Rucker in September. The group was too large and unwieldy, so a smaller, more select group, which included Lockard as the AMEDD representative, was identified and sequestered at Fort Monroe, Virginia, for several weeks to discuss the issues in focus teams. She was one of six colonels on the Fusion team. Her Proponency deputy, Joy, was assigned to the doctrine and training team where he worked as the only MEDEVAC person with several other aviators and a few ground officers. Of the 43 members of the overall group, they were the only MEDEVAC personnel formally assigned.[8]

Word of Task Force Aviation quickly spread through the MEDEVAC community. Several senior cohorts who wanted to be apprised of developments contacted Lockard. As a requirement for her assignment to the group, she signed a nondisclosure agreement. Consequently, although she called on her compatriots for information and advice on several occasions, she withheld discussing the task force's developments with them.

She had many other experts within the MEDEVAC community, including Lt. Col. Pete Smart, on whom she called for assistance. Smart had recently left his position as the Commander of the 45th Med Co at Ketterbach, Germany, and had moved to the Army Aviation and Missile Command at the Redstone Arsenal at Huntsville, Alabama. He was the director of the Utility Helicopters Project Office and gave her data on the composition and projected structure of the MEDEVAC fleet.[9]

Maj. Bill Goforth was also available to assist. Goforth, another career MEDEVAC officer, worked in the Army National Guard (ARNG) Surgeon's Office as its senior evacuation staff officer and executive officer. He was aware of the transformation issues and unit size reduction proposals and examined them from the ARNG perspective, ever mindful that the 16 MEDEVAC companies in the ARNG were a key part of the overall MEDEVAC force. Already ARNG MEDEVAC units were used in Bosnia, Kosovo, Afghanistan, and Iraq, and as backfill at several bases for active duty units deployed overseas. Goforth knew that any significant changes resulting from the ATI would have a great impact on the ARNG force.[10]

Maj. Jon Fristoe, the aviation staff officer in the Force Management Division on the OTSG staff, assisted Lockard on the task force. Following his tour as the commander of the 236th in Germany, Fristoe attended the Army Command and General Staff College at Fort Leavenworth, Kansas, and then reported for his staff tour.

Lockard got to know him well because he was the primary action officer for many of the issues that she tracked as the MEPD director. He had already written several of the preliminary plans for the reduction of the MEDEVAC units to as few as eight aircraft. When the ATI process started, Fristoe was concerned. He had not found any solid historical data about MEDEVAC unit operations. His instincts told him that such data were probably critical to any rational discussions of MEDEVAC matters with aviation officers. But he concluded that no process or methodology existed whereby the Department of the Army staff was informed of what was going on with the MEDEVAC units. He found an expectation that—when necessary—the MEDEVAC units "would just be there." As a former commander, he intuitively knew that the units were trained and ready to perform. However, he did not find any enthusiasm on the Army staff to modernize the MEDEVAC UH-60 fleet or any strategic analysis ongoing to determine the required size of the MEDEVAC fleet to support current or projected Army operations as directed by the wide array of contingency plans.[11]

Lt. Col. Randall Anderson, a MEDEVAC officer serving as the Aviation Staff Officer in the OTSG, had completed an excellent MEDEVAC study in May 2002. The Army G-3 directed the study under the auspices of the earlier ATI to determine which CONUS Army training sites still required Army MEDEVAC coverage and how many aircraft were necessary to provide coverage at each site. The plan also suggested alternative methods to provide quality of care and draft a CONUS installation prioritization list for the Army G-3. However, it only looked at units in the United States rather than units overseas or the overall concept of MEDEVAC operations.[12]

The exhaustive Anderson study scrutinized the previous three years of domestic MEDEVAC operations. A prioritized list of 18 forts and training sites requiring MEDEVAC support and a baseline for installation MEDEVAC coverage was developed. Such peacetime coverage required 128 aircraft, with three basing courses of action, and a four-aircraft detachment option presented. This study did not consider obligations under the Military Assistance to Safety and Traffic (MAST) program that were still in effect at several locations but steadily reduced as civilian companies took over the mission.[13]

Fristoe unsuccessfully tried to find the necessary operational data to initiate a larger strategic effort. He was determined to assist on the aviation task force as best he could and collected operational and safety data. Coincidentally, he knew Golson from his deployment with the 236th to Kosovo.[14]

Lockard, Joy, and—periodically—Fristoe attended the meetings at Fort Monroe. All aviation communities were represented:

- Attack forces;
- Scout units;
- Cargo; and
- MEDEVAC.

The list of issues ranged from air traffic control to logistics, training, and unit organization. Lockard also noticed that at many smaller meetings only select individuals were invited. She sensed that other agendas were being discussed. Aware of the long history of attempts by aviation to control MEDEVAC, she reviewed some of the history from Vietnam and the attempts made during the creation of the aviation branch, which she discussed with Col. (ret) Tom Scofield. She became aware that some aviation brigade commanders in Iraq complained through safety reports that the MEDEVAC units there were not properly tied in with their units and the medical chain of command did not provide proper command oversight for their flight operations. The report suggested that the MEDEVAC units should align under the control of aviation brigade commanders.[15]

Thurman had a few private meetings with Lockard where she clearly presented a strong case for maintaining MEDEVAC as it was with the 15-ship companies. Her deputy, Joy, had a different opinion. In his MEDEVAC assignments both in units and as an observer/controller at the Joint Readiness Training Center, he had developed a strong belief that the MEDEVAC units needed to be under aviation control. He had long talks with the aviators on his committee who concurred. When he made his views known to Lockard, she told him that he could have his own opinions, but during these meetings he represented the AMEDD and needed to maintain the AMEDD position.

Subsequently, Thurman heard of Joy's discussions with his committee compatriots and approached him directly for his opinion. As per Lockard's instructions, Joy gave him the AMEDD position. The General waved him off. "I know the AMEDD's position," he said, "I want to know what you think." Joy told him:

> My position on it was that it needed to be up under the aviation brigade... Arguments can be given for both sides of it. My personal view of it is that we hold that aviation brigade commander responsible for everything that flies. Therefore, if that's the case, and they are looked at and he is responsible for that, what does the MEDEVAC do that is so special that that aviation brigade commander cannot oversee? And really, it is nothing. If you look at what a MEDEVAC pilot does, and what a lift pilot does, there is no difference. They transport items from point A to point B. What makes the MEDEVAC different is that mission equipment package that is in the back of the aircraft. And it is that medic and the equipment that is on board that aircraft that makes it special.

> Otherwise, the pilots up there are no different. We put warrant officers in the front of the aircraft and go off single ship and perform that mission and they have no additional training other than their flight training. That's no different than a lift unit can do.[16]

Thurman thanked him and walked away. He discussed it with Sinclair and then decided to include Joy's concept as a proposal that all MEDEVAC units be reorganized as divisional assets along the lines of the 50th Med Co (AA) assigned to the 101st Airborne Division. Under the modular concept, all divisions would expand to four brigades. Each brigade could have an Forward Support MEDEVAC Team (FSMT) of three aircraft and crews that could then form a habitual relationship with them. A restructured 12-ship MEDEVAC company could be assigned as a subordinate unit to the general support aviation battalion (GSAB) and under aviation control.[17]

When Lockard learned what had happened, she had a firm conversation with Joy. She also immediately argued against the proposal. To Thurman and the others on the working group, she pointed out that a pure divisional/brigade allocation left no units to provide area general support. She questioned how pure divisional units could provide all of the CONUS support that the MEDEVAC units provided. She discussed the evolving doctrine that required MEDEVAC to be available for a much larger patient base, such as joint/coalition forces, Department of Defense personnel, contractors, and local populations as opposed to just providing for the parent divisions. She highlighted all of the almost uncounted missions that MEDEVAC units performed domestically, such as the hugely successful MAST program. How would all of that be provided for with small units focused on a divisional identity? She patiently explained to them the key role that the helicopters and crews played in the medical continuum of care. She buttressed all of her points with reports from the 36th and 56th Medical Battalions and the 50th, 54th, 57th, 82d, 126th, 159th, 507th, 571st, and 1042d Medical Companies detailing their experiences in ongoing operations in Iraq and Afghanistan. She was now deeply concerned that the path that the working group was drifting toward would restructure the MEDEVAC force into one incapable of meeting current or projected mission requirements.

Lockard also showed that the concept of the GSAB was flawed. Under the current 15-ship Medical Force 2000 structure, an air ambulance company could essentially operate independently as long as it could locate with a larger aviation unit for logistics support. In being assigned to a GSAB, the MEDEVAC company's support elements would be dramatically reduced, and it would not be able to deploy independently. It would need to deploy with the GSAB properly to operate. Lockard argued vehemently against these proposals. She said:

This was briefed over and over again, yet the aviation community really felt that they could put their arm around us and do a lot more of the management, consolidate the maintenance, do some other type of organizational structure changes that would work better for us all, and keep the modularity or the transformation going ahead.

…I can give them all of these "what if" situations and I can create so many vignettes and give them examples of how successful MEDEVAC has been and how well we worked together in Somalia—that I wasn't *assigned* to aviation, I was *attached* to the maintenance and logistics. But I had the operational control by the medical field because we knew where to go when. We were tied at the hip to the evacuation process from the guy on the ground to the aid station to the hospital. We weren't just an aviation element calling a taxicab.[18]

Lockard asked Heintz for his thoughts on how to proceed. He believed that the study group had purposely been stacked with aviators who both outnumbered and outranked the MEDEVAC attendees. He also felt that Cody, the G-3 on the Department of Army staff, supported moving MEDEVAC into aviation and closely watched the efforts of Task Force Aviation through his close relationship with Sinclair. Cody had served in the 101st Division on several tours, including as the division commander, and thought the example set by the "Eagle Dustoff" was the proper way to organize MEDEVAC. Heintz, in turn, did all he could as the consultant to explain the issues to The Surgeon General and his contacts throughout the MEDEVAC community in an attempt to sway the arguments. Heinz had even suggested to the Surgeon General that failure to fight this proposed change to doctrine was tantamount to abdicating fundamental Title 10 responsibilities to properly and responsibly clear the battlefield. Heintz also enlisted the support of MEDEVAC Medal of Honor recipient, Maj. Gen. (ret) Pat Brady, to petition the senior Army leadership to reconsider these recommendations.[19]

The aviators on the working group listened politely to Lockard, but the 12-ship proposal under GSAB and aviation was written into the transformation package. She noticed that she was being left out of more and more meetings and—on several occasions—was told that she was "too parochial" in her views.

Fristoe also became involved as much as he could in the discussions. As a relatively young officer, he did not have much influence with the group. He was challenged on several occasions to produce hard data showing the efficacy of the 15-ship company or to buttress the Lockard's arguments. He could not find the information and concluded that it did not exist. Fristoe remembered that "Every time we brought up a course of action or potential change, anything at all, the response was 'until and unless you have the data, you are being parochial. You need to just get on board, just be part of the team.'" In a more candid moment, an aviation colonel pulled him aside and told him:

> You guys are doing the right things. What's not happening is your leadership isn't engaged. You're right; you guys got the mission right. It's just that your leadership is not engaging; that's why you are losing this battle. But we are not going to say anything; we have our marching orders.[20]

Neither he nor Lockard could do anything about that. She did feel that the working group had been stacked to achieve a preordained outcome. But she did persevere. In another session, Lockard pointed out that recent events in Iraq reconfirmed that MEDEVAC was communications intensive. Every patient had a unique condition requiring different and perhaps specialized medical care that could require intense and focused communications that had no business being passed through aviation C2 channels because the pure volume of calls could block out all else.

Both she and Fristoe also realized that the reassignment of the MEDEVAC companies to the GSABs would eliminate the rationale for the medical evacuation battalions. They tried to argue the key role that the battalions played in orchestrating the overall evacuation process and providing for medical regulation. Again, however, they were dismissed as being too parochial. Sinclair believed that recent operations in Iraq showed that the MEDEVAC units did not have the necessary connectivity under the medical evacuation battalions to maintain the situational awareness to operate over the modern battlefield. The personnel billets in the medical evacuation battalions could be reprogrammed into the proposed new aviation force structure.[21]

Sinclair also believed that the MEDEVAC company commanders exercised far too much launch authority and were not in compliance with Army standards. He said:

> Per Army Regulation 95-1, an extremely high risk mission has to be approved by a general officer; high risk has to be approved by an O-6. In the MEDEVAC world, they were delegating that down to captain level. I understand that they have experience but there was a lot of concern because as a result, you had, for example, these single ship MEDEVAC missions going out into combat areas where there was heavy fire.[22]

One of the aviation officers also suggested that all 67Js should be "re-branched" into aviation with a specific 15 series AOC sub-identifier. Lockard and Fristoe responded vigorously and argued vehemently for the 300 plus 67J MEDEVAC officers and the unique training and knowledge of both medicine and aviation that they possessed. Fristoe recalled:

> There was discussion about just making [the 67J] a 15 Series with additional skill identifier for MEDEVAC, but we carried the day because the way we are tracked in the Medical Service Corps, we all have secondary [area of occupational concentrations]. They can be logisticians, they can be comptrollers, they can be health care administrators, they can be all sorts of stuff. The AMEDD's position was: "We can't afford to lose that; those secondary AOC [area of occupational concentration] areas of expertise and functionality within the structure." The whole health care system would collapse if we just all of a sudden one day said, "All of you [67Js] now belong to aviation."[23]

Lockard had a one-on-one discussion with now Maj. Gen. Thurman and obtained his support to keep the 67Js unique and in command of the companies. Deputy Surgeon General, Maj. Gen. Kenneth Farmer, who also discussed this issue with Cody, supported Lockard in this effort. However, the question of career development opportunities for the 67Js as aviators beyond company command if the medical evacuation battalions were inactivated was not discussed.

Fristoe sculpted a concept to assign the MEDEVAC companies to the aviation brigades as separate units that would have retained the unit structure and autonomous operations capability. As such, the companies would have retained their distinctive "AA" suffix unit identification codes that allowed them to be individually tracked by the AMEDD. Fristoe felt that this was absolutely critical for continued medical oversight of the units, but did not get support from senior medical officers to fight for this issue.

Lockard took a different tack and suggested that the best way to integrate MEDE-VAC into aviation was to attach rather than organically assign the MEDEVAC companies to the aviation battalions and brigades. She stressed that it was simply the best way to combine the best of medicine and aviation. In analyzing this action, Fristoe did not think it was a viable option. Sinclair listened to the presentations, but neither suggestion was accepted.[24]

Reluctantly, Lockard realized that among the aviation officers who ran the task force a historic assumption that MEDEVAC belonged under aviation existed. The opportunity to absorb it when the branch was created was missed. She later lamented that:

> I think it has been a theme. If you go back in time with Tom Scofield, all the way back to when they wanted us to be in aviation branch, there has always been a certain intent by the aviation community that MEDEVAC needs to belong to aviation. Some people will say they agree with it and some will say "No, don't." But I will say the current leadership that we had during the current transformation process versus the leadership that we had during the '80s had a different opinion and the current leadership felt strongly that MEDEVAC should be part of aviation, and that aviation branch guys can command a MEDEVAC company. MEDEVAC should just be one of the many missions associated with aviation. Just like picking up bullets and supplies and milk and water. And that they can manage it; they can operate it; they can send it out where they need to; they can command and control it. …In some people's minds, they think that this would be more efficient—to have MEDEVAC under aviation. …It looks great on Power Point slides.[25]

Still not ready to concede, Lockard pointed out that making the MEDEVAC units letter companies under aviation battalions required them to give up their medical identities and lineages. The MEDEVAC veterans groups had also heard about this potential change and were distressed about such a dramatic step. Fristoe raised this issue more than once. He and Lockard were again told that they were being "parochial" and that the redesignation of the companies as aviation units was not a subjective decision, but just the way the Army organizes and operates. The same thing was happening to most of the air cavalry units that were also being realigned under aviation. The new designations would be determined by the Army Center for Military History that maintained unit lineages and designations. This was a bitter pill to swallow because—as separately identified companies—most of the units had long and distinguished heritages reaching back to Korea. All of that would end as the MEDEVAC units inactivated and their personnel and equipment were reassigned to letter companies in the GSABs.[26]

Lockard and Fristoe frequently briefed the Surgeon General, Lt. Gen. James Peake or his deputy, Farmer. Peake's attitude was, "If it isn't broke, why fix it?" On a few occasions, he and Farmer weighed in as they could on the issues, although they were dealing with other huge battles concerning transformation initiatives for other medical units and ever increasing numbers of critically wounded soldiers filling Army hospitals. As she continued to struggle with the working group, Lockard was overwhelmed with a growing sense of inevitability about the outcome. The 12-ship company under GSAB and aviation control stayed in the aviation transformation package with all of the other decisions about the reorganization of attack, lift, cargo, and scout aviation units. All of that then became subsumed in the overall modularity package.[27]

Report

The Army Aviation Task Force Study Report was completed and submitted in early November 2003. The report, which exceeded 140 pages, was restricted in distribution and included numerous recommendations that affected the entire aviation community. Only a few pages addressed MEDEVAC. The results were as Lockard had feared.

In response to the Chief of Staff's tasking, the Aviation Task Force conducted a comprehensive review and assessment of aviation forces, considered different courses of action, and developed recommendations for the development of a new aviation modernization plan to support the Army as it continued to transform into the future force. One of the recommendations was to "Consolidate Aviation Proponency for MEDEVAC aircraft and make MEDEVAC units organic to the Aviation UA [units of action] with an SRC of 01." That recommendation would presumably improve capabilities, flexibility, maintenance, safety, standardization, airspace management, and resourcing. AMEDD would retain proponency for special mission equipment. MEDEVAC companies would reduce from 15 to 12 aircraft and be removed from the medical chain of command. Proposed personnel reductions could reduce the MEDEVAC company to as few as 50 soldiers. The heritage MEDEVAC units would be inactivated and their assets and personnel would be used to create new companies that would then be identified as subordinate letter companies of GSABs.[28]

Decision

In reviewing the report, Schoomaker approved much of it, including the MEDEVAC portion, stating that, "Army aviation has more potential than any other branch—we just have not maximized its potential. My commitment to you is we are going to make Army aviation the best damn outfit on the battlefield. We owe it to our soldiers, our Army, and the nation." The report reaffirmed the restructuring of MEDEVAC units with 12 aircraft and their reassignment from medical to aviation command. It also directed the task force to develop an implementation plan and develop a charter for overall MEDEVAC proponency.[29]

The Surgeon General, Lt. Gen. Peake, was not happy with the result. At Lockard and Fristoe's suggestion, he met with Thurman and Sinclair on 18 December. A subsequent memorandum from Peake to Thurman, with a copy to Cody, captured the issues:

- Proponency;
- Future structure design;
- Mission; and
- Resourcing implications.

Peake agreed to share proponency, with the AMEDD responsible for doctrine, organization design, force structure development, AMEDD personnel management, and the issues that were fundamental to the mission set for patient evacuation. Aviation would be the proponent for aviation training, aircraft procurement and modernization, airspace coordination, maintenance, logistics, safety, and standardization.

Operationally, the MEDEVAC companies had to be fully integrated into the aviation scheme of maneuver to operate safely and with the same standards as the aviation troops. Organization of the units and proper command and control required another look. The MEDEVAC companies needed to remain as SRC 08 [medical] units versus SRC 01 [aviation] units. Placing the MEDEVAC units under the aviation brigades addressed the support requirements, but there still needed to be medical command and control in the linkage because MEDEVAC clearly remained a part of the integrated medical support to the force.

Peake addressed the 50th Med Co (AA) of the 101st Division as an outstanding example of a unit directly supporting a division. He also pointed out that it relied on varying levels of aeromedical evacuation support from corps-level assets at different phases of current operations, especially for missions outside of division boundaries or for support of joint or coalition partners. He also, again, pointed out that direct support units could not provide general support to other units at the same time. Other SRC 08 MEDEVAC units not under division control could provide for all of these needs.

Peake did not support the 12-ship proposal for the four-brigade division. He did support procuring a new light utility helicopter to be assigned to Table of Distribution and Allowances units so the UH-60s could be freed up for assignment to Modified Table of Organization and Equipment units. He also asked if UH-1s could be used in Kuwait—again—to free up UH-60s for service in the higher threat areas.

He once again stressed the critical role that MEDEVAC played in the continuum of care and mentioned that the U.S. Army MEDEVAC force was always in high demand and the envy of the world.[30]

Implementation

Task Force Aviation now switched functions and transformed into a series of implementation conferences. Lockard, Joy, and Fristoe stayed engaged as Medical and Aviation Branch staffs began to work through the various residual issues.

Still not satisfied with the flow of events, Peake wrote a memorandum for Gen. Jack Keane, the Army Vice Chief of Staff, on 5 February 2004. Keane had supported keeping MEDEVAC under the AMEDD. In Peake's memorandum to Keane he expressed his continuing concerns about MEDEVAC, emphasizing that, "The mission of clearing the battlefield and providing en route care is intrinsically and fundamentally a medical mission and not simply transportation. It is integral to maintaining the continuity of care, and its retention within the medical battlefield operating system supports the principles of unity of effort and command."[31]

Peake indicated that since the Medical Reengineering Initiative of the 1990s FSMTs were formed and deployed far forward to support maneuver elements or in general support for echelons above division in support of joint/combined tasking or even domestic support operations. Current MEDEVAC company structure provided a small support package to go with each FSMT. Under the GSAB, those packages would be lost and such support would have to come out of the battalion. If the battalion was supporting multiple aviation operations, then MEDEVAC support could suffer.

Under the proposed plan, overall theater coordination of MEDEVAC would also suffer because there would be no one headquarters like the existing medical (evacuation) battalions to provide it. The proposed reorganization would necessitate the creation of a medical operations cell to augment the aviation brigade staff to provide for overall coordination and synchronization so that casualties could be moved, tracked, and regulated as expeditiously as possible.

Peake also indicated that no evidence suggested that flight safety would improve with the reassignment of MEDEVAC units to aviation. He cited statistics for fiscal year 2003 showing that the Army rotary-wing community suffered Class A, B, and C accidents at significantly higher rates than the MEDEVAC community, specifically:

Rate of Accidents per 1,000 Flight Hours in UH-60A/L Aircraft

		MEDEVAC	**Nonmedical**
Overall			
	Class A	.03067	.11873
	Class B	.01533	.07476
	Class C	.09200	.29024
Operation IRAQI FREEDOM			
	Class A	.08880	.37802
	Class B	.00000	.11937
	Class C	.08880	.37802[32]

Peake was very passionate about MEDEVAC for personal reasons. As a young lieutenant in Vietnam, he had been wounded and then evacuated by a MEDEVAC helicopter and he retained vivid memories of that event. In a later interview, Peake recalled that as he was being flown out, he could still remember the calming effect of the morphine and the smell of the secretions from the patient in the rack above as they dripped down onto him. As he watched the ATI process move forward, though, he finally conceded that, "I don't have any heartburn about it [MEDEVAC] being part of the aviation brigade."[33]

For the most part, his concerns were disregarded, as Task Force Aviation continued to transform aviation. On 4 March 2004, Thurman briefed the results of his overall review of Army aviation to the Tactical Air and Land Forces Subcommittee of the Committee on Armed Services of the U.S. House of Representatives.

Citing his derived tasking from Schoomaker, he explained the results of his review and stated:

> We need to have trained, standardized modular units that are fully connected to the combined arms team and joint forces…Army aviation is a unique combat element whose requirements extend across all Joint Functional and Operating Concepts. The task force analyzed required capabilities from Joint doctrine down to company level in order to develop a basic building block for units. These company building blocks permit the creation of a truly capable Aviation Unit of Action (UA) with standardized formations. Aviation UAs are multifunctional aviation brigades that will support four to five brigade combat teams. The Aviation UA incorporates the lessons learned from recent operations and corrects deficiencies in our current structure by moving aviation assets closer to the warfighter.

> The Aviation UA is able to organize by task, purpose, and mission…Combat medical evacuation aircraft are directly organic to the aviation brigade commander to better support our forces…We developed a Brigade Aviation Element (BAE) organic to every ground maneuver unit equipped with long range joint communications packages to better synchronize and deconflict airspace for responsive planning and execution of combat operations.[34]

Included in the briefing were the plans to include within each divisional aviation brigade a GSAB that included the 12-aircraft MEDEVAC company equipped with UH-60s that would be modernized as the overall aviation fleet was modernized. ARNG divisions would also convert to the 12-aircraft companies, although many would be equipped with UH-1s, and overall plans were not yet firm.[35]

Three weeks later, Fristoe briefed the plan for transforming the MEDEVAC company to the implementation committee. Heretofore, the company had 15 aircraft, organized into three FSMTs with three aircraft each, and an area support section of six aircraft. The FSMTs would directly support tactical units while the area support section would provide back-haul or area coverage on a general support basis, or could provide spare aircraft for the FSMTs if one of their assigned machines was down for maintenance. The company also had its own refueling trucks and troops and an Aviation Unit Maintenance section that could perform all unit level maintenance and provide small support teams to move forward with the FSMTs. The unit was manned with 10 officers, 26 warrants, and 113 enlisted troops. Its basis of allocation was one company per division.

The proposed 12-ship company was much leaner. Still allocated as one per division, it provided three aircraft each for four FSMTs that would directly support the four Brigade Combat Teams being fielded by each division. It did not have an area support section, and its total manning was only 85 soldiers, consisting of 10 officers, 25 warrants, and 50 enlisted troops. The company no longer had refueling trucks or troops or an Aviation Unit Maintenance section; both would have to be provided by the parent GSAB.[36]

Still working with the ARNG Command Surgeon, Goforth watched the unfolding ATI process with some dismay. He was beginning to understand the significant challenges that the process presented to the ARNG MEDEVAC community. The realignment of units from 15 to 12 aircraft would cause wholesale reorganization issues for almost all ARNG units as they realigned their company commands and detachments to meet federal and state missions. Many MEDEVAC units were commanded and staffed with aviation officers on waivers instead of 67Js because of personnel recruiting challenges. Many of those officers were receiving bonuses for their MEDEVAC duty. Goforth was concerned that these bonuses might now be at risk. These issues and many more would have to be resolved as ARNG units were activated for overseas duty and backfill at CONUS bases for deploying active duty units.[37]

Through the spring months, Lockard and her compatriots continued to work with the implementation committee as they slowly worked through the intricate details. In March, she prepared a package for Cody requesting that the AMEDD be allowed to retain proponency of the MEDEVAC units and the 67Js and 91Ws. He approved the requests that meant that the MEDEVAC units would continue to be identified as SRC 08 instead of SRC 01 units and the AMEDD could properly manage its specialized personnel.[38]

In May, the committee crafted a compromise charter agreeable to the AMEDD and the Aviation Branch/U.S. Army Aviation Center (USAAVNC). The document delineated responsibilities for each organization, specifically:

AMEDD

1. Develop the organizational design (SRC 08) air ambulance organization to support command and control and evacuation requirements. Present change to design within the Force Design Update process.
2. Develop medical doctrine that supports the Combat Health Support System to include roles and responsibilities in joint and coalition environments.
3. Retain personnel proponency for AMEDD personnel (91W and 67J MOS/AOC). Command aeromedical evacuation companies with O4/67J. Establish training and medical mission manpower requirements.
4. Develop field manuals supporting integrated health care operations in a joint, interagency, multinational theater of operations.
5. Be responsible for AMEDD-specific mission/equipment package development and training. Coordinate with the USAAVNC and vice versa, regarding materiel requirements (airframe, medical and nonmedical support, communications requirements).
6. Conduct the essential medical training course (2CF7) for aeromedical evacuation personnel. Include in the course the training on appropriate subjects in medical evacuation doctrine for commissioned, warrant, and noncommissioned officers.
7. Develop an Aeromedical Evacuation Operational and Organizational Plan that fully integrates medical evacuation operations within the Aviation Operational and Organizational Plan across all echelons of care.

USAAVNC

1. Integrate medical doctrine into USAAVNC Operational and Tactical Doctrine and Operational and Organizational Plan for full-spectrum operations.
2. Develop aviator and nonrated crewmember training programs and associated training documents except for those skills specific to AMEDD personnel.

3. Provide leadership development of Aviation Branch Military Occupational Skill/Career Management Field (less 91W & 67J).
4. Determine (proponent-specific) materiel requirements and input to modernization strategies/plans for aviation systems. Implement emerging aircraft requirements to include AMEDD and medical mission support/ equipment package requirements.
5. Incorporate aeromedical evacuation organizations, medical doctrine, and operations into all aviation safety and standardization documentation and training.
6. Develop appropriate aviation field manuals outlining/supporting integrated aviation operations.
7. Develop operational and organizational plans that integrate aviation operations within the full spectrum of operations. Implement AMEDD employment concepts for aeromedical evacuation ensuring the continuity of health care functions and medical base operating systems from the tactical to strategic levels (levels 1–5).
8. Coordinate with other Army proponents providing vision and set the foundation for aviation operations within the Army.[39]

The charter went through a few more iterations before it was finally approved by Gen. George Casey, the Army Vice Chief of Staff, on 14 May 2004.[40]

In April, Peake tried to raise once more the contentious issue of unit identification and status reporting. Statutorily, he was still obligated to maintain visibility of the readiness of his medical units. Aviation had agreed to allow the MEDEVAC companies to retain their SRC 08 designations. However, the decision to reorganize and identify the units as letter companies of the GSABs was final. His request was not honored. The units would be inactivated and re-constituted as letter companies of the battalions even though they would still be coded as SRC 08 units.[41]

Post-Decision Debate

In July 2004, Lt. Col. (P) Dave MacDonald joined the OTSG staff as the Deputy Chief of the Force Management Division, with a follow-on assignment to replace Lockard as the Director of the MEPD. Unlike her though, he would move to Fort Rucker.

Settling into his assignment on the OTSG staff, he reviewed the progress of the ATI and felt compelled to write a magazine article about the dramatic changes about to unfold. Titled "Is MEDEVAC Broke?" his article took that open-ended and oft-repeated question and turned it on its head, stating peremptorily, "The perception that the MEDEVAC system is broken is misguided and unfortunately shared by many non-medical military professionals who do not understand the medical evacuation system. The fact is MEDEVAC professionals have executed their missions superbly, despite being under-resourced since aviation became a branch of the Army in 1983."[42]

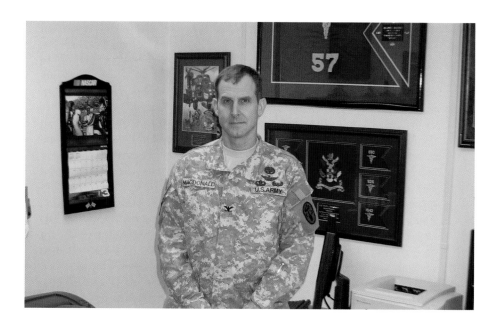

Col. Dave MacDonald in 2006.
Source: Author

He explained that MEDEVAC had proven to be a combat multiplier in every military action since Vietnam. From Operation URGENT FURY to IRAQI FREEDOM, it had proven itself a key component of a world class medical system that supported the young men and women sent into harm's way and was now seeing a 97% plus survival rate for wounded soldiers. MacDonald highlighted the role that MEDEVAC units played in supporting almost every humanitarian and peacekeeping operation that the United States supported, and indicated that in many cases, MEDEVAC teams were the first elements deployed. He also mentioned the almost continuous involvement of MEDEVAC units in domestic relief operations, base support, and the historical support for the still ongoing MAST program. MEDEVAC units did all of this while flying a mixed fleet UH-1 and UH-60 helicopters, maintaining an accident rate well below the Army average, and receiving a preponderance of commendable ratings on Army Resource Management Survey inspections.

Why then, he queried, was there such a negative perception of MEDEVAC? He offered two reasons:

1. There was a widespread misunderstanding of the MEDEVAC system and a misapplication of MEDEVAC assets by both the Army and the joint community. To support this, he stated that both communities consider MEDEVAC to be a solely Army asset designed to support primarily Army missions and other service components secondarily. The reality was that

Army MEDEVAC was a core competency that supported the full spectrum, interdependent, joint and coalition fight in a theater of operations as defined by current joint and service doctrine. Its patient load could consist of joint or coalition forces troops, displaced civilians, enemy prisoners of war, or personnel from interagency, nongovernmental, or civic organizations. Army MEDEVAC was part of the intra-theater joint patient movement system, as directed by Joint Publication 4-02.2. This misunderstanding resulted in the failure of planners to integrate Army MEDEVAC into the theater joint patient movement plan. Consequently, Army planners only focused on Army requirements while overlooking the larger theater requirements. This disconnect appeared in both Operation ENDURING FREEDOM and Operation IRAQI FREEDOM (OIF).[43]

2. There was continual controversy over who should own and control MEDEVAC assets between Army aviation and AMEDD. This political posturing had been ongoing since the Aviation Branch was formed in 1983. Army leaders then recognized the inherently joint nature of MEDEVAC, and while the units had to coordinate and integrate airspace usage with both the Army and Air Force components, ultimate control of the mission had to remain under AMEDD to ensure evacuation (as part of the joint health care continuum) remained responsive to the needs of the wounded soldier or patient. Not understanding the evacuation part of the care continuum, senior Army aviation commanders attempted to reverse that decision, and this conflict has migrated down the command chain to tactical commander resulting in the misapplication of MEDEVAC assets.[44]

To correct these two problems, MacDonald suggested that the Army needed clearly to recognize that MEDEVAC was a joint asset that served the intra-theater joint patient movement system. Joint leadership needed to establish MEDEVAC requirements under the Joint Operations Planning and Execution System and request funding through the Joint Requirements Oversight Council as a separate funding line in the Army aviation budget.[45]

The January 2005 edition of the *Army Aviation Magazine* carried a quick response from Col. Bill Forrester, Chief of Staff, U.S. Army Aviation Center at Fort Rucker. Forrester had served with Sinclair as the commander of the 159th Aviation Brigade of the 101st Division during OIF. Without addressing MacDonald's specific criticisms in any methodical way, Forrester mentioned that the modern battlefield was now a complex place, and, "The days of receiving a call for help and blindly launching in haste to save lives are truly over." He stated that MEDEVAC had a history of being logistics poor and always needed the fuel, maintenance support, intelligence, and tactical and operational awareness best supplied by the aviation battalions and brigades. The Army aviation plan to integrate fully the medical evacuation mission with the commander's scheme of maneuver and link them in through the brigade aviation elements was well founded from lessons learned from earlier conflicts and analysis of future fights. It was time to move into the future as a team, and not keep a parochial point of view.[46]

As Heintz had requested, Brady, perhaps the patriarch of the MEDEVAC veterans, had followed the transformation efforts and increasingly fractious debate and had been active behind the scene contacting senior officers. In reading Forrester's comments he felt compelled to respond in an open forum.

Responding also in the *Army Aviation Magazine,* he stated, "There is not enough room in this magazine for me to say all that came to mind when I read Col. Bill Forrester's letter... [that] MEDEVAC … is not on track." He recalled his own experiences in Vietnam and had to wonder if the spirit of Charles Kelly was even being considered as MEDEVAC was being transformed. Lambasting Forrester for saying that MEDEVAC crews were prone to "blindly launching in haste," he indicated that Forrester's reference to "haste" suggested rash action. Brady turned the reference into a positive notion of rapid to swift action. He then completely reversed the argument back against Forrester by saying:

> The most serious 'rash action' that can occur during patient evacuation is when anything or anyone interferes with the patient's needs and the swiftness of evacuation. In his entire dissertation of bureaucratic changes, Col. Forrester does not mention patient needs once. And that is the question that should be at the foundation of any changes to the method of Dustoff…

> Col. Forrester opines that the aviation battalion is the answer to Dustoff missions, mission understanding, maintenance, and operational awareness. I never met a non-Dustoff aviator who understood my mission better than I did. But more importantly, what does assigning Dustoff to the aviation battalion do for patient's needs? I would bet that it will not add to the swiftness of launch, essential in life saving…Is Dustoff not performing? Have patient needs changed?

> If Col. Forrester represents current attitude, I sense the beginning of the end of Dustoff and I fear the patient will be the worse for it.[47]

This three-legged discourse was a recapitulation of the classic debate about MEDEVAC. Is it medicine or aviation? MacDonald, in arguing about the expanded patient load directed by joint doctrine and ongoing operations, addressed the larger medical imperative. Forrester, in arguing about the exigencies of operating over the modern battlefield and addressing the logistic needs of the MEDEVAC units, argued about the pressing realities of the physics of aviation. Brady brought the debate to a higher level. He slid by both of their arguments and asked plaintively, "What about the patients needs? Have patient's needs changed?" To him, the argument was misplaced. It all had to be about doing what was best for the patients out there who needed to be cared for. That simple but powerful and even eloquent statement came from a man who knew intuitively and instinctively what MEDEVAC was all about and had perfect moral authority to make it.

However, the decisions had been made, and the transformation committee continued to meet and work through the issues. The template for the new GSAB was drafted. The Table of Organization and Equipment (SRC 01305G100) called for 531 soldiers organized into a headquarters and headquarters company, a command aviation company equipped with eight UH-60s, a heavy helicopter company equipped with 12 CH-47s, a MEDEVAC helicopter company assigned 12 aircraft, an intermediate maintenance company, and a forward support company. The additional personnel for these units were drawn in part from the manpower positions taken from the MEDEVAC companies. It was commanded by an aviation branch lieutenant colonel.

One of the first units to be so reformed was the 2d Battalion, 4th Aviation Regiment, assigned to the Aviation Brigade of the 4th Infantry Division at Fort Hood, Texas. Its MEDEVAC company was designated Charlie Company of the 2d/4th (C/2d/4th). It would be formed from the personnel and equipment taken from the soon to be inactivated 507th, which had so ably supported the 3d Infantry Division in the attack to Baghdad.[48]

Lockard realized that the fight was lost, and she just had to live with the decision. Subsequently, she moved into another job in Health Care Operations until retiring in 2006. MacDonald replaced her as the Director of the MEPD. Shortly after leaving Task Force Aviation, Joy returned to Fort Rucker and submitted his retirement papers. Lt. Col. Glen Iacovetta replaced Joy. Iacovetta inherited numerous issues generated by the ATI. Joy finally hung up his uniform on 1 December 2004 convinced that it was he more than anyone else who facilitated the transfer of MEDEVAC from medicine to aviation.[49]

The response within the MEDEVAC community was predictable. Those still serving were shocked and dismayed but resolved to carry on and do what they were told. But the seeds of bitterness were spread far and wide.

The Death of Maj. Gen. Spurgeon Neel

As these events occurred, the MEDEVAC community suffered a personal loss on 6 June 2003, the 59th anniversary of the allied landings on Normandy Beach in France in World War II, when retired Maj. Gen. Spurgeon Neel, widely recognized as the "Father of Army Aviation Medicine," and unarguably the patron saint of MEDEVAC, died of complications from pneumonia in San Antonio, Texas. He was survived by his wife of 63 years, Alice Neel. Widely recognized for his pioneering work in and tireless advocacy for MEDEVAC, he had also been the first Army Aviation Medical Officer and first commander of the Health Services Command. After his retirement, he remained active in Army medical affairs and was inducted into the U.S. Army Aviation Hall of Fame and the DUSTOFF Hall of Fame. He was buried under a bright Texas sun in the Fort Sam Houston National Cemetery, amidst a very large gathering of family, friends, and admirers.[50]

Unit Transformation Plans

After Schoomaker approved the plan for the aviation transformation, the Army staff published the list of estimated dates for inactivation of the legacy units and activations of the new units as 12-ship companies.

Unit	Inactivation Date	Activate as Unit/ /battalion/regiment	Location
377th	16 May 05	C/2d/52d	Korea
507th	16 Jun 05	C/2d/4th	Fort Hood
542d	16 Feb 07	C/6th/101st	Fort Campbell
57th	30 Sep 07	C/1st/52d	Fort Wainwright
498th	16 Jul 06	C/2d/3d	Fort Stewart
82d	16 Jul 07	C/2d/501st	Fort Riley
50th	16 Feb 07	C/7th/101st	Fort Campbell
571st	16 Jun 06	C/2d/227th	Fort Hood
54th	16 Jun 06	C/3d/82d	Fort Bragg
159th	16 Sep 07	C/3d/10th	Fort Drum
236th	16 Oct 06	C/1st/214th	Landstuhl
45th	16 Mar 07	C/5th/158th	Wiesbaden
68th	16 Jun 06	C/3d/25th	Wheeler

The five U.S. Army Air Ambulance Detachments at Forts Rucker, Drum, Irwin, Polk, and Soto Cano, Honduras, would remain as they were. The actual dates of inactivation and activation were preliminary and varied as operations continued in Kosovo, Iraq, and Afghanistan.[51]

The ARNG units would also transform and relinquish their heritage unit identities. Proud designations such as the 24th, 86th, 112th, 126th, 149th, 717th, 1042d, etc., would likewise be replaced with Charlie Company designations of GSABs. For them, too, the actual dates varied, and many would also change missions as regularly happened with ARNG units. Additionally, detachments from individual states would be realigned into new pairings to make up the 12 aircraft UH-60 companies.

Unit/battalion/regiment	Activate on	State(s)
C/2d/104th	1 May 06	West Virginia, Tennessee
C/2d/149th	1 Jun 05	Texas, Oklahoma
C/1st/111th	2 Oct 05	Florida, Arkansas
C/3d/238th	1 Jun 05	New Hampshire, Michigan
C/1st/189th	1 Jun 05	South Dakota, Montana
C/1st/168th	1 Jun 05	California, Nevada
C/2d/211th	1 Oct 05	Minnesota, Iowa
C/3d/126th	1 Jun 05	Vermont, Massachusetts
C/1st/126th	1 Oct 05	Maine
C/2d/238th	1 Oct 05	Indiana, Colorado
C/1st/169th	1 Oct 05	Maryland, Pennsylvania, Kentucky
C/5th/169th	1 Oct 07	Wyoming, Arizona
C/1st/171st	1 Oct 07	New Mexico, Kansas
C/7th/158th	1 Oct 07	Oregon
C/2d/135th	1 Oct 05	Nebraska, Colorado[52]

Four ARNG legacy units would maintain their heritage designations and re-main equipped with UH-1Vs. They would remain as the base generation force and would eventually be reequipped with a new light utility helicopter yet to be selected and procured. The four ARNG legacy units were:

Unit	State(s)
148th Med Co	Washington, DC, Delaware
249th Med Co	New York, Rhode Island, New Hampshire
812th Med Co	Louisiana, California, New Mexico
832d Med Co	Wisconsin, Georgia, North Dakota[53]

The ARNG units were equipped with 180 UH-60s — mostly -As but with a few -Ls, and -Qs — and almost equaled the 18 active duty units equipped with 192 UH-60s and 26 UH-1Vs. Additionally, consideration was given to reactivate several U.S. Army Reserve (USAR) MEDEVAC units based on demographic studies and the availability of new UH-60Ms.[54]

From their introduction into the MEDEVAC force in the 1950s, the Reserve Component units remain a vital part of the MEDEVAC community. They were not used in Vietnam, but they provided great service in all subsequent conflicts, the MAST program, innumerable natural disasters, and as backfill for active duty units. They are an integral part of the great MEDEVAC heritage.

Moving On

Most officers within the MEDEVAC community watched the developments with transformation very closely, realizing that it would dramatically affect their careers and possibly personal lives. When Lt. Col. Bob Mitchell's tour as the ex-ecutive officer of the 1st Medical Brigade at Fort Hood ended in the summer of 2004, he took command of the 36th Medical Battalion (Evacuation) collocated at Fort Hood. The implementation committee was grinding through all of the steps necessary to carry out the transformation. As Mitchell watched, he realized that The Surgeon General would lose control of all of the MEDEVAC companies. He had hoped that the medical evacuation battalions would possibly be rolled up under the aviation brigades but was saddened to see that they would instead inactivate or transform to something else. Yet he had seen early on when he served with the standardization and evaluation team at Fort Rucker that MEDEVAC in-tuitively needed to be better aligned with aviation because of its need for opera-tional and logistical support that could only be provided by larger aviation units.

He recalled that, "From my perspective ... I was on a Department of the Army level inspection team. I can speak for them. I have grown up in this field where we just don't do things with the aviation side. And I don't understand that."[55]

He also felt that all of the key decisions had been made too quickly without considering the current combat deployment cycle for MEDEVAC companies and

GSABs. The companies and battalions that absorbed them were on different deployment schedules, and it would take several iterations of deployments to realign them so that they could deploy together.[56]

His battalion deployed to Iraq in December 2004 and replaced the 429th Medical Battalion (Evacuation), a USAR unit from Savannah, Georgia. Located at Tikrit, the 36th battalion was the only evacuation battalion in the country and provided general area support and command and control of the three residual MEDEVAC companies and two ground ambulance companies. The battalion worked closely with three different aviation brigades that had the MEDEVAC companies located with them.

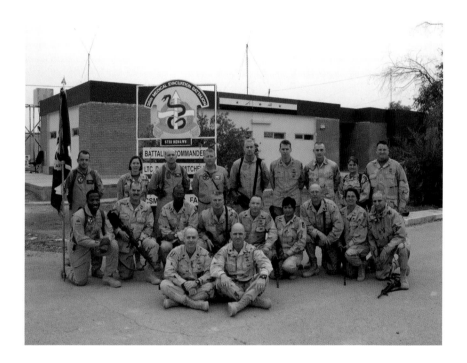

Commander and staff of the 36th Medical Battalion (Evacuation) in Iraq in 2005.
Back row, left to right: Maj. Bill Howard, 50th Med Co (AA), Capt. Anne Garcia, 141st Med Co (GA), Maj. Terry McDowell, 498th Med Co (AA), Maj. Keith Farrar, 1159th Med Co (AA), Maj. Eric Rude, 571st Med Co (AA), Maj. Pete Lehning, 54th Med Co (AA), Capt. Craig Strong, 313th Med Co (GA), Capt. Nancy Ginas, Capt. Ron McBay, 128th Med Co (GA).
Middle row, left to right: 1st Sgt. Norris Thomas, 50th Med Co (AA), 1st Sgt. John Stonoha, 141st Med Co (GA), 1st Sgt. Alonzo Dixon, 498th Med Co (AA), 1st Sgt. Raymond Persinger, 1159th Med Co (AA), 1st Sgt. Joseph Cevesco, 571st Med Co (AA), 1st Sgt. Ruth Byner, 54th Med Co (AA), 1st Sgt. Mark Carlson, 313th Med Co (GA), 1st Sgt. Jennifer Pirtle, 1st Sgt. Eddie Henshaw.
Front row, left to right: Cmd. Sgt. Maj. Brian Fahl, 36th Med Bn, Lt. Col. Robert Mitchell, 36th Med Bn.
Source: Lt. Col. Robert Mitchell

Shortly after arriving, Mitchell met with all three aviation brigade commanders to determine whether any issues existed that required his attention. He also met with his MEDEVAC company commanders and explained that he expected them to work closely with the brigades. He directed them to place liaison officers in the brigade tactical operations centers and also attend their intelligence and standardization briefings and the daily battle update briefings. He said to his commanders, "If you are operating in their sector, you are going to listen to what they have to say. You have two daddies here. So balance them out commanders. You figure it out."[57]

To another MEDEVAC commander, he was more specific. "I want the 1st Cav [aviation brigade] to think they own you. That's the only way we can win this thing and do it right." The commander followed his orders, and Mitchell noticed that the brigade commander was—within a few weeks—"doing cheetah flips" about how the MEDEVAC unit was well organized and disciplined.

Mitchell had another reason for pushing his MEDEVAC commanders to develop stronger relationships with the aviation brigades and their assigned GSABs. He knew that when his battalion left Iraq in late 2005, it would not be replaced. Instead, the companies would then be formally assigned to those brigades and battalions. The overall theater MEDEVAC program would be overseen and coordinated by Lt. Col. Bill Goforth, who was assigned to the G3 on the staff of the Multinational Corps Iraq.[58]

Mitchell had his reservations about transformation but knew that the Army had made its decision and it was time to carry on. His 21 years as a warrant officer and then MEDEVAC officer had taught him that all of the issues would be resolved. He was well familiar with the arguments on both sides, but his bottom line was well formed. "This is about the soldier on the ground that is counting on somebody getting in there and getting him out. If we don't do that and do it right… somebody has got to be able to answer for that. [We will do] whatever it takes to make sure that this is done right." Pat Brady could not have said it better.[59]

Unit Inactivations

Then the MEDEVAC companies began to transform to their new configurations and identities. The proud 507th at Fort Hood was the first. On schedule in June 2005, the unit formed up for the inactivation ceremony. By now, the news of the transformation of MEDEVAC had spread throughout the Dustoff veterans' community. They were not in favor of such a dramatic change, especially the change in unit designations from their heritage designations to the relative anonymity of the Charlie Company of the whatever. They rallied to lobby as they could against the transformation. But it was just wasted effort.

They also showed up to witness the ceremonies. As the maroon guidon of the 507th Med Co (AA) was furled for the last time and cased, and the blue guidon of the Charlie Company, 2d Battalion, 4th Aviation Regiment, was unfurled, a low moan rolled through the veterans. To them, it was the personification of their worst dream. Their beloved MEDEVAC was finally being consumed by Army aviation. It was something that they and their predecessors had fought since the very beginning, all the way back to the bitter conflict in Korea. They now knew that the battle was lost. It was a bitter pill to swallow.[60]

Operations

MAST

When the MAST program was first initiated, its original intent was to demonstrate the efficacy of aeromedical evacuation to the civilian community with the fervent hope that private companies would assume the task. The response was slow but inevitable. One example sprang forth in Missouri. In 1985, Colin Collins started Air Evac Lifeteam in the small town of West Plains. It eventually grew into an organization of more than 1,300 employees in 11 states, utilizing 64 operational sites that served more than 600 hospitals. Its fleet of 85 Bell 206 Long Ranger helicopters was rated as some of the safest and most reliable general aviation aircraft in the world. Since its founding, the company transported more than 120,000 patients. It is a testimony to the trailblazing efforts of the Army MEDEVAC community that set the example and the vision of Neel.[61]

As the operational tempo for Army MEDEVAC units increased after the events of 9/11, those units that had not been replaced by civilian agencies slowly backed away from their MAST commitments. In 2005, the controlling Army Regulation for MAST, Army Regulation 500-4, was not renewed, and Headquarters, Department of the Army, sent a field message stating:

> "Current Wartime sourcing requirement and the operational tempo of the Army's MTOE [Modified Table of Organization and Equipment] aeronautical evacuation assets exceed their capacity to perform installation MEDEVAC support. U.S. Army CONUS MTOE MEDEVAC installation support ceases O/A 1 Jun 05 or upon the demobilization of Reserve Component MEDEVAC assets currently providing support."[62]

Exceptions were granted for the Table of Distribution and Allowances U.S. Army Air Ambulance Detachment units at Fort Drum, New York; Fort Rucker; the National Training Center at Fort Irwin, California; the Joint Readiness Training Center at Fort Polk, Louisiana; and a few other training sites that these units directly supported. This directive did not direct the termination of MAST for the units in Hawaii and Alaska because they were not CONUS-based.

Under Army Regulation 95-1, Army MEDEVAC helicopters could still be used to transport civilian personnel when they were involved in rescues or were involved in major disasters or catastrophes that required lifesaving aeromedical evacuation.

The intent was clear. MAST, so long a customer of MEDEVAC services and the trainer of many MEDEVAC crewmembers, was slowly being overcome by events and supplanted by overriding priorities. It was not being terminated, but most effectively curtailed or perhaps more accurately—suspended—and the program's potential for future service to the nation remains.

However, since its initial prototype flying in July 1970, the MAST program has been phenomenally successful. The MEDEVAC companies and detachments who flew the mission — active, USAR, and ARNG — logged more than 55,000 missions and more than 116,000 flight hours, carrying almost 52,000 patients and rescuees. It is a great part of the MEDEVAC legacy.[63]

Central America

In Honduras, the 1st Battalion, 228th Aviation Regiment, continued to serve as the U.S. Army aviation component of Joint Task Force (JTF) Bravo and occupied new permanent facilities built after Hurricane Mitch devastated the area. The attached MEDEVAC U.S. Army Air Ambulance Detachment was reequipped with new UH-60L aircraft and continued to support the task force in a multitude of missions:

- Support for counter drug operations;
- Civic action projects;
- Relief operations for natural disasters; and
- Classic patient recoveries and transfers.

Operations there by the men and women of the detachment are ongoing.[64]

Hurricane Katrina

Background. The next challenge for MEDEVAC came from another completely different quarter. The traditional beginning of the United States hurricane season is 1 June. All southeastern states have—at one time or another—been pummeled by these devastating storms and have developed contingency response plans in conjunction with various federal agencies and the military services.

The summer of 2005 was an average season with 10 named storms by mid-August. Using weather satellites in geosynchronous orbit over the Atlantic Ocean, The National Hurricane Center began tracking a tropical depression well east of Puerto Rico in mid-August. By 24 August, it drifted west to the Bahamas and formed into a tropical storm named Katrina.

Continuing to strengthen into a category 1 Hurricane with sustained winds exceeding 75 mph, it crossed southern Florida on the 26 August, causing localized flooding, some damage to buildings and homes, and 14 deaths. It then slowly traversed the Gulf of Mexico—gaining strength—on a generally westerly track. By 28 August, the storm was almost due south of New Orleans and had strengthened to a category 5 storm with winds exceeding 155 mph. All Gulf Coast states closely watched the storm and activated command centers and National Guard units. On 28 August, the storm turned to a northerly track and seemed to be headed directly for New Orleans. Top winds were 175 mph and recorded lowest air pressure was 902 millibars (1,013 is normal), one of the lowest recorded readings ever.[65]

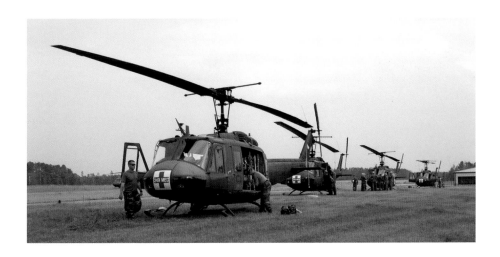

Helicopters and crews from the 249th Med Co (AA), New York and Rhode Island ARNGs deployed to support recovery operations after Hurricane Katrina.
Source: Maj. Mike Charnley

As he watched the storm closely the State Army Aviation Officer for Louisiana, Col. Barry Keeling, began pre-positioning aviation assets on 25 August and directed his flying units to form a team of four UH-60s and two UH-1s to be

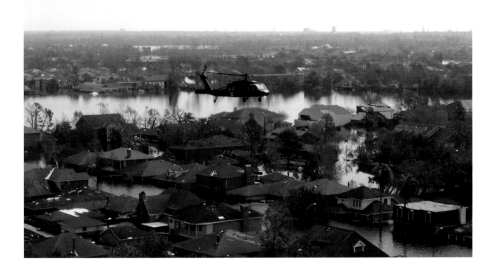

Arkansas ARNG UH-60 over New Orleans after Katrina.
Source: U.S. Army

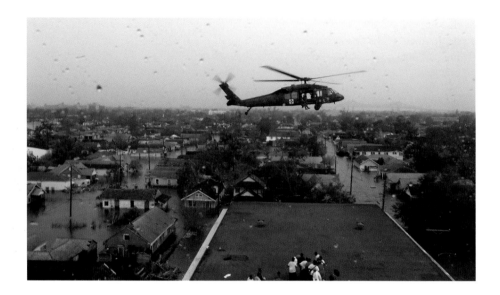

Rooftop recovery by an Arkansas ARNG MEDEVAC UH-60 after Hurricane Katrina.
Source: U.S. Army

available to fly in the wake of the storm for immediate rescue operations. The next day he activated several command centers and established Task Force Eagle. It consisted of all state aviation and aviation support assets, and had the capability to command and control deployed ARNG units from other states. He also directed the full manning of all affected command centers and the deployment of fuel and support equipment to the Baton Rouge and Hammond Airports. The state also had flight facilities at Lakefront Airport and Jackson Barracks, both located on the north side of New Orleans. However, if massive flooding were to occur, neither might be usable.[66]

Keeling also requested aviation support from other states under the provisions of the Emergency Management Assistance Compact (EMAC). Created by Public Law 104-321, the EMAC was an agreement among 48 states, Washington, DC, Puerto Rico, and the Virgin Islands to provide assistance across state lines when any type of disaster occurs. It was first used effectively in Florida in 2004 when that state was swept by four hurricanes. Within hours of receiving Louisiana's request for help, several states activated their Army Guard units for deployment.[67]

Federal agencies and the military services were also beginning proactive actions to deal with the looming storm. First U.S. Army headquartered at Fort Gillem on the southeast edge of Atlanta, Georgia, primarily trained units for overseas deployment and utilization. Headquarters U.S. Army had also assigned First Army a secondary mission to be prepared to support disaster relief operations in the eastern half of the United States. The commander, Lt. Gen. Russell Honore, and his staff had been monitoring the storm for several days. On 25 August, he directed the activation of the command crisis action team at Fort Gillem and the deployment of Defense Coordinating Elements, with senior Defense Coordinating Officers to Florida, Alabama, and Mississippi. Additionally, Honore made contact with the Adjutant Generals of the National Guard forces of Louisiana, Mississippi, Alabama, and Florida, to begin the steps necessary to coordinate the flow of federal aid into the states.[68]

All aviation units from the Louisiana ARNG, including the 812th Med Co (AA) with 12 UH-1V aircraft, were activated for the storm response. Initially, they worked primarily out of their flight facility at Esler Field near Pineville—in the middle of the state—but also operated from the Baton Rouge Airport and the Hammond Airport just north of Lake Pontchartrain. The 812th and its state brother unit, the 1st Battalion, 244th Aviation Regiment, were experienced in hurricane response, having been called out many times for the storms that either threatened or hit the Louisiana coast each summer and fall. Contingency plans were robust and well practiced.

On 28 August, Keeling deployed a special reaction team to the Superdome in New Orleans. This team acted as a forward command and control center for operations in and around the city. It was fully trained, having deployed six times already to the Superdome in support of civil authorities, two of which were for hurricanes threatening the city. Additional personnel, assets, supplies, food, and water were also deployed to the Superdome, the Naval Air Station at Belle Chasse, and the other sites activated earlier. By that afternoon, evacuees began to flock to the various centers and an estimated 2,500 were already at the Superdome.[69]

The storm made landfall near the mouth of the Mississippi River at 0500 on 29 August as a category 4 storm with maximum sustained winds of 150 mph. Six hours later, winds lessened to 125 mph sustained as the storm eye passed just a few miles east of New Orleans and slammed into southern Mississippi.[70]

The storm devastated the area. New Orleanians and suburb residents were ordered to evacuate, and the roads were packed as the populace fled to higher ground. But tens of thousands had also been trapped in the city. They sought cover from the hurricane winds and more than eight inches of rain at preplanned public shelters like the Superdome in the middle of the city, where an estimated 10,000 to 12,000 had gathered.

The worst was yet to come. As the storm moved off to the north and the citizens stepped outside to survey the damage, several key levees that could no longer hold back the storm surge and the massive amounts of rain broke almost simultaneously, and the city flooded. Within hours, whole neighborhoods were under water, in some places as much as 20 feet deep. Looting erupted, and police and national guardsmen tried to restore order.[71]

Sixty miles to the northeast, the Mississippi coastline had also been devastated. Ships and boats were swept up out of the harbors by the wind and storm surge and scattered through the cities and towns along the coast destroying structures wholesale. Even huge floating casinos were pushed up on the shore. More than 100 deaths were reported in the first few hours, including 30 at one apartment complex that was smashed by storm surge. All roads and rail lines were blocked, all area airports were out of commission, and the electrical power grid and all phone service was completely disrupted.[72]

As the storm passed New Orleans, President George W. Bush signed a Declaration of Major Disaster that authorized federal assistance for Louisiana, Mississippi, and Alabama. Headquarters Northern Command directed both First and Fifth Armies to begin crisis response operations. Honore ordered his forward headquarters to move to Camp Shelby, Mississippi.

Response

As the winds died down, military forces in the area sprang into action. Helicopters from the 812th and 1st Battalion, 244th Aviation Regiment, were airborne from Baton Rouge. Several aircraft from the 812th had also pre-positioned at New Iberia located 60 miles west of New Orleans. From there, these aircraft intended to launch into the devastated area behind the storm as soon as it was safe to fly. The next morning before sunrise, an 812th crew composed of pilot Capt. Ryan Faulk, copilot 1st Lt. Stuart Maxwell, crew chief Sgt. Jeremy Miller, and medic S.Sgt. David Jacob launched from Iberia for rescue duties in New Orleans. They logged 11.5 hours in their hoist equipped UH-1V as they responded to the desperate scenes below that day. Unable to land because of the flooding, they hoisted 30 stranded people from the roofs of homes, apartments, and cars. That total included a family with six children and several wheelchair-bound elderly. To facilitate the recoveries, Jacob went down on the hoist several times to help the frightened rescuees. All were then flown to recovery centers where they received water, food, and necessary assistance.[73]

The Louisiana ARNG facilities at the Lakefront Airport and Jackson Barracks—both on the north side of New Orleans—were completely flooded and unusable. To the men and women of the Louisiana units, it was more than a mission—it was personal. "I was thinking about my community, New Orleans, my home. I was taking care of the people who are from here," said S.Sgt. Eugene Bordelon, a UH-60 crew chief.[74]

Helicopters of all services joined them as soon as they arrived as did any civilians who could get airborne to conduct immediate search and rescue operations. They joined a growing fleet of boats, both military and civilian, beginning to motor through the city. Recovery centers were activated at the Naval Air Station just south of New Orleans and the international airport on the west side of the city. Rescued personnel were dropped at these two sites or at the Superdome in the middle of the city. Navy SEABEE units located in the area also used their heavy equipment to clear roads and secure live electrical lines. All public utilities were nonfunctional as were all land phone and cell phone systems.[75]

By 1800, several state command and control elements were consolidated at the Superdome as a key part of Task Force Eagle. The "Eagle's Nest," as the command center was called, began an earnest effort to gain some control over 150 plus helicopters operating over the city and suburbs. Maj. Matt Brocato, the S-3 of the 1st Battalion, 244th Aviation Regiment, was in the Eagle's Nest with liaison officers from several services. With several operable radios of varying capability, they—defacto—began tasking any helicopters that they could contact for rescue missions. Crews from their own units who were familiar with the city were given street addresses to fly to. Crews from other units were given geographical coordinates. Brocato and his team improvised a simple expedient for determining the location coordinates. When given an address for rescue, they logged on to the *Google Earth* website and obtained the converted coordinates that were then passed to the crews. Countless rescues were mounted this way. At one point, Brocato received a huge list of 911 calls for assistance. When the storm raged through the city, all of the cell phone repeater towers were knocked out. However, the calls had all been logged onto the receiving system. When the overall cell phone system was restored, all of those calls were forwarded in a continuous stream. Brocato was presented this huge list and began systematically using it to dispatch the helicopters.[76]

At one point, a controller in the Eagle's Nest received a call from a retired Army colonel in Mississippi. An elderly lady trapped in her home in New Orleans had contacted the colonel. A crew was dispatched and flew to the home. They did not see the woman. Upon checking, they determined that the woman could not walk. The crew landed the helicopter a block away in a parking lot. The crew chief and medic proceeded to the house, found the woman, and then got her aboard the helicopter for recovery. Such events—although varied in detail—were very common.[77]

Within two days the team in the Eagle's Nest had begun to work out an overall rescue and recovery plan, and began distributing the equivalent of an air tasking order to all units to better coordinate the effort. The next morning, Louisiana ARNG engineers turned the Superdome parking lot into a massive heliport, and helicopters began to move 24,000 accumulated evacuees out of the city and shuttle in arriving support personnel. Later that day, Northern Command directed First Army to lead the recovery effort and to establish JTF-Katrina. Honore complied, designating himself as the commander. Under the EMAC agreement, all ARNG aircraft in Texas, Louisiana, Mississippi, Alabama, and Florida were declared immediately available for disaster relief. Many were airborne within four hours of Katrina's passing, and in conjunction with aircraft from all military services and other governmental agencies, they converged on the disaster area, over-flying massive ground convoys of active duty, ARNG, USAR, engineer, military police, medical, and other assorted support and even combat units, plus comparable elements from the other military forces and governmental agencies. As they arrived they were organized under a series of task forces. Active forces and activated Federal Reserve forces were under the operational control of JTF-Katrina. National Guard units were under the operational control of the State National Guard to which they deployed. Honore and his staff had the huge challenge of coordinating the actions of all of the disparate task forces.[78]

On 31 August, Honore made his first visit to New Orleans. Surveying the death and destruction, he immediately determined that his mission priorities were as follows:

1. Search and rescue;
2. Life sustainment;
3. Medical support established in every parish (county); and
4. Communications.[79]

MEDEVAC Units

Literally while the General was speaking, the 498th Med Co (AA) deployed a team from its home base at Fort Benning, Georgia. Its six UH-60s, eight crews, and 28 support personnel arrived at the main airport at Baton Rouge, Louisiana, 35 miles northeast of New Orleans. All aircraft were equipped with hoists and all aircrew members were trained to use night vision goggles. However, the unit had recently returned from its second deployment to OIF, and none of its crews was qualified for or current for over-water operations.

Immediately upon arriving, they met with representatives of the 1st Battalion, 244th Aviation Regiment, of the Louisiana ARNG who were running aviation operations there under Task Force Eagle. Once briefed, the 498th crews launched and proceeded to New Orleans to commence search and rescue operations. The crews adjusted aircraft and crew schedules to maintain 24-hour operations. During the first week of recovery operations the crews performed 108 hoist rescues and 178 rescue missions, recovering 822 personnel. Additionally, they performed 65 resupply missions and moved 58 nonmedical personnel.[80]

Some of the missions flown were very challenging. On one mission, survivors were trapped in a building that was almost completely submerged. The only access was through a skylight. The medic used a jungle penetrator to break out the skylight to gain entrance and then evacuate the family. On another mission, a crew was operating at night with night vision goggles when a small light was spotted leaking out of a building almost completely submerged except for the roof. The flight medic was lowered by hoist onto a partly submerged balcony. He extracted the survivors and helped them to be hoisted aboard.[81]

The second week was not nearly as intense as the first seven days. Most missions flown were support sorties for the now massive ground elements and units in the area. The 498th returned to home station on 16 September as primary search and rescue operations terminated. The unit had flown 365 hours in the operation and recovered 917 personnel.

Much of what the unit did was ad hoc and required tactical and administrative flexibility. The 498th had neither an "official" assignment to nor connection with the 1st Battalion, 244th Aviation Regiment, but developed an excellent working relationship with it and other units at the Baton Rouge Airport to accomplish the mission. All unit commanders and supervisors were stretched to the maximum because they had to perform their supervisory duties in addition to flying missions.[82]

Joining the various elements at Baton Rouge was another aviation team from the 2d Battalion, 4th Aviation Regiment (GSAB), from Fort Hood. It included an

HH-60L from the C Company (formerly the 507th Med Co [AA]), which provided general support with the rest of the battalion. Capt. Cory Boudreau was the small MEDEVAC detachment leader. He recalled the team's first mission:

> On 2 September, CW2 Roderick Peterson and I departed Baton Rouge Airport en route to the Superdome. As we transited east along Lake Pontchartrain, the damage looked minimal until we crossed over I-10. We were both amazed at the water level and destruction. Houses were underwater as far as we could see. After the initial shock, we continued to the Superdome... There were numerous fires and more helicopters than we could count... There was no common air to air frequency to deconflict aircraft. Everyone was just under the rule of see and avoid... On our way to the Superdome, we saw hundreds of civilians with "HELP" signs written on their roofs and people who had cut through their roofs in order to escape... Nobody on board had ever seen anything like this and weren't sure what to do. There were so many we didn't know who to choose. We finally just ... found [a needy person] and began hoisting. We sent [S.Sgt.] Gregory Givings, flight medic, down to get a woman who was sitting on the corner of her roof. She had cut out just enough room for herself to stand up and be seen. She was very distraught and very excited to see Greg... We just crept along until we saw another person and started hoisting until we had a full aircraft. Once full, we were like "where do we take them?" There was no real plan. We just watched other aircraft and had heard through some of the traffic ... about a place called the "Clover Leaf." It was the intersection of the highway that looked like a cloverleaf and was the dropoff point closest to the area we were operating. I thought we had seen the worst until we saw the cloverleaf. It looked like a refugee camp. I can't recall how many people were there but there were hundreds. The amount of people carrying their only belongings and the amount of trash made it look like a third world country...We did 25 live hoists and rescued 19 personnel. The hoisting was very demanding due to the congestion of aircraft, flying debris and trash, power lines, and the lack of any landing areas if something in fact did go wrong...[83]

Boudreau and his small detachment operated until 9 September. They did 57 live hoists in the first 72 hours and saved 70 people before returning to home station to rejoin their unit as it prepared for deployment to Iraq.[84]

Detachment 1 of the 146th Med Co, Tennessee ARNG, sent a small team of 11 personnel and two UH-60Q aircraft. Arriving on 2 September, they also staged out of Baton Rouge and joined the effort over New Orleans and the local area.[85]

At Fort Polk in western Louisiana, the effects of the storm had been minimal. MEDEVAC crews from the U.S. Army Air Ambulance Detachment were called upon for some local patient transfers. Prudently, though, the unit prepared for heavier duty. On 1 September, the unit was directed to deploy to the Hammond Airport, east of Baton Rouge. Upon arrival, the commander, Maj. Ed Zarzabal, set up a hasty command center, and crews immediately launched and headed for New Orleans, not knowing what to expect. Pilot CW3 Lori Russell remembered, "I felt nervous anticipation ...not quite as many butterflies as a mission where gunfire may come into play (although there was a rumored possibility here), but the unknown always makes you a little more tense. As we flew into the [Super] Dome, you could see aircraft swarming everywhere you looked, like mosquitoes buzzing around. The next thing that hit you was the stench ... a mix of rot and garbage in stagnant sewer water."

Russell and her crew flew several missions that day to pinpoint the problems and challenges and the location of the delivery and casualty collection points for those rescued and recovered. Using conventional city maps, they literally flew down the avenues and streets to specific addresses to make recoveries. Every power line, pole, antenna, and tree was a threat. The ground and water were littered with loose material that was easily disturbed by the downwash of the helicopter blades. Many recoveries were by hoist. On several occasions, Russell and her crew had to improvise landing procedures in a field or on a roof to collect those needing recovery. It was a long and challenging day.[86]

CW2 Jerry Eads led another crew. Experiencing similar challenges, he and his crew recovered more than 500 individuals from the flooded areas. They were perched on top of buildings, highway overpasses, and—in a few cases—in trees and on top of vehicles.[87]

MEDEVAC assets also gathered at the Naval Air Station, New Orleans, located 10 miles south of the city near the suburb of Belle Chasse. On 8 September, the "Eagle Nest" command center was moved there too, and all residual aviation recovery operations consolidated at the base. One of the key officers in the operation, Lt. Col. Garrett Jenson of the Louisiana ARNG, said, "This unprecedented historic joint service effort played a vital role in assisting the rescue of 60,000 displaced citizens from New Orleans." The *USS Iwo Jima* docked on the Mississippi River in downtown New Orleans and also served as an additional rescuee dropoff point.[88]

The 1022d Med Co (AA), Wyoming ARNG, was busy at its home station at Cheyenne preparing for deployment to Egypt to support Operation BRIGHT STAR when the call came to assist for Katrina. It took a day to straighten out the necessary orders for the change of mission. They self-deployed four of their UH-60s to the Naval Air Station at Belle Chasse. As soon as the helicopters refueled, the crews launched to join the ever expanding rescue effort. Wyoming Air National Guard C-130s flew in its support gear.

With limited command and control over the city (just the area immediately around the Superdome), the crews intuitively joined the effort. It was "just mass confusion," one pilot noted as he watched the gaggle of helicopters over the city. As the crews found somebody needing recovery, they did so, primarily by hoist, and delivered them to the recovery facility at the main airport on the west side of the city. The unit remained until 20 September.[89]

Alerted under the EMAC agreement, the 149th Med Co (AA) of the Texas ARNG deployed three UH-60A aircraft, crews, and support personnel as part of a larger state aviation task force to Baton Rouge on 30 August. Initially assigned to the Louisiana ARNG, the unit fell in under Task Force Eagle and flew rescue missions one hour after arriving. Within the first 24 hours, crews rescued 732 stranded persons. The unit aircraft were not equipped with hoists, and all recoveries in the flooded areas were made off rooftops, bridges, and highway overpasses.

Within the first week, the unit crews recovered more than 2,500 people. They also provided general aviation support and transported food and supplies, and— even on a few missions—dropped sandbags to staunch flooding. They also flew a few actual MEDEVAC missions, transporting five critically wounded civilians and two patients suffering cardiac arrest. The detachment returned to its home base near San Antonio on 20 September.[90]

On 31 August, the 24th Med Co (AA), Nebraska ARNG, deployed two UH-60s, three crews, and a small maintenance team to the Naval Air Station at Belle Chasse. The unit fell in on the large helicopter force gathering there and quickly joined into the effort. Equipped with hoists, the unit was very busy the first week, steadily receiving taskings from the Eagle's Nest. After two weeks, crews swapped out their crews. The operations tempo steadily declined, however, and on 30 September, the unit returned home.[91]

On 2 September, the 832d Med Co (AA), Wisconsin ARNG, mobilized as part of a larger state task force. It deployed 38 soldiers and three UH-1V aircraft to Camp Beauregard, near Alexandria, Louisiana. Operating from there and the Naval Air Station at Belle Chasse, the unit detachment remained for four weeks, swapping out personnel at the two-week point. The crews flew 331 hours, rescued or evacuated 133 persons (59 by hoist), transported 210 other personnel and 13 animals, and delivered more than 17,000 pounds of food and water.[92]

The crews dealt with some unusual challenges during the recoveries. One mission flown by an 832d crew highlighted this experience. CW3 William Richey and CW2 Doug Determan were the pilots. Flying over the city, their crew chief, Sgt. Eric Leukert, spotted a man in a boat. The man appeared to be exhausted and signaled that he wanted to be picked up but he was tied to a pole under some high-tension power lines. Leukert signaled to the man to move away from the wires. Determan spotted a flooded vehicle not far away. He hovered over it and had Leukert lower the medic, S.Sgt. Patrick Deuberry, onto the roof of the vehicle. Determan then used the rotor wash of the helicopter to push the boat over to the vehicle. When the man was safely with Deuberry, Determan resumed his hover over them and Leukert hoisted both into the aircraft. They then delivered the very appreciative man to the recovery center set up at the New Orleans Airport and resumed their mission.[93]

Other MEDEVAC elements supported rescue and recovery operations in Mississippi. Just recently released from active duty and a long tour at Fort Bragg, the 249th Med Co (AA), New York ARNG, deployed six of its UH-1s, crews, and support personnel to Camp Shelby, near Gulfport, Mississippi, in early September. The 249th worked with Task Force 185th Aviation from the Mississippi ARNG to perform search and recovery missions. They flew logistical support missions throughout Mississippi, delivering food, ice, water, and infant supplies to various local distribution points. They also flew medical teams to towns isolated by damaged roads and bridges. As the immediate needs abated, four aircraft and crews returned home on 15 September, while the other two crews and support personnel remained to the end of the month.[94]

On 1 September, the 148th Med Co, Georgia ARNG responded to the EMAC request. The unit already had two UH-1Vs, crews, and support personnel at Hagler Army Airfield located at Camp Shelby, Mississippi, supporting summer training for ARNG and USAR units. The 148th was under the operational control of Lt. Col. Paul Frazier, the airfield commander. Frazier established a de facto command center to coordinate the aerial rescue efforts taking place in Mississippi being mounted by aircraft staging out of Hagler, the airport at Jackson, and eventually, the airport at Gulfport when it was reopened.[95]

CW4 Jim Brennan was one of the 148th pilots. He was an old hand at hurricane response, having flown support for Florida in September 2004, when Hurricane Charley came ashore near Fort Myers. He and the other crewmembers repositioned to Jackson, Mississippi, to ride out Katrina, and then returned when the storm had passed. The unit dispatched four more UH-1Vs and crews. Three aircraft and crews stayed at Camp Shelby and the other three went to the Naval Air Station at Belle Chasse. Each of the teams supported task forces in their areas. Initially, the crews at Belle Chasse performed hoist rescues and recovered about 120 people. The Shelby crews primarily conducted search missions or delivered supplies, equipment, and personnel. Overall, the unit crews accomplished approximately 1,500 personnel evacuations before returning home on 20 September.[96]

Detachment 1 of the 148th Med Co (AA), Washington, DC ARNG, deployed six UH-1 helicopters and 19 soldiers to the Baton Rouge Airport and joined Task Force Eagle. Under the command of 1st Lt. Florian Heithier, the crews flew rescue and recovery missions and rescued seven persons in the first three days. The crews also made many reports of floating bodies. Those recoveries were passed off to teams in boats. After three days, they moved their operation to the Naval Air Station at Belle Chasse, seven miles south of the downtown New Orleans area, and were joined by Lt. Col. Maureen Bellamy and several other troops as replacements for soldiers who had initially deployed. When settled there, the crews flew actual MEDEVAC missions, ferrying patients between medical facilities as they reopened. The unit also kept two aircraft on MEDEVAC alert as required for classic medical response. The unit redeployed at the end of September to its home base at Fort Belvoir, Virginia.[97]

Hurricane Rita

Mother Nature struck again on 24 September when Hurricane Rita swept ashore just south of Houston. The storm was not as strong as Katrina, and the damage was not as severe. Yet, preventive actions had to be taken. JTF-Rita was established with the Fifth U.S. Army, commanded by Lt. Gen. Robert Clark, as the lead command. Texas activated 10,000 Guardsmen for state duty and also requested aid under the EMAC agreement. Some elements assigned to JTF-Katrina were transferred to JTF-Rita and repositioned as necessary. The 149th Med Co (AA), Texas ARNG, was activated again on state orders and deployed to Ellington Air Force Base near Houston. Four helicopters, crews, and support personnel from the 498th Med Co (AA) from Fort Benning joined the 149th at Ellington. The 149th provided general support for the directed evacuation of the area by transporting food and water to predesignated rest stops along the main highways. The unit also flew numerous missions evacuating infirm elderly patients from retirement homes to hospitals further inland.[98]

In support, JTF-Katrina was directed to conduct search and rescue operations as far west as the Texas-Louisiana border. Helicopter units still in Louisiana, including the 812th and 832d Med Cos (AA), responded with helicopter and crews repositioned at Lafayette. Several helicopters were assigned the gruesome task of hunting for and in some cases, recovering caskets that had been blown from the above ground cemeteries so common to the area.[99]

To relieve departing units, in late September, the 112th Med Co (AA), Maine ARNG, deployed a detachment of three UH-60s and 15 personnel for 30 days of duty. The 112th also based at the Naval Air Station at Belle Chasse and provided general support for residual operations.[100]

Results

The national response to Katrina and lesser Rita was unprecedented. The military portion of that was the largest Department of Defense domestic response since the Civil War. Within hours of the realization that Katrina would hit Louisiana, 2,500 Guardsmen were on state-ordered active duty. Within 24 hours of Katrina's landfall, 8,500 Guardsmen and 1,000 active duty troops were in the disaster area. At its peak on 11–12 September, 50,116 Guardsmen and 22,670 active duty personnel from all services served with countless personnel from other governmental agencies and even other nations to help the residents of the stricken areas to begin to recover.

For the first several days, search and rescue was the priority mission. A nominal command and control system was established by the Task Force Eagle personnel at the Superdome and subsequently moved to the Naval Air Station at Belle Chasse. That only applied to helicopters immediately in that area. Most crews acted intuitively and did what needed to be done for those in such distress below. Overall, the collective rescue forces that responded to the disaster rescued 33,544 personnel.[101]

More than 400 helicopters sent to the disaster area performed much of the rescues. The numbers for the collection of units that operated as Task Force Eagle were more descriptive. The helicopters and crews of the task force flew 3,307 hours, rescued or evacuated 60,091 personnel, and carried 3,016 tons of cargo of all classes. The hometown 812th Med Co logged 204 hours in the first seven days performing 144 hoist recoveries and the overall recovery of 482 evacuees. Those numbers also included 2,514 patients who were medically evacuated out of medical facilities threatened or damaged by Katrina. Most were carried by the MEDEVAC units.[102]

However, the congressionally mandated bipartisan review of the response to Katrina criticized the overall effort noting that, "Search and rescue operations were a tremendous success, but coordination and integration between the military services, the National Guard, the Coast Guard, and other local, state, and federal rescue organizations was lacking."[103]

Those totals included the efforts of the MEDEVAC units that operated more as aviation than medical elements. Three active duty and eight ARNG Guard units responded to the disaster with detachments of varying size. All integrated with aviation units because of the absolute lack of any usable surviving infrastructure.

The crews all noted the deficiencies reported above as they flew through the chaos and mayhem that reigned over the stricken area. However, their professionalism enabled them to run a mishap-free operation. No data exist that shows the number of rescues or evacuations that the MEDEVAC units and personnel exclusively logged. The MEDEVAC units' contribution, however, was true to their mission and purpose as defined by doctrine, convention, and heritage.[104]

Organization

Medical Evacuation Proponency

Just a few weeks before Hurricane Katrina, MacDonald replaced Lockard as the director of the MEPD at Fort Rucker. As he watched the horrific events occurring along the Gulf Coast and tracked the actions of the MEDEVAC forces among the larger military and national response, he conducted a review all of the issues facing the community. Operationally, the long MAST commitment was suspended, but his units were engaged in Central America, Kosovo, Iraq, and Afghanistan. Developments in the longer war on terror just five years into the new millennium suggested the good potential for other actions in other arenas.

The Army faced an extended high operations tempo, and MacDonald saw the stress it put on the MEDEVAC force. Organizationally, the ATI was a *fait acompli*. The units shed their heritage identities and reformed within the aviation battalions. MacDonald had to stay engaged with his counterparts in Army aviation as they worked through all of the issues in the Transformation Charter. However, he was under no illusions regarding the struggle's difficulty. He easily recognized what had happened in ATI. The aviation commanders had imposed on the MEDEVAC community the format used by the 50th Med Co in the 101st. Although that may have made great sense from a tactical unit perspective, it encumbered the MEDEVAC community's ability to respond to joint or combined needs or be used as an operational or strategic asset. MacDonald remembered, too—somewhat regrettably—that it was he and Heintz who had initially authored chapter 9 of the 101st Division *Gold Book,* which specified that format and its operational procedures. MacDonald later recalled:

> If you understand how ... aviation saw us, how we would best be structured, it smacks of the *Gold Book,* and it is déjà vu forming because how they structure aviation now is exactly how it was structured in the 101st. When you look at the leadership that has done Army aviation transformation, and you look at the right shoulder patches, you can understand why some of those decisions were made.[105]

MEDEVAC doctrine would need to be rewritten under the joint doctrine structure and format to reflect its newer deeper integration into aviation. MacDonald explained it all in a 30-slide "Quad Charts" Briefing.

Using that as his analysis tool, he then determined what the MEPD focus would be during his watch. His focus included the following:

1. Guide the development of evacuation doctrine;
2. Oversee the transformation of MEDEVAC;
3. Advise during the development of new equipment, aircraft, and vehicles; and
4. Work on personnel solutions for MEDEVAC troops.[106]

All of this would have to be done while the Army itself was going through great change, but the Army has always experienced change. In fact, it seems sometimes that the only thing that is constant is change itself.

* * * *

It was the new millennium. Events of the previous decade had suggested that the Army needed to transform from a ponderous armor-heavy division structured force to a lighter, more mobile force built around autonomous brigades. A new chief of staff embraced that need, and following on the actions of his predecessors, attempted to focus the process and increase the pace of change. Those efforts collided with world events as a lurking enemy dragged the United States into a global war on terror. That struggle has led to the dispatch of U.S. Army forces to several more theaters in ongoing operations. These two parallel and challenging developments plus dramatic events at home have put great strain on Army.

The MEDEVAC community has not been immune to that strain. True, the long commitment to the MAST mission was effectively suspended, but the MEDEVAC force endured the stress of its wholesale reorganization under the ATI, and Hurricane Katrina showed that domestic crises can occur at any time. More ominously, though, the long-term duration of the war on terror is worrisome. No end is yet clearly evident.

The MEDEVAC community will adjust and adapt as transformation occurs and the campaigns continue. It has before, and it will do so again. The reason is fundamentally simple. The men and women of MEDEVAC are masters of both aviation and medical service. They will support their soldiers in harm's way as they always have. That is their legacy and enduring mission.

Chapter Eleven
Warriors of Compassion

"This unit as it stands this day has been forged in the fire of compassion, in the adversity that faces every American soldier in the toil of war."
Charles Kelly Jr.[1]

T he history of MEDEVAC is a long and fascinating tale. It sprang forth from initial incidental uses in World War II, inception in the minds of men like Chauncy Dovell and Spurgeon Neel, and then validation in the frozen fields of Korea. Its evolution continued in Vietnam, through the cold war and subsequent hot actions in Grenada, Panama, Kuwait, Afghanistan, and Iraq, plus its creative and continued use for all manner of domestic taskings. MEDEVAC has become a staple of overall Army operations in defense of the United States and its interests.

The Medical Versus Aviation Debate

This medical versus aviation debate has raged since the earliest days in Korea. The collected history clearly shows that MEDEVAC is not simply one or the other; it is both. It is the classic combination of two things for a larger and better good. Medicine gives it its moral imperative to move patients through the medical system rapidly to get the care that each uniquely needs. The ever improving helicopter provides the ability to overcome many traditional surface obstacles to facilitate that move. Again, it was Neel who understood this and said, "There is a very interesting togetherness between medicine and aviation with which I have been fascinated over the years." He saw them as great management tools that allowed the wounded soldier/casualty to be taken to the medical facility and the doctor best prepared to deal with that soldier's specific needs.[2]

However, helicopters are complicated vehicles with large logistical and administrative needs. They are constrained by the physics of flight, and their use must be overseen by soldiers who understand that there are places where helicopters cannot go for many reasons. Those commissioned and warrant officers and soldiers who have been most successful in MEDEVAC have been those who have developed themselves through a diversity of assignments in both fields. They have learned to focus on what is best for those soldiers or patients in the field who need their services. It is interesting that these same successful individuals—in most cases—served their first Army assignments in medical units seeing Army medicine at the "retail" level before becoming aviators. For most of them, this was a positive and foundational experience.

MEDEVAC *is* a child of those two parents: medicine and aviation. One MEDEVAC commander said, "The MSC officer is, in fact, a dual branch [medical and aviation] officer. He has to be proficient in both branches or he cannot effectively operate on the battlefield... The MEDEVAC officers are the marriage counselors who hold it all together."[3]

To those who had argued that "Aeromedical evacuation is an *aviation mission* that entails *the movement of patients*," the actions of men such as Charles Kelly, Patrick Brady, Mike Novosel, Louis Rocco, and so many others counterargued and proved through their actions that no, aeromedical evacuation was really "a *medical operation* that entails the *use of aircraft*." The long historical trail of this mission shows that the first definition is CASEVAC. The second is MEDEVAC. Additionally, the history shows that it should be favored as a medical vice aviation operation.[4]

Risk Assessment

As a corollary to the above, the commanders of MEDEVAC units have developed a keen ability to balance the needs of the two specialties through structured risk assessment procedures, while clearly placing the priority on the patient's medical concerns. It has been a common and powerful component of their effective mentoring, a ubiquitous virtue within the MEDEVAC community.

Vietnam veterans such as Maj. Gen. Patrick Brady and Brig. Gen. Jerry Foust also emphasized quick reaction times whenever a MEDEVAC request was received, and they optimized their launch procedures to do so. After Vietnam, they taught that methodology and sense of urgency to the younger troops. One of those was Bill Thresher, who remembered Brady telling him the following:

> "You can't train people to do unsafe things by avoiding them. You have to manage the risk with which you train people to do those dangerous things.... You have to train to do dangerous things . . . but you have got to be able to mitigate the risks ...in a way that you are ... approaching it professionally."[5]

In later years, Thresher mentored younger troops like Dave MacDonald and Pete Smart who then applied those principles when they were MEDEVAC commanders, learning how to carefully balance the medical risk to the patient with the operational risk of the mission. They and several other commanders described in detail the procedures that they used with their aircrews to facilitate expeditious launch. They authorized their subordinate commanders and even pilots in command to launch under specified conditions, and then they established communications procedures so that they or even higher commanders were quickly reachable if launch conditions had significantly changed. It empowered the aircrews and kept launch times to a minimum.

The MEDEVAC pilots were aware that many commanders within the aviation community were uncomfortable with this authorization. The aviation commanders maintained launch authority firmly with battalion or even brigade commanders. However, their mission parameters were starkly different. In most cases, aviation missions were scheduled in advance, and the crews had plenty of time to plan their mission. MEDEVAC missions were not specifically planned. They were reactive to events in the field that then required MEDEVAC support. The crews had to be as prepared as possible and adaptive to changing situations. Smart saw this clearly. He remembered the following:

> I came from the aviation community myself and a lot of times I consider myself more from the aviation side. But those [aviation] guys …the people who have never flown MEDEVAC out there don't realize the intricacies of the work that we do and the responsibilities that our [pilots in command] have out there by themselves. The assault guys… they've got 72 hours to plan the mission that's going to last for 45 minutes. We have 45 minutes to plan a mission that might last 72 hours.[6]

The MEDEVAC crews prided themselves on being responsive and chaffed at indecision. They remembered Neel's admonition uttered way back in Korea that, "Speed of evacuation is most important in the severely wounded…. A man dies in so many minutes, not over a distance of so many miles. Any measure that will reduce the time lag between wounding and treatment will reduce both the mortality and morbidity of war wounds."[7] They grew frustrated when they were under aviation command and suffered extensive launch delays. Consider this quote from an after-action report from Afghanistan:

> One specific incident involved a patient with a through-and-through gunshot wound [GSW] to the chest. The casualty was conscious, alert, and oriented, two and one half hours post injury under the care of a physician assistant and senior 18D at the area operations base….the CASE-VAC arrived approximately three hours post injury with a physician and blood products. The casualty expired just prior to the arrival of the CASEVAC aircraft.[8]

To a MEDEVAC troop, this was absolute heresy. After this incident, an anonymous MEDEVAC soldier stated the following:

> How quickly should MEDEVAC respond? Simple. We should respond at the speed of blood, because if that soldier out there who needs our services bleeds out before we get there, we have failed, and it does not matter if this is for medical or aviation reasons.

However, no amount of medical imperative can override the immutable laws of physics. There are still places in this world where helicopters cannot go. MEDEVAC and aviation commanders must carefully weigh the medical risk and operational risk to do what is best for the soldiers.

Why Do They Do It?

It is a powerful and resonating question. Beyond the discussion of organization, operations, and doctrine, why do the soldiers do it? The answer seems simple, "It's the right thing to do," the soldiers say. (This was a common refrain among all interviewees.) Pfc. Ray Leopold, a medic with the 28th Infantry Division in World War II, gave it a more timeless dimension when he said, "It is never pleasant to do the work of a medic. But it's one of the essentials of civilized behavior."[9]

This history suggests, however, that there is more to it. The *logos* of MEDE-VAC, the history of how it is done, is clear. But what is the *pathos* behind the propensity or—better yet—passion to execute MEDEVAC?

Losses in war are expected. All planners know when they plan military operations that soldiers will be wounded and some will die. Guidance for the calculation of projected casualties is replete in medical doctrine. As part of the overall plan, sub-plans are developed to handle the casualties.

All commanders wrestle with mission accomplishment versus cost. They know that in imposing America's will in a war, campaign, or battle, there will be a "butcher's bill" to be paid. That paradox or dilemma is ingrained in the Army creed, "I will always place the mission first," and "I will never leave a fallen comrade."[10]

Lt. Gen. David D. McKiernan, commander of V Corps in Operation IRAQI FREEDOM, addressed this when he wrote the following:

> As a commander, I have the responsibility of sending the sons and daughters of America into harm's way knowing full well it can lead to their death or serious injury. I also have an unwavering moral obligation to do everything possible to … prevent the loss of the lives of those fine men and women who voluntarily serve their country…[11]

The noted author, Rick Atkinson, traveled with Maj. Gen. David Petraeus when he commanded the 101st Division in Operation IRAQI FREEDOM. He said of the man: "I never sensed that personal ambition eclipsed his visceral awareness that 17,000 lives were in his hands, and that no occasion could be more solemn or profound for a commander than ordering young soldiers to their deaths."[12]

The American people know, too, that in war losses will occur. They are prepared to accept them, provided that the cause is worth fighting for. "As much as I don't want my dad to fight, I am willing to give him to you," wrote one young girl to President George W. Bush, just before he dispatched American troops to Afghanistan.[13]

Although casualties can be expected, America does not give easily or blithely of those losses. "The Army has long been the strength of the Nation," wrote Army Chief of Staff Gen. George Casey. "Our soldiers and their families epitomize what is best about America." Speaking about those who have been wounded, he stated, "We will also ensure that our wounded warriors receive the care and support they need to reintegrate effectively into the Army and society."[14]

In parallel, the nation expects its wounded men and women to receive the best care available as expeditiously as possible. "Our wounded soldiers deserve nothing less than the best health care this country can provide," said Congresswoman Louise Slaughter at a congressional hearing.[15]

U.S. Marine Corps Gen. James Jones, the past commander of the U.S. European Command, gave a more focused reason when he said, "The military must have a 'social contract' with the troops, and must never see them as expendable."[16]

The latest and best technology will be used to provide that care, and the MEDEVAC fleet is the hard physical representation of that "social contract." That fleet is a combination of the best of aviation joined with soldiers who harbor a sympathetic consciousness of others' distress together with a desire to alleviate it. There is a word for such an emotion. It is called compassion.[17]

The men and women of MEDEVAC are warriors of compassion. In Vietnam, one soldier wrote of them, "To the wounded soldier, DUSTOFF was his salvation in the form of an olive drab Huey emblazoned with bright red crosses. Whatever else might fail him—and in this brutal, unforgiving war, much did—DUSTOFF never would."[18]

That bond is just as valid today. That is why the MEDEVAC crews want to respond at the "speed of blood." Capt. Justin Avery of the 82d Med Co in Operation IRAQI FREEDOM said, "We were out there to support those ground soldiers and make sure they got back home alive if at all possible."[19]

The thank-you notes arrive in many forms, like this email sent to CW2 Gerald McGowen, a MEDEVAC pilot recently assigned to the 50th Med Co (AA):

> "Hi, my name is S.Sgt. Olson. On 27th Oct of 03, you flew a MEDEVAC out of Tel A Far [sic]. I was wounded in an ambush there. I am at Walter Reed still, but I am recovering. Thanks to you and your dedication to your job I am still alive and I try to live every day to its fullest. Thanks again and God Bless all of you. Good Luck and God speed to whichever way life takes you. Yours in service, S.Sgt. Joshua Olson.[20]

Sometimes the simplest rewards are the sweetest.

Inactivation of the 57th Med Co (AA) "The Originals"

It was a cold crisp February morning when veterans and friends from far and wide gathered with the soldiers of the 57th Med Co (AA) at their hangar at Fort Bragg, North Carolina, for the inactivation of "The Originals," as they proudly displayed on their unit patch. That company was the most blooded air ambulance unit. More than any other, it personified the spirit of MEDEVAC. Now, it would be inactivated and its colors retired as directed by the Aviation Transformation Initiative.

A dinner was held the previous evening at the NCO Club. Members of the unit from three different generations gathered and mixed easily. The stories from Vietnam, Military Assistance to Safety and Traffic duties, Grenada, Desert Storm, Bosnia, Iraqi Freedom, and so many stateside exercises and missions flowed. There were too many to capture.

Tom "Egor" Johnson addressed the evening crowd. Johnson, a former crew chief with the unit with two tours in Vietnam, spoke of Maj. Charles Kelly and the battles that he and his troops fought to establish MEDEVAC and protect its unique status. He saw in those currently serving, the same dedication to mission that he and his contemporaries had experienced. In reflecting on conversations that he had had with them that evening, he said, "What I heard from [today's] crews is the same ... desire to save the patient on the battlefield." He reminded them that the 57th—the "Original Dustoff"—had set the standard for MEDEVAC. It had never let its patients down. He saluted those still serving as the final 57th crews and finished by saying to them, "You have held the tradition and legacy to a very high standard. Major Kelly on high looks down and I guarantee is proud of each and every one of you. And I salute you."[21]

The inactivation ceremony was the next morning. Lt. Col. Scott Putzier, the commander of the parent 56th Multifunctional Medical Battalion, welcomed the XVIII Airborne Corps commander, Lt. Gen. Lloyd J. Austin III, and a large collection of veterans and family. After introductory remarks, Putzier was followed by a video historical presentation of the unit's stellar accomplishments, including being awarded a Presidential Unit Citation, six meritorious Unit Commendations, and the Vietnam Cross of Gallantry with Palm Device.

The next speakers were the members of the "last" 57th MEDEVAC crew. Each explained his or her duties.

The pilot in command, CW2 Kevin Moore said, "I am the pilot in command. My responsibility is the safety of the crew, patients, passengers, and the overall success of each mission. I understand that our mission is of the utmost importance to the combat readiness of any unit. I am an American soldier and I will not fail."

Pilot 1st Lt. Rebecca Joseph said, "I am the pilot. I act with the awareness that every second is critical to saving a life. To quote Kelly, 'No compromise, no rationalization, no hesitation, fly the mission.' I am an American soldier and I will not fail."

She was followed by the crew chief, Sgt. Josh Touchton, who said, "I am the crew chief. I will ensure that my aircraft is maintained and ready. I will provide security for my aircraft and the other members of my crew during missions and will provide support to the flight medic with any assistance necessary. I am an American soldier, and I will not fail."

Lastly, the flight medic, S.Sgt. Shawn McNabb, spoke. "I am the flight medic. My primary responsibility is the casualties on my helicopter. I will sacrifice everything for my patient's survival. I have to be the best medic on the battlefield. I will strive to provide the best care possible to those entrusted to my skills. I am an American soldier and I will not fail."

The company commander, Maj. Brady Rose, then called the unit to attention and called for the casing of the unit guidon. As it was being passed forward, the narrator, Capt. Pete Hudgins, said, "...Though today, we are seemingly ending an era by casing this unit guidon, it does not mean that the 57th Medical Company (AA) will simply go away, for its accomplishments, its soldiers, and its outstanding lineage and honors will be forever recorded in not only MEDEVAC history, but in military history."[22]

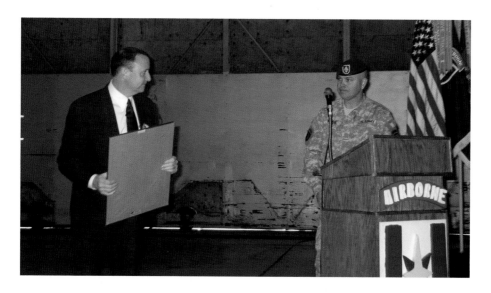

Mr. Charles Kelly Jr., and Maj. Brady Rose at the unit inactivation ceremony in 2007.
Source: Author.

Then, as the guidon was being slowly and carefully encased, he read the inactivation order, "By authority of Army Regulation 71-32 Paragraph 7-14: the 57th Medical Company (Air Ambulance) is hereby inactivated."[23]

Putzier returned to the podium to introduce Mr. Charles Kelly Jr., who paused momentarily and then began.

> Good morning. My father was Major Charles Kelly. I carry his name; I speak for him today. It's an honor to be here because in my opinion, you are the finest example of men and women who exist in the Army today. We are at war and you are operating at peak performance in a profession that few understand or appreciate outside the military community. You're cohesive, dedicated, selfless; you are the standard bearer for Army Air Medical Evacuation.

> In the movie *Enter the Dragon* Bruce Lee's nemesis says, "We forge our bodies in the fire of our will." This unit as it stands this day has been *forged in the fire of compassion*, in the adversity that faces every American soldier in the toil of war. We are at war. Americans are dying almost daily. The 57th Medical [Company] becomes inactivated today. I guess somebody decided it was time to reinvent the wheel. With my apologies to anyone on the wrong side of that decision, I cannot agree. It is a bad idea, because it is too risky right now. "If it ain't broke, let's don't fix it." We are in the middle of a war. Now I understand we must reorganize and streamline this Army. Change is the only thing that is constant in this world and our armed forces will have to operate differently in the future.[24]

Kelly then went on to share some personal history about his father. He held few actual memories of him since he had been a young lad when his father left for war. However, in later years he had read all of his father's papers and records and came to know him well as a true hero of MEDEVAC.

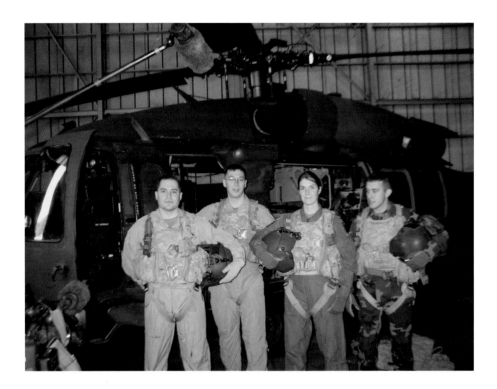

The "Last" 57th Med Co MEDEVAC crew: CW2 Kevin Moore, S.Sgt. Shawn McNabb, 1st Lt. Rebecca Joseph, Sgt. Josh Touchton.
Source: Author.

Kelly talked of his father's travails in Korea and exposed many of his faults. "He was not a perfect man," he said openly. He spoke of his father's dogged determination, strict standards, and devotion to his men and the troops in the field. He spoke of the battles that his father fought to keep his helicopters under medical control when other commanders wanted them for other missions. He spoke of how his father agonized about caring for so many soldiers throughout a country the size of south Vietnam with just five aircraft. He spoke tenderly of a father that he deeply respected, loved, and still missed.

Then he continued:

> But to me, the 57th represents the father that I did not know. I know him now from those who served with him and from his writings and I see in your eyes, the dedication of professional soldiers that is born from history, compassion, personal courage, and discipline.

> And today, I can say to you, ...the men and women of the 57th, the last of the originals, that you are a shining example of that standard. You have upheld that tradition set by those who came before you. I daresay, even improved upon them. My father would be very, very proud of you. I thank you on behalf of him and my family.

I encourage you to face the future as the excellent soldiers that you are. Let adversity and fear, if it exists in you, not weaken you but make you stronger. Let those things continue to forge you into a better soldier, a better aviator, with an even stronger mind and spirit than you already have.

The 57th is inactivated today but you are the originals, the last of the best. Carry that with you wherever you go in whatever you do because one day, one of you may be seated at the table where these policy decisions will be made. I look forward to the reactivation ceremony then.

And so here we are, tomorrow is a new day. The pages are blank. The next chapter is yours to write. If there is weakness in this new system, root it out. If you face adversity or frustration, let it make you stronger. When you feel fear, remember that fear is the furnace that can destroy you or forge you into a sword of steel with a razor's edge—a mighty weapon to overcome your enemy with. Your enemy is death itself. That's why you fly...You will not fail. You are the originals. You are the heart and soul of Dustoff. You are soldiers. Thank you and God bless you on your journey through this Army and through this life. Keep the faith.[25]

And with that, it was done. The festivities lasted for an hour or so.

Then the veterans and guests left, and commander and soldiers began disbursing the personnel and equipment to other units and jobs. The MEDEVAC units would now be known by other titles and designations. Their unit heritages would derive from another strain of warriors.

Regardless, the MEDEVAC spirit would be the same because the propensity to care for the men and women of America who volunteer to travel in harm's way to protect the nation and its interests is fundamental to the American way of war. American soldiers are the blood of the nation. Americans owe it to the soldiers to care for them when they fall with every tool available. It is the bond Americans have with them.

The men and women of MEDEVAC are the keepers of that bond, so clearly defined by Maj. Charles Kelly so long ago...

...when I have your wounded.

* * * *

From its humble beginnings in Burma through Korea and the bitter experience of Vietnam, the rebuilding years and Military Assistance to Safety and Traffic, through conflicts in places like Grenada, Panama, Kuwait, Iraq, Somalia, Bosnia, the horror of 9/11, Afghanistan, and Iraq again, the men and women of MEDEVAC took an unproven concept and developed it into a system that saves lives. The MEDEVAC community is a national treasure, and its men and women are the constant face of hope in so many scenes of chaos. They were and are the warriors of compassion.

Theirs is a monumental accomplishment and has generated a proud heritage—the kind that could attract a young lieutenant like Andrew Russ or Rebecca Joseph, an earnest warrant officer like Kevin Moore, a dedicated crew chief like Josh Touchton, or a focused medic like Shawn McNabb. (Note: S.Sgt. Shawn McNabb was killed in action in Afghanistan on 26 October 2009.) It will be their heritage too, for in their time and place, they will be called upon to add to it in their own measure and create that next chapter of this enduring legacy.

List of MEDEVAC Units

Note: Prior to their assignment as aeromedical units, many existed with other specializations and designations. As medical units, all had subidentifiers. Companies and separate platoons were designated as (AA) for air ambulance, any aircraft. Medical detachments were designated as (HA) for helicopter ambulance, any aircraft, or (RA) for UH-1 aircraft, or (RG) for UH-60 aircraft. Another designation (RC) was used for a short time for units assigned for crash and rescue duties.

Korea Era

1st Helicopter Detachment
— 8190th Army Unit
— 37th Medical Detachment (HA)
— 47th Medical Platoon (AA)

2d Helicopter Detachment
— 8191st Army Unit
— 49th Medical Detachment (HA)

3d Helicopter Detachment
— 8192d Army Unit
— 52d Medical Detachment (HA)

4th Helicopter Detachment
— 8193d Army Unit
— 50th Medical Detachment (HA), Air Ambulance Platoon, 326th Medical Battalion, Delta Company, 326th Medical Battalion,
— 50th Medical Company (AA)

1st Helicopter Ambulance Company (Provisional)

Post–Korea

15th Medical Detachment (HA/RA/RG)
21st Medical Platoon (AA)
32d Medical Detachment (HA)

36th Medical Detachment (RA/RG)   – U.S. Army Air Ambulance
                                                 Detachment Fort Polk, Louisiana

36th Medical Battalion (Evacuation)
45th Medical Company (AA)
47th Medical Detachment (HA)
52d Medical Battalion (Evacuation)
53d Medical Detachment (HA)
54th Medical Detachment (HA/RA)   – 54th Medical Company (AA)
56th Medical Detachment (HA)   – 56th Medical Platoon (AA)
56th Medical Battalion (Evacuation)
57th Medical Detachment (HA/RA/RG)   – 57th Medical Platoon (AA) – 57th
                                                 Medical Company (AA)

58th Medical Detachment (HA)
58th Medical Battalion (Evacuation)
61st Medical Battalion (Evacuation)
63d Medical Detachment (HA/RA/RG)
68th Medical Detachment (RA/RG)   – 68th Medical Company (AA)
78th Medical Detachment (RA)
82d Medical Detachment (HA/RA)   – 82d Medical Company (AA)
85th Medical Battalion (Evacuation)
132d Medical Detachment (RC)
151st Medical Detachment (RA)
159th Medical Detachment (RA/RG)   – 159th Medical Company (AA)
212th Medical Detachment (RA)
214th Medical Detachment (RC/RG)
218th Medical Detachment (RC)
229th Medical Detachment (RA)   – U.S. Army Air Ambulance
                                                 Detachment, Fort Drum, New York
236th Medical Detachment (RA/RG)   – 236th Medical Company (AA)
237th Medical Detachment (RA)
247th Medical Detachment (RA/RG)   – U.S. Army Air Ambulance
                                                 Detachment, Fort Irwin, California

254th Medical Detachment (RA)
274th Medical Detachment (HA)
283d Medical Detachment (RA/RG)
377th Medical Company (AA)
421st Medical Company (AA)   – 421st Medical Battalion
                                                 (Evacuation)

431st Medical Detachment (RA)
436th Medical Detachment (HA Provisional)
498th Medical Company (AA)
507th Medical Company (AA)
542d Medical Company (AA)
571st Medical Detachment (RA)   – 571st Medical Company (AA)

587th Medical Detachment (RA)
658th Medical Detachment (AA)   – 658th Medical Company (AA)
                                          (Provisional)
Air Ambulance Platoon, 15th Medical Battalion

Army Reserve

136th Medical Detachment (RA)
145th Medical Detachment (RA)
273d Medical Detachment (RA)
312th Medical Detachment (RA)
316th Medical Detachment (RA)
317th Medical Company (AA)
321st Medical Detachment (RA)
336th Medical Detachment (RA)
341st Medical Battalion (Evacuation)
343d Medical Detachment (RA)
345th Medical Company (AA)
347th Medical Detachment (RA)
348th Medical Detachment (RA)
354th Medical Detachment (RA)
364th Medical Detachment (RA)
374th Medical Detachment (RA)
412th Medical Detachment (RA)
423d Medical Detachment (RA)
429th Medical Battalion (Evacuation)
872d Medical Detachment (RA)   – 872d Medical Company (AA)
989th Medical Detachment (RA)
990th Medical Detachment (RA)
991st Medical Detachment (RA)

Army National Guard

Note: These units are organized under the 54 individual National Guard organizations. All have lineages that evolve from previous units of all Army branches. Unit redesignations are common and occur yearly. Any unit may have existed for decades, at one time as an infantry unit, then transportation, then aviation, then medical, etc. See Appendix B for an example.

24th Medical Company (AA) Nebraska
86th Medical Company (AA) Vermont
104th Medical Company (AA) Maryland
107th Medical Company (AA) Ohio
110th Medical Battalion (Evacuation) Nebraska

112th Medical Company (AA) Maine
121st Medical Company (AA) Washington, DC
123d Medical Company (AA) Mississippi
126th Medical Company (AA) California
133d Medical Company (AA) Alabama
142d Medical Detachment (HA/RA) North Dakota
146th Medical Detachment (HA/RA) West Virginia
148th Medical Company (AA) Georgia
151st Medical Battalion (Evacuation) Georgia
157th Medical Detachment (HA/RA) Colorado
172d Medical Company (AA) Arkansas
198th Medical Company (AA) Delaware
199th Medical Company (AA) Florida
397th Medical Detachment (HA/RA) New Hampshire
400th Medical Detachment (HA/RA) Washington, DC
441st Medical Detachment (HA/RA) Kentucky
470th Medical Detachment (HA/RA) Kentucky
659th Medical Detachment (HA/RA) South Carolina
670th Medical Detachment (HA/RA) Tennessee
681st Medical Company (AA) Indiana
717th Medical Detachment (HA/RA)   - 717th Medical Company (AA) New Mexico
812th Medical Detachment (HA/RA)   - 812th Medical Company (AA) Louisiana
813th Medical Detachment (HA/RA) Louisiana then Minnesota
832d Medical Company (AA) Wisconsin
841st Medical Detachment (HA/RA) Wisconsin
867th Medical Detachment (HA/RA) Missouri
868th Medical Detachment (HA/RA) Missouri
920th Medical Detachment (HA/RA) Kansas
986th Medical Detachment (HA/RA)   – 986th Medical Company (AA) Virginia
997th Medical Company (AA) Arizona
1022d Medical Detachment (HA/RA)   -1022d Medical Company (AA) Wyoming
1042d Medical Detachment (HA/RA)   - 1042d Medical Company (AA) Oregon
1058th Medical Detachment (HA/RA) South Dakota
1059th Medical Detachment (HA/RA) Massachusetts/New Hampshire
     - 1059th Medical Company (AA) Massachusetts/New Hampshire
1085th Medical Detachment (HA/RA)   - 1085th Medical Company (AA) South Dakota
1133d Medical Company (AA) Alabama

1136th Medical Detachment (HA/RA) Texas
1150th Medical Detachment (HA/RA) Nevada
1159th Medical Company (AA) New Hampshire
1187th Medical Company (AA) Iowa
1214th Medical Company (AA) North Dakota
1250th Medical Company (AA) Utah
1255th Medical Company (AA) Nevada
1259th Medical Company (AA) South Carolina
1267th Medical Company (AA) Missouri
1297th Medical Detachment (HA/RA) Alaska

Post–Transformation (Planned)

Charlie Company, 5-158 General Support Aviation Battalion (GSAB)
Charlie Company, 1-214 GSAB
Charlie Company, 3-10 GSAB
Charlie Company, 2-52 GSAB
Charlie Company, 1-52 GSAB
Charlie Company, 7-101 GSAB
Charlie Company, 2-3 GSAB
Charlie Company, 2-1 GSAB
Charlie Company, 3-82 GSAB
Charlie Company, 6-101 GSAB
Charlie Company, 3-25 GSAB
Charlie Company, 2-227 GSAB
Charlie Company, 2-4 GSAB

US Army Aviation Detachment   – Fort Rucker
US Army Aviation Detachment   – Fort Drum
US Army Aviation Detachment   – Fort Irwin
US Army Aviation Detachment   – US Army South
US Army Aviation Detachment   – Fort Polk

Army National Guard

Charlie Company, 2-104 GSAB
Charlie Company, 1-111 GSAB
Charlie Company, 1-189 GSAB
Charlie Company, 2-211 GSAB
Charlie Company, 2-149 GSAB
Charlie Company, 3-238 GSAB
Charlie Company, 1-168 GSAB
Charlie Company, 3-126 GSAB
Charlie Company, 1-126 GSAB

Charlie Company, 1-169 GSAB
Charlie Company, 1-171 GSAB
Charlie Company, 2-238 GSAB
Charlie Company, 5-159 GSAB
Charlie Company, 7-158 GSAB
Charlie Company, 2-135 GSAB
121st Medical Company (AA)
249th Medical Company (AA)
812th Medical Company (AA)
832d Medical Company (AA)

Sources: Hough, *United States Army Air Ambulance;* Anderson, *The DUSTOFF Report;* Briefing by Lt. Col. James Schwartz, DASG-HCO.

Typical History of an ARNG MEDEVAC Unit

The 112th Med Co (AA), Maine ARNG, traces its origin as a unit back to 22 June 1927, when it was organized in Gardiner, Maine, as Headquarters Company, 1st Battalion – 103d Infantry Regiment. As a member of the 103d, it inherited a rich tradition in military history because the 103d was one of the oldest and most famous fighting forces in the history of the United States.

On 1 February 1929, the unit was redesignated "Mike" Company, 103d Infantry Regiment, and was known as the top machine-gun company in the entire regiment.

As part of one of the three regimental combat teams in the 43d Infantry Division, "Mike" Company was mobilized and sailed 1 October 1942 from San Francisco, California, and arrived in Auckland, New Zealand, on 22 October 1942. The unit later landed and defended the central part of the New Caledonia Island until February 1943. The unit received its first battle casualties while occupying the Russell Islands. Throughout its tour in the Pacific Islands the unit took part in the battle of the Munda airstrip and in the New Georgia Island Group, and in July of 1943 it helped repulse a formidable Japanese offensive on New Guinea.

"Mike" Company was officially returned to National Guard status on 17 April 1946. In March of 1959 the proud company was reorganized and designated "Aviation Troop, 103d Armored Cavalry Regiment." It was equipped with OH-13 Sioux helicopters.

In 1960 the unit was redesignated the Aviation Company, 103d Armored Cavalry Regiment. In June 1961, it was again reorganized as the 112th Aviation Company (Fixed wing, light transport). The company traded its OH-13 Sioux Helicopters for U-1A Otter fixed wing aircraft. Unit strength at this time was about 5 pilots and 45–50 enlisted personnel.

The unit was further reorganized in March of 1963 when it became the 112th Aviation Company (CORPS ARTILLERY). It was the most combat ready unit in the Maine Army National Guard for that year.

After a short period of stability, the company was redesignated and federally recognized as the "112th Medical Company (Air Ambulance)" on 13 November 1967. Its headquarters was in Gardiner, Maine, with its flight facility at the Augusta Airport.

The 112th moved to Bangor, Maine, in July of 1968 and took up residence in the original Army Aviation Support Facility that was dedicated on 23 July 1977. Aircraft and maintenance were located in the old hangar, building 254, from July 1968 to July 1977. The unit Headquarters and Operations were located in building 255, now the Band Armory.

The 112th moved up on the hill to the current armory in the summer of 1980.

The 112th has gone through several airframes over the years, including the CH-34 Choctaw and OH-23 Raven. In 1972 the 112th received its first UH-1H Huey and they continued to arrive until there were a total of 25 Hueys in the unit, six for each of the four flight platoons, and one for the Company Headquarters. The unit now had slots for 53 pilots, and a total of 142 personnel.

The 112th has saved many persons since receiving the UH-1H helicopter. One program, the Maine Incubator Transfer Service for Infant Emergencies (MITSIE) flew more than 400 premature babies. During the 1970s and 1980s the 112th gained a reputation as one of the most mission capable MEDEVAC companies in the entire U.S. Army. During this period the company participated in numerous exercises including "REFORGER," "WINGED WARRIOR," and many MEDEVAC support missions throughout the United States and foreign countries, performing hundreds of real world rescues.

On 6 December 1990, the 112th was again called into active federal service in support of Operation DESERT SHIELD/DESERT STORM. It deployed to Germany to support MEDEVAC operations in the European theater and remained in Europe up through and including Operation PROVIDE COMFORT. Distinguishing itself as reliable and highly mission capable, 112th was praised by General Crosby Saint, the commander of all U.S. Army forces in Europe.

The company returned to the United States and was released from active federal service on 4 September 1991.

From January 1994 through June 1994, 3 aircraft and 15 personnel deployed as MEDEVAC Support of Task Force Dirigo, an engineer mission to build roads, bridges, and schools near Salama, Guatemala.

From 1993 through 1997 the company underwent a total of five U.S. Army Aviation evaluations where it was validated as combat ready and deemed capable of performing its mission worldwide. As a result the 112th was designated as a "Force Support Package" and was selected to begin receiving the UH-60 "Blackhawk" helicopter in 1997. The program required the unit to maintain a high state of readiness and be prepared to mobilize and integrate with active duty counterparts on very short notice, a responsibility still taken very seriously today.

The first two Blackhawks to enter the state arrived in August of 1997.

From 19 August 1999 until 31 March 2000, 77 unit members successfully deployed to Bosnia-Herzegovina, where they provided MEDEVAC and peacekeeping support to the Stabilization Force 6 mission.

On 10 February 2003, the 112th was activated and mobilized through Fort Drum, New York, in support of Operation IRAQI FREEDOM. The unit arrived in Kuwait on 29 March and was based there with forward support medical teams at several locations throughout Iraq until April 2004. The unit flew more than 3,600 hours and evacuated more than 1,000 patients. The unit received the Master Readiness Award for the Highest Operational Readiness of any aviation unit in theater.

In the summer of 2005, 3 aircraft and 15 crewmembers voluntarily deployed to Louisiana in support of Hurricane Katrina relief efforts. They operated out of Belle Chasse Naval Air Station, where they augmented the 812th Med Co (AA) of the Louisiana ARNG.

Over the years the 112th has provided medical and aviation support to many organizations, both domestic and foreign. Unit members and equipment have frequently been called to other states and even other countries including Germany, Panama, Guatemala, Japan, Newfoundland, Bosnia-Herzegovina, Kuwait, Iraq, and most recently Louisiana.

Within Maine, the 112th is often requested to assist in search and rescue for lost persons, emergency medical evacuations, and medical assistance and rescue to accident victims in remote areas of the Maine wilderness.

(112th Med Co Unit History provided by 2d Lt. Jasmine Chase, Unit Historian, Maine ARNG)

Appendix C
MEDEVAC Losses Post–Vietnam Era through Operation IRAQI FREEDOM 1

UH-1 Aircraft

Date	Location	Unit	Crewmembers killed	Cause
15 Mar 75	Germany	421st	WO1 Desmond Downey CW2 John Johnson SP5 Earl Rankhorn SP5 Harvey Salas	Crash
13 Jul 77	Korea	377th	Capt. William Lashley CW2 James Miles S.Sgt. Horace Robinson Unknown	Crash
4 Jan 78	Tennessee (MAST)	326th Bn	Capt. John Dunnavant Capt. Terry Woolever Sgt. Floyd Smith Lt. Col. Ray Maynard Four Unknown	Crash
4 Mar 80	Kentucky (MAST)	326th Bn	WO1 Sheryl Siroonian Three Unknown	Crash
4 Sep 82	Colorado (MAST)	571st	Maj. Richard Bulliner Capt. William Inklebarger Pfc. Mark Welch S.Sgt. Gregg Penn	Crash
17 Sep 84	Indiana	412th USAR	Capt. Tom Heaverin CW2 Robert Machholz	Crash

6 Feb 87	Georgia (MAST)	498th	1st Lt. Jim Belcher CW2 Kevin Killman Sp4c. Jerome Brachel Sfc. Doyle Cannon	Crash
23 Nov 90	Oklahoma	374th USAR	CIV Philip Walker	Crash
14 Dec 90	Texas	1267th Missouri ARNG	1st Lt. Peter Rose CW2 Carol McKinney Sgt. Dallas Cooper	Crash
7 Feb 91	S. Arabia	229th	CW3 Richard Lee	Crash
27 Feb 91	Iraq	507th	1st Lt. Daniel Graybeal WO1 Kerry Heine S.Sgt. Mike Robson	Shot down
13 May 91	Honduras California ARNG	126th	1st Lt. Vicki Boyd Capt. Sashai Dawn S.Sgt. Linda Simonds	Crash
1 March 97	Indiana	681st	CW2 Thomas Miller	Crash

http://www.armyaircrews.com/huey.html (accessed 2 April 2008)

UH-60 Aircraft

Date	Location	Unit	Crewmembers killed	Cause
28 Aug 88	Germany	236th	Capt. Kim Strader	Ground accident
30 Nov 89	Panama	214th	S.Sgt. Adrian Rosado	Water crash
19 Jan 91	S. Arabia	236th	S.Sgt. Garland Hailey	Crash
12 Mar 91	Iraq	36th	1st Lt. Joseph Maks CW2 Patrick Donaldson Spc. Kelly Phillips Sgt. Mike Smith	Crash
9 May 03	Iraq	571st	CW2 Hans Gukeisen CW3 Brian Van Dusen Cpl. Richard Carl	Combat loss

http://www.armyaircrews.com/blackhawk.html (accessed 2 April 2008)

Abbreviations and Acronyms

A2C2	Army airspace command and control
AA	Air Ambulance
ABIP	Aviation Branch Implementation Plan
ACLS	Advanced cardiac life support
ACR	Armored cavalry regiment
AD	Armored Division
ADA	Air defense artillery
AFB	Air Force Base
AHR	Attack Helicopter Regiment
AHS	Academy of Health Services
AMEDD	Army Medical Department
AMES	Army Medical Evacuation System
AMS	Army Medical Service
AOC	Area of occupational concentration
ARI	Aviation Restructuring Initiative
ARMS	Aviation Resource Management Survey
ARNG	Army National Guard
ARS	Air Rescue Squadron
ARVN	Army of the Republic of Vietnam
ATI	Aviation Transformation Initiative
ATLS	Advanced trauma life support
AU	Army Unit
AVIM	Aviation intermediate maintenance
AVUM	Aviation unit maintenance
AXP	Ambulance transfer point
BAE	Brigade aviation element
BCT	Brigade combat team
BIAP	Baghdad International Airport

C2	Command and control
CALL	Center for Army Lessons Learned
CASH	Combat Army Surgical Hospital
CAT	Crisis action team
CD	Cavalry Division
CEOI	Communications electronic operating instructions
CHS	Combat health support
C/JFLCC	Combined/Joint Force Land Component Command
CMF	Contingency Medical Force
CMTC	Combat Maneuver Training Center
CONUS	Continental United States
COSCOM	Corps Support Command
CSAR	Combat Search and Rescue
CSH	Combat Support Hospital
CTC	Combat training center
CTF	Combined task force
DAART	Downed aircraft or aircrew recovery team
DASC	Direct air support center
DCE	Defense coordination element
DCO	Defense coordination officer
DCSOPS	Deputy chief of staff for operations
DCSPER	Deputy chief of staff for personnel
DISCOM	Division Support Command
DMOC	Division medical operations center
DOD	Department of Defense
DOMS	Director of Military Support
DOT	Department of Transportation
EAC	Echelon above corps
EMAC	Emergency Management Assistance Compact
EMT	Emergency medical technician
ESSS	External stores support system (UH-60)
FARP	Forward arming and refueling point
FASCOM	Field Army Support Command
FC	Field Circular
FEAF	Far East Air Force
FECOM	Far East Command
FHP	Force health protection
FLIR	Forward Looking Infrared
FLOT	Forward Line of Troops
FM	Field Manual
FOB	Forward Operating Base
FORSCOM	U.S. Army Forces Command
FSMT	Forward Support MEDEVAC Team
FST	Forward surgical team

FTX	Field training exercise
GPS	Global positioning system
GSAB	General Support Aviation Battalion
HCA	Humanitarian civilian assistance
HF	High frequency
HSS	Health service support
HSSALB	Health service support to AirLand Battle
ID	Infantry Division
IFOR	Implementation Force, Bosnia
ISAF	International Security Assistance force
JAAF	Joint Army Air Force
JFLCC	Joint Forces Land Component Command
JFS	Joint force surgeon
JNA	Yugoslav National Army
JOC	Joint operations center
JOPES	Joint Operation Planning and Execution System
JP	Joint Publication
JPMRC	Joint patient movement requirements center
JROC	Joint Requirements Oversight Council
JRTC	Joint Readiness Training Center
JTF	Joint task force
JVX	Joint vertical aircraft experimental
KFOR	Kosovo Force
KIA	Killed in action
KKMC	King Khalid Military City, Saudi Arabia
KLA	Kosovo Liberation Army
LHX	Light helicopter experimental
LSA	Logistics support area
MASCAL	Mass casualty event
MASH	Mobile Army Surgical Hospital
MAST	Military Assistance to Safety and Traffic
MAW	Marine Aircraft Wing
MDW	Military District of Washington
MEB	Marine Expeditionary Brigade
MEDCOM	Medical Command
Med Co (AA)	Medical Company (Air Ambulance)
MEDDAC	Medical Department Activity
Med Det (HA)	Medical Detachment (Helicopter Ambulance)
Med Det (RA)	Medical Detachment UH-1
Med Det (RC)	Medical Detachment (Crash Rescue)
Med Det (RG)	Medical Detachment UH-60
MEF	Marine Expeditionary Force
MEU	Marine Expeditionary Unit
MEPAO	Medical Evacuation (Air/Ground) Proponency Action Office

MEPD	Medical Evacuation Proponency Directorate
METT-TC	Mission, enemy, terrain, troops, time, civilian considerations
MFO	Multinational force and observers
MF2K	Medical Force 2000
MHS	Military health system
MNB	Multinational brigade
MND	Multinational division
MND-N	Multinational division - North
MOASS	Mother of all Sandstorms (in Iraq, 24–25 March 2003 during Operation IRAQI FREEDOM)
MOOTW	Military operations other than war
MOS	military occupational specialty
MRI	Medical Reengineering Initiative
MSC	Medical Service Corps
MSPR	Medical System Program Review
MTF	Medical task force
NATO	North Atlantic Treaty Organization
NCO	Noncommissioned officer
NTC	National Training Center
NVGs	Night vision goggles
OPCON	Operational control
OPMS	Officer personnel management system
OTSG	Office of The Surgeon General
QRF	Quick reaction force
PDF	Panamanian Defense forces
PET	Patient evacuation team
RCT	Regimental combat team
RIF	Reduction in Force
RL	Readiness level
ROTC	Reserved Officers' Training Corps
RSOI	Reception, staging, onward movement, and integration
SAR	Search and Rescue
SC	Specialty code
SFOR	Stabilization Force, Bosnia
SIPRNET	SECRET Internet Protocol Router Network
SOP	Standard operating procedure
SPINs	Special instructions
SRC	Standard requirements code
SRT	Special reaction team
TDA	Table of distribution and allowances (organizations that are part of the base infrastructure of an Army garrison)
TF	Task Force
TFME	Task Force Medical Eagle (deployment to Bosnia)

TFMF	Task Force Medical Falcon (deployment to Kosovo)
TO&E	Table of Organization and Equipment
TOC	Tactical operations center
TPMRC	Theater patient movement requirements center
TRADOC	U.S. Army Training and Doctrine Command
TROAA	TRADOC Review of Army Aviation
TTP	Tactics, techniques, and procedures
UA	Unit of action
UE	Unit of employment
UN	United Nations
UNMIK	United Nations Mission, Kosovo
UNOSOM	United Nations Operation in Somalia
UNPROFOR	United Nations Protection Force
USAAAD	U.S. Army Air Ambulance Detachment
USAAVNC	U.S. Army Aviation Center
USAR	U.S. Army Reserve
USAREUR	U.S. Army Europe
USASAM	U.S. Army School of Aviation Medicine
USASCV	U.S. Army Support Command Vietnam
USASGV	U.S. Army Support Group Vietnam
USCENTCOM	U.S. Central Command
USNORTHCOM	U.S. Northern Command
USSOCOM	U.S. Special Operations Command
USSOUTHCOM	U.S. Southern Command
VNAF	Vietnamese Air Force
ZOS	Zone of separation, Bosnia

Endnotes

Preface

1. Oral History Interview with Maj. Gen. Spurgeon Neel, John W. Bullard, U.S. Air Force, Fort Sam Houston, TX, 3 March 1977, 29.
2. U.S. Army FMI 4-02.2 (Final Draft), 30 June 2006, 1-7.
3. Ibid.

Chapter One
An Honorable Heritage

1. Dorland, Peter, and Nanney, James. *Dust Off: Army Aeromedical Evacuation in Vietnam.* Washington, DC, Center of Military History United States Army, 1982, 37.
2. 2d Lt. Andrew Russ interview, 24 September 2006.
3. Ibid.
4. Fardink, Lt. Col. Paul. "Amazing Men," *Army Aviation Magazine,* 29 February 2000, 27.
5. Ibid., 27.
6. Guilford, Lt. Col. Fredrick R., and Soboroff, Capt. Burton J. "Air Evacuation: An Historical Review," *Journal of Aviation Medicine,* 8, December 1947, 602.
7. Ibid., 604.
8. Ibid., 605.
9. Lawrence, Lt. Col. G.P. MC. "The Use of Autogiros in the Evacuation of Wounded," *Military Surgeon,* 73(6), December 1933, 319.
10. Fardink, 6.
11. Van Wagner, Maj. R.D. *1st Air Commando Group: Any Place, Any Time, Anywhere.* Maxwell Air Force Base, AL: Air Command and Staff College, 1986, 40, 92.

12. Ibid., 81, 91.
13. Wells, Maj. Kristin L. "Luck of the Irish," *The Retired Officer Magazine,* October 1986, 36.
14. Ibid., 36. (This mission is noted as both the first helicopter rescue and first helicopter MEDEVAC, although technically since Harmon did not have a medic onboard, it would now be considered CASEVAC. Both the MEDEVAC and rescue communities celebrate it as a key event in their respective heritages.)
15. Van Wagner, 93.
16. Smith, Robert Ross. *United States Army in World War II, Triumph in the Philippines,* Office of the Chief of Military History, Department of the Army, Washington, DC, 1961, 421. http://www.centenialofflight.gov/essay/Rotary/MASH/HE12G7.htm
17. The History of Aeromedical Evacuation in the Pacific Theater During World War II, document #UH215 L746H, 1945, 40; Operation Ivory Soap, PowerPoint Presentation, n.d., sent to the author by Mr. Dan Gower, Dustoff Association, 17 December 2008.
18. Holley, Irving B., Jr. *The United States Army in World War II, Special Studies, Buying Aircraft: Materiel Procurement for The Army Air Forces,* Office of the Chief of Military History, Department of The Army, Washington, DC, 1964, 551.
19. Kitchens, Dr. John W. "Cargo Helicopters in the Korean Conflict, Part 2 of 2," *U.S. Army Aviation Digest,* November/December 1952, 39.
20. Maj. Gen. (ret) Spurgeon Neel, U.S. Air Force Oral History interview by John Bullard, 3 March 1977, Brooks Air Force Base, TX, 2.
21. Greenwood, John T., and Berry, F. Clifton Jr. *Medics at War: Military Medicine from Colonial Times to the 21st Century.* Annapolis, MD: Naval Institute Press, 2005, 119.
22. U.S. Army Field Manual 8-10, Medical Service of Field Units, 22 March, 1942, 6, as quoted in Wagner, Donald, O. *The System of Field Medical Service in Theaters of Operations: Its Principles and the Types of Units Authorized.* Unpublished manuscript, September 1959. NARA, RG 112, Stack 390, Box 287, HU 314.7.
23. Marion, Forrest L., Lt. Col. *That Others May Live: USAF Air Rescue in Korea,* Air Force History and Museums Program, Washington, DC, 2004, 2.
24. Dorland, 11.
25. History, Headquarters 8055th MASH, APO 301, 1 October–31 October 1950, NARA, Record Group 407, Stack 270, Box 23.
26. Futrell, Robert F. *The United States Air Force in Korea 1950–1953.* Washington, DC, Office of Air Force History, United States Air Force, 1983, 586.
27. Ibid., 586.
28. Ibid., 590. As can be seen by these events Air Force Rescue and Army MEDEVAC are close cousins. In addition to Harmon's rescue in World War II, both communities claim some of these same Korea events as part of their own heritage. Many years later an Air Force Rescue unit, the 33d Expeditionary Rescue Squadron, would be dispatched for MEDEVAC duty in Afghanistan in 2005.
29. Ibid., 589; Marion, 10.
30. Kirkland, Richard G., *MASH Angels, Tales of the First Air Evac Helicopters.* Professional Press, Chapel Hill, NC, 2004, 44.
31. Driscoll, Col. Robert S. "U.S. Army Medical Helicopters in the Korean War," *Military Medicine,* 166, April 2001, 291.
32. Ibid., 291.
33. Ibid., 291.
34. Hamner, Capt. Louis. "Helicopters in the Medical Service," *Military Bulletin, U.S. Army Europe,* 11(7), July 1954, 157; Neel, Lt. Col. Spurgeon H., "Helicopter Evacuation in Korea," *U.S. Armed Forces Medical Journal,* VI(5), May 1955, 693. (Neel, Helicopter Evacuation)

35. Driscoll, 291.
36. Hamner, 158, Directory and Station List of the United States Army, June 1953.
37. Maj. Gen. (ret) Spurgeon Neel, Senior Officers Oral History Program interview by Lt. Col. Anthony Gaudiano, Carlisle Barracks, PA, 1985, 47. (Neel/Gaudiano); Neel, Lt. Col. Spurgeon H., "Medical Considerations in Helicopter Evacuation," *U.S. Armed Forces Medical Journal*, 5(1), February 1954, 220.
38. Neel/Gaudiano interview.
39. Ginn, Richard V.N. Col. (ret). *The History of the U.S. Army Medical Service Corps.* Washington, DC: Office of the Surgeon General and Center of Military History, 1997, 251.
40. Cowdrey, Albert E. *The Medics' War.* Washington, DC: Center for Military History United States Army, 1987, 165; Driscoll, 292.
41. Driscoll, 295.
42. Cowdrey, 165.
43. Driscoll, 292.
44. Ibid., 293.
45. Ibid., 293.
46. Ibid., 293.
47. Marion, 15.
48. Cowdrey, 165, 199; Dorland, 14.
49. Driscoll, 294.
50. History, Headquarters 1st Helicopter Ambulance Company, Command Report for June 1953. NARA, Record Group 407, Stack 270, Box 23.
51. Kitchens, Dr. John W. "Cargo Helicopters in the Korean Conflict, Part 2 of 2," *U.S. Army Aviation Digest*, November/December 1952, 36–37; Neel, Helicopter Evacuation, 697.
52. Maj. Gen. (ret) Spurgeon Neel, U.S. Air Force Oral History interview by John Bullard, 3 March 1977, Brooks Air Force Base, TX, 19. (Neel/Bullard)
53. Neel, Helicopter Evacuation, 698–701.
54. Marion, 17.
55. Smith, Allen D., Col., "Air Evacuation–Medical Obligation and Military Necessity," *Air University Quarterly Review*, Maxwell AFB, AL, Summer 1953, 99.
56. Marion, 18.
57. Driscoll, 295.
58. Cowdrey, 167, 342.

Chapter Two
From Korea through Vietnam

1. Neel, Maj. Gen. Spurgeon, *Vietnam Studies: Medical Support 1965–1970*. Washington, DC: Department of the Army, 1991, 59. (Neel, Vietnam Studies)
2. Lam, Lt. Col. David M. "From Balloon to Blackhawk, PART IV," *U.S. Army Aviation Digest,* September 1981, 45.
3. Directory and Station List of the United States Army, June 1954, December 1954.
4. Neel, Lt. Col. Spurgeon H. "Aeromedical Evacuation," *Army Magazine,* April 1956, 33. (Neel, Aeromedical Evacuation)

5. Geiger, Lt. Col. Victor Geiger, MS. "Views from Readers," *U.S. Army Aviation Digest,* May/June 1991, 51.
6. Neel/Bullard interview, 25, 83–85, 94.
7. History of the 54th Medical Detachment, 6 January 1958, MEDEVAC Files, Office of Medical History, Falls Church, VA.
8. Directory and Station List of the United States Army, April 1955, December 1955.
9. Cook, John L. *Rescue Under Fire: The Story of Dust Off in Vietnam.* Atglen, PA: Schiffer Military/Aviation History, 1998, 24.
10. Hough, Mark, M. *United States Army Air Ambulance,* Bellevue, WA: Vedder River Publishing, 1999, 8.
11. Ibid., 5, 210.
12. Col. (ret) Doug Moore interview, 31 October 2006.
13. Newsletter – The American Helicopter Society, July 1961, 57th Med Co (AA) File, MEDEVAC Historical File, Office of Medical History, Falls Church, VA.
14. Directory and Station List of the United States Army, October 1960; Hough, 5.
15. United States Army Medical Service Combat Development Group Project NR AM-SCD 56-6, Aeromedical Evacuation Final Report, December 1959. M-41566-NC (AMSCD 56-6), 2.
16. Ibid., 2–8
17. Ibid., 9–11.
18. Ibid., 11.
19. Ibid., cover letter.
20. Field Manual 8-55, 23 October 1960, 172–175.
21. Hough, 227, 232; Historical data for the 24th Med Co (AA), supplied by Col. Tom Schuurmans, Nebraska ARNG, MEDEVAC Unit files, Office of Medical History, Falls Church, VA.
22. Directory and Station List of the United States Army, October–December 1961.
23. Currie, Col. James T., and Crossland, Col. Richard B. *Twice the Citizen: A History of the United States Army Reserve, 1908–1995,* Office of the Chief, Army Reserve, Washington, D.C., 1997, 137; Doubler, Col. Michael D. *I am the Guard: A History of the Army National Guard, 1636–2000*, Department of the Army, Washington, DC, 2001, 251; Directory and Station List of the United States Army, December 1961, June 1962; Historical data for the 24th Med Co (AA), supplied by Col. Tom Schuurmans, Nebraska ARNG, MEDEVAC Unit files, Office of Medical History, Falls Church, VA.
24. Cook, 29; Cosmas, Graham A. *MACV The Joint Command in the Years of Escalation 1962–1967,* Center for Military History, United States Army, Washington, DC, 2006, 54.
25. Dorland, 117–118.
26. Cook, 46.
27. Dorland, 24–26.
28. Ibid., 76.
29. Directory and Station List of the United States Army, December 1962, June 1963.
30. Cook, 86.
31. Dorland, 77.
32. Cook, 93.
33. http://www.transchool.eustis.army.mil/lic/documents/OCOT_Interviews/klingenhagen.htm; Ginn, 322.
34. Dorland, 26–27; Ginn, 322.

35. Dorland, 28–29
36. Ibid., 118.
37. Directory and Station List of the United States Army, December 1963.
38. Dorland, 30–31.
39. Ibid., 35, 53.
40. Ibid., 37.
41. Directory and Station List of the United States Army, December 1964.
42. Ginn, 337.
43. Moore interview.
44. Col. (ret) Jim Truscott interview, 5 January 2007.
45. Dorland, 39; Truscott interview.
46. History, Headquarters 15th Medical Battalion, 1st Cavalry Division, 1 January–31 December 1968, 10 January 1969. NARA RG 112, Stack 390, Box 1, Aeronautical Units, 15th Medical Battalion.
47. Cook, 80; Ginn, 339.
48. Cook, 82.
49. Dorland, 49.
50. Cook, 84.
51. Dorland, 52.
52. Ibid., 44.
53. Moore interview.
54. Directory and Station List of the United States Army, June 1966; Moore interview; Army Medical Profiles: Col. Douglas E. Moore U.S. Army, Office of Medical History, Office of the Surgeon General, Alexandria, VA, January 2004, 62.
55. Pamphlet, *421st Medical Company,* March 1966, MEDEVAC Files, Office of Medical History, Falls Church, VA.
56. Truscott interview.
57. Dorland, 54.
58. Ibid., 78.
59. Cook, 90.
60. Ibid., 91.
61. Ibid., 81.
62. Moore interview.
63. Truscott interview.
64. Directory and Station List of the United States Army, December 1967.
65. Directory and Station List of the United States Army, December 1967; Brig. Gen. (ret) Jerome Foust interview, 21 February 2007.
66. *Jane's All the World's Aircraft, 1962/63,* Great Missenden, England, 1963, 178–179; *Jane's All the World's Aircraft, 1964/65,* Great Missenden, England, 1965, 182–183; *Jane's All the World's Aircraft, 1970/71,* London, England, 1971, 274–276; Cook, 24, 39.
67. Dorland, 69; Moore interview.
68. Directory and Station List of the United States Army, December 1968.
69. MFR, DASG – HCA files, 16 August 1968, Office of Medical History, Falls Church, VA.
70. Historical data for the 24th Med Co (AA), supplied by Col. Tom Schuurmans, Nebraska ARNG, MEDEVAC Unit files, Office of Medical History, Falls Church, VA.
71. DASG-HCA files, MFR 29 January 1970, Office of Medical History, Falls Church, VA.
72. Dorland, 63.

73. Ibid., 44; Neel, Maj. Gen. Spurgeon. *Vietnam Studies: Medical Support 1965–1970.* Washington, DC: Department of the Army, 1991, 18. (Neel, Vietnam Studies)
74. Directory and Station List of the United States Army, December 1968, April 1969; Hough, 134.
75. *Dustoff Association Newsletter,* Summer 1999, 9.
76. Pamphlet, *Dustoff Europe,* 1969, MEDEVAC Files, Office of Medical History, Falls Church, VA.
77. Dorland, 95; "Dustoff" Newsletter, 50th Med Det (RA) June 1968, 50th Med Co History, Fort Campbell, KY.
78. USARV Aviation Operational Procedures Guide, 1 June 1970, page 5-1, MEDEVAC Files, Office of Medical History, Falls Church, VA.
79. Dorland, 100–101.
80. Ibid., 96.
81. Ibid., 102–105.
82. Truscott interview.
83. Field Manual 8-10, April 1970, 1–1.
84. Field Manual 8-10, April 1970, 2–1.
85. Field Manual 8-10, April 1970, 4–4.
86. Field Manual 8-35, December 1970, 1.
87. TOE 8-660H, 17 April 1970, Box 228, Office of Medical History, Falls Church, VA.
88. TOE 8-137H, 23 May 1972, Box 224, Office of Medical History, Falls Church, VA.
89. Field Manual 8-15, September 1972, 2–23.
90. Directory and Station List of the United States Army, October 1971.
91. Foust interview.
92. Col. (ret) Art Hapner interview, 23 March 2007.
93. Dorland, 113.
94. Ginn, 328.
95. Dustoff Association Newsletter, Fall 1997, 1.
96. Dorland, 118–119.
97. Ibid., 119.
98. Neel, Helicopter Evacuation, 698; Dorland, 120.
99. Cook, 147.
100. Ibid., 147.
101. Neel/Bullard interview; Ginn, 321.
102. www.dustoff.org.
103. Neel, Vietnam Studies, 59.
104. Ginn, 322.

Chapter Three
Quiet Years, 1973–1980

1. Annex B1, MAST Military Assistance to Safety and Traffic, Appendices to Report of Test Program by the Interagency Study Group, March 1971, Box HCO-FD (AVN) Office of Medical History, Falls Church, VA.
2. Stewart, Dr. Richard. *American Military History Volume II, The United States Army in a Global Era, 1917–2003.* Washington, DC: Center for Military History, 2005. (*American Military History Volume II*), 369.

3. Col. (ret) Frank Novier interview, 18 February 2007.
4. Novier interview.
5. *"Culture, et cetera," Washington Times,* 2 February 2007, A2.
6. Ginn, 375.
7. Col. (ret) William Thresher interview, 23 October 2007.
8. Ibid.
9. Ibid.
10. Dell, M. Sgt. Nat. "The Future is Now," *Soldiers Magazine,* August 1973, 5.
11. Maj. Gen. (ret) Pat Brady interview, 15 February 2007.
12. Moore interview; Moore, Lt. Col. Douglas, "Air Ambulance Support for the Combat Division," unpublished paper, Command and General Staff College, Fort Leavenworth, KS, June 1974.
13. *American Military History Volume II,* 373.
14. Dell, M.Sgt. Nat. "Toward a Professional Army," *Soldiers Magazine,* August 1973, 5.
15. Foust interview.
16. *American Military History Volume II,* 374; Currie, Col. James T., and Crossland, Col. Richard B. *Twice the Citizen: A History of the United States Army Reserve, 1908–1995,* Office of the Chief, Army Reserve, Washington, DC, 1997, 246.
17. *American Military History Volume II,* 374.
18. Moore interview.
19. Ginn, 379.
20. Ibid., 398.
21. Directory and Station List of the United States Army, September 1973.
22. Department of the Army Force Accounting System Active Army Troop List, June 1974, June 1975, October 1979, December 1980.
23. Truscott interview.
24. Hapner interview.
25. Currie, Col. James T., and Crossland, Col. Richard B. *Twice the Citizen: A History of the United States Army Reserve, 1908–1995,* Office of the Chief, Army Reserve, Washington, DC, 1997, 176–179; Doubler, Col. Michael D. *I am the Guard: A History of the Army National Guard, 1636–2000,* Department of the Army, Washington, DC, 2001, 278.
26. *American Military History Volume II,* 376.
27. Hough, 205–226.
28. Hough, 227–272.
29. Letter from Dr. Charles Atkinson, to Col. Neel, 16 February 1968, and response 26 February 1968, MAST Files, Office of Medical History, Falls Church, VA.
30. Neel, Col. Spurgeon. "Army Aeromedical Evacuation Procedures in Vietnam," *JAMA,* 204(4), April 22, 1968, 99.
31. Sears, "An Air Medical Evacuation System for Highway Accident Victims," Arizona State University, June 1968, iii, Item 2, MAST Book 2 of 2, U.S. Army Aviation Museum Archive, Fort Rucker, AL.
32. Letter from Maj. Gen. Winston P. Wilson, Chief, National Guard Bureau, Item 3, Mast Book 2 of 2, U.S. Army Aviation Museum Archive, Fort Rucker, AL.
33. Historical data for the 24th Med Co (AA), supplied by Col. Tom Schuurmans, Nebraska ARNG, MEDEVAC Unit files, Office of Medical History, Falls Church, VA; MEMORANDUM FOR the Secretary of the Army From the Secretary of Defense, 12 August 1969, Item 3 MAST Book 2 of 2, U.S. Army Aviation Museum Archives, Fort Rucker, AL.

34. MEMORANDUM SUBJECT: Results of MAST Study Group Meeting 13 May 1970, Item 5 MAST Book 2 of 2, U.S. Army Aviation Museum Archive, Fort Rucker, AL.

35. Annex E, MAST Military Assistance to Safety and Traffic, Appendices to Report of Test Program by the Interagency Study Group, March 1971, 12–13, Box HCO-FD (AVN), Office of Medical History, Falls Church, VA.

36. Ibid.

37. Ibid.

38. Ibid., 16–24.

39. Ibid., 3–5.

40. Pettyjohn, Lt. Col. Frank S., M.D. *Review of the U.S. Army Aeromedical Research Laboratory Conference on Aeromedical Evacuation, 15–16 January 1974.* U.S. Army Aeromedical Research Laboratory, Ft. Rucker, AL. August 1974, iii.

41. Annex B1, MAST Military Assistance to Safety and Traffic, Appendices to Report of Test Program by the Interagency Study Group, March 1971, Box HCO-FD (AVN) Office of Medical History, Falls Church, VA.

42. "Over Two Decades of Service: An Update on MAST," no author, 1987, Box HCO-FD (AVN), Office of Medical History, Falls Church, VA.

43. Ibid.

44. Pettyjohn, 5.

45. Hough, 20, 49, 66, 72, 95, 124, 127, 206.

46. Foust interview.

47. Col. (ret) Dan Gower interview, 21 February 2007.

48. Ibid.

49. "Baby Born During Mast Flight," *Army Aviation Digest,* September 1976.

50. "The MAST Program," *U.S. Army Aviation Digest,* October 1976, 8, and March, 1977, 12.

51. Hough, Mark, 81, 88, 89; Halloran, Barney, "Red Hot Mission," *Soldiers Magazine,* January 1973, 17.

52. "Dustoff: Med Choppers Ready Anytime," *Medical Bulletin of the U.S. Army, Europe,* January 1976, 25.

53. Wood, Maj. William C. "MEDEVAC on the European Battlefield," *U.S. Army Aviation Digest,* August 1977, 5.

54. Truscott interview.

55. *American Military History Volume II,* 377.

56. *American Military History Volume II,* 380–384.

57. Ibid., 378, 388, and *Annual Report - The Surgeon General of the United States Army, Fiscal Years 1976–1980,* 141.

58. Field Manual 8-35, January 1977, 1-1.

59. Field Manual 8-35, January 1977, 5-3.

60. Field Manual 8-35, January 1977, 5-2.

61. Field Manual 8-10, 2 October 1978, i, and 2-1.

62. Field Manual 8-10, 2 October 1978, 1-9, 1-10.

63. Field Manual 8-10, 2 October 1978, 2-4, 4-3.

64. MAST File, Office of Medical History, Falls Church, VA.

65. 326th Med Bn Quarterly Historical Summary, 1 January–31 March 1978, 7 April 1978, Historical Files, 101st ABN Div, Fort Campbell, KY.

66. Foust interview.

67. Brady interview.

68. Truscott interview.
69. Neel/Bullard interview, 37.
70. Ibid.
71. Thresher interview.
72. Col. (ret) Scott Heintz interview, 16 September 2007.
73. *Annual Report - The Surgeon General United States Army, Fiscal Years 1976–1980,* 257, 258.
74. Neel/Gaudiano interview, 90.
75. Col. (ret) Pauline Lockard interview, 14 March 2007.
76. Lt. Col. Pete Smart interview, 6 March 2007.
77. Moore interview.
78. Moore, Douglas E., Col. (ret). "The Mount Saint Helens Search and Rescue Effort May 18–29, 1980," unpublished paper.
79. Ibid.
80. *American Military History Volume II,* 391–392.
81. Department of the Army Force Accounting System Active Army Troop List, December 1980.
82. MAST File, Office of Medical History, Falls Church, VA.
83. "MAST Anniversary," *U.S. Army Aviation Digest,* July 1980, 7.
84. *American Military History Volume II,* 393.
85. Ginn, 398.

Chapter Four
New Challenges: Near and Afar, 1981–1990

1. MEMORANDUM FOR the Chief of Staff, Army, SUBJECT: Aviation Branch Composition – Action Memorandum, 13 Apr 1983, MEDEVAC File, Notebook AVN BR vs 67J, Office of Medical History, Falls Church, VA.
2. *American Military History Volume II,* 393.
3. Hapner interview.
4. Ibid.
5. Ibid.
6. Col. (ret) Tom Scofield interview, 30 March 2007.
7. 326th Medical Battalion Quarterly History, 1 October 1980 to 30 September 1981, 101st ABN Division History Office, Fort Campbell, KY; Scofield interview; Novier interview
8. Lockard interview; Scofield interview.
9. Novier interview.
10. Ibid.
11. After Action Report AHUAS TARA II, Box 157E, Office of Medical History, Falls Church, VA).
12. Foust interview.
13. Ibid.
14. Col. Dave MacDonald interview, 14 September 2006.
15. *American Military History Volume II,* 379.
16. Field Manual 8-35, 22 December 1983, 5-12.

17. Field Manual 8-55, 15 February 1985, 1-1, E-1.
18. Pratt, Capt. Bob. "USAR Unit Aids in D.C. Aircraft Recovery Operations," *Army Reserve Magazine*, Spring 1982, 33.
19. "Sinai 'Nomads,'" *Army Aviation*, 28 February 1997, 43.
20. Knisely, Col. Benjamin. "Army Medical Department Aviation and Its Relationship to the New Army Aviation Branch," unpublished paper, Army War College, April 1985.
21. Letter from Maj. Gen. (ret) George Putnam 4 March 2004, Msg from HQDA Wash DC, dtg 132225Z Apr 79, Subject: Commissioned Officer Aviation Management, Aviation Branch Implementation File, Aviation Library, Fort Rucker, AL.
22. MFR, Subject: General Officer Aviation Branch Composition Meeting 7 April 1983. MEDEVAC File, Notebook AVN BR vs 67J, Office of Medical History, Falls Church, VA.
23. MEMORANDUM FOR Deputy Chief of Staff for Personnel, SUBJECT: Inclusion of Medical Service Corps (67J) Aviators in the Aviation Branch, 7 April 1983, MEDEVAC File, Notebook AVN BR vs 67J, Office of Medical History, Falls Church, VA.
24. Scofield interview.
25. MEMORANDUM FOR Deputy Chief of Staff for Operations and Plans, SUBJECT: TRADOC Proposal to Centralize Aviation Proponency and Form an Aviation Branch, 8 April 1983, MEDEVAC File, Notebook AVN BR vs 67J, Office of Medical History, Falls Church, VA.
26. MEMORANDUM FOR the Chief of Staff, Army, SUBJECT: Aviation Branch Composition – Action Memorandum, 13 Apr 1983, MEDEVAC File, Notebook AVN BR vs 67J, Office of Medical History, Falls Church, VA.
27. "Army Aviation Branch Implementation." *U.S. Army Aviation Digest*, August 1983, 2.
28. Knisely, Col. Benjamin. "Army Medical Department Aviation and Its Relationship to the New Army Aviation Branch," unpublished paper, Army War College, April 1985.
29. Ginn, 398.
30. Lockard interview.
31. Scofield interview.
32. Thresher interview; Greenwood, 159.
33. Truscott interview.
34. Kruse, Lt. Col. William R. "Separate but not Apart," *U.S. Army Aviation Digest*, September 1985, 38.
35. Ginn, 376, 398; Knisely, Col. Benjamin, "Army Medical Department Aviation and Its Relationship to the New Army Aviation Branch," U.S. Army War College, April 1985: Jablecki, Maj. Joseph S., "AMEDD Aviation Update," *U.S. Army Aviation Digest*, July 1988, 6.
36. Story, Maj. Dennis C., "Aviation Medicine, Its Origins and a Training Perspective," *U.S. Army Aviation Digest*, July 1988, 2–5.
37. Ibid.
38. MacDonald interview.
39. McAndrews, Kevin, "Helicopter crew seeks gubernatorial rider," *The Prairie Rider*, June 1986, 1; Historical data for the 24th Med Co (AA), supplied by Col. Tom Schuurmans, Nebraska ARNG, MEDEVAC Unit files, Office of Medical History, Falls Church, VA.
40. Lockard interview.
41. Ibid.

42. Ibid.
43. Gower interview.
44. Ibid.
45. Ibid.
46. Heintz interview.
47. Lt. Col. Bob Mitchell interview, 19 March 2007.
48. Ibid.
49. Ibid.
50. Department of the Army Force Accounting System Active Army Troop List, June 1986.
51. "Over Two Decades of Service: An Update on MAST," no author, 1987, Box HCO-FD (AVN), MAST Files, Office of Medical History, Falls Church, VA.
52. Nomination Package for Mr. Craig Honaman to the DUSTOFF Association Hall of Fame, 16 April 2007, Box HCO-FD (AVN), Office of Medical History, Falls Church, VA.
53. Hapner interview.
54. Ginn, 423; *American Military History Volume II*, 396.
55. Hapner interview.
56. Peake, Col. James B., "Message to Warfighters: Historical Perspective on Combat Medicine," Army War College, 17 March 1988, 18.
57. Richards, Lt. Col. Donn R. "Medical Trends: An Evaluation of Medical Care Given in Vietnam, Grenada, Panama, and Desert Storm," U.S. Army War College, April 1999, 19.
58. Hapner interview
59. "Dustoff Europe," *Medical Bulletin of the U.S. Army, Europe*, July 1984, 23.
60. *Dustoff Follies Notebook,* unpublished, in six volumes and still being used, Hohenfels Dustoff Alert Facility, Germany.
61. Furbish, Maj. Bruce G. "Dustoff Panama," *U.S. Army Aviation Digest,* November 1982, 38.
62. Department of the Army Force Accounting System Active Army Troop List, June 1984.
63. History of JTF-Bravo, NARA, RG 338, file 870-5b-6/36.
64. Ginn, 399.
65. 1st/228th Aviation Battalion, Fort Kobbe, Panama, Annual Historical Review, 1 October 1988–30 September 1989, NARA, RG 338, file 870-5c-57/4; Lt. Col. Vinny Carnazza interview, 27 September 2006.
66. Jacobs, Lt. Col. Bill M. "Winged Warriors' in Central America," *U.S. Army Aviation Digest,* November/December 1993, 34.
67. Greenwood, 156; FC 8-45, October 1986, front page.
68. FC 8-45, October 1986, 1–5.
69. FC 8-45, 2–6.
70. FC 8-45, 4–-10.
71. FC 8-45, 5–2.
72. FC 8-45, 5–5.
73. Greenwood, 157.
74. "Joint Services Operational Requirement for the Advanced Vertical Lift Aircraft (JSX JSOR)," April 1985, MEDEVAC Files, Box HCO-FD (AVN), MEDEVAC Files, Office of Medical History, Falls Church, VA.
75. MFR, V-22 Joint Working Group Meeting, 4 March 1976, MEDEVAC Files, Box

HCO-FD (AVN), Office of Medical History, Falls Church, VA.

76. "Army XXI Aviation: Time for the V-22," *Army Magazine,* 1 Nov 1999, "Fact Sheet" Subject: V-22 (Osprey) Program, Purpose: To inform the CG TRADOC about the rationale of the SECDEF and HQDA in their decision to cancel the V-22 Program." 11 May 1989. From Historian, U.S. Army Aviation Center, Fort Rucker, AL.

77. Novier interview; Heintz interview.

78. Risio, Maj. Andrew. "421st Medical Evacuation Battalion History and Accolades," *Army Medical Department Journal,* October/November/December 2005, 11; Hapner interview; Novier interview.

79. Risio, Maj. Andrew. "421st Medical Evacuation Battalion History and Accolades," *Army Medical Department Journal,* October/November/December 2005, 9; Department of the Army Force Accounting System Active Army Troop List, December 1988.

80. Hapner interview; Jackson, James O. "West Germany Hellfire from the Heavens," *Time Magazine*, 12 September 1988.

81. Hapner interview; Department of the Army Force Accounting System Active Army Troop List, June 1989, June 1990.

82. Lt. Col. John Lamoureux interview, 24 May 2007.

83. Heintz interview.

84. Thresher interview.

85. Smart interview.

86. Ibid.

87. MacDonald interview.

88. Smart interview, Thresher interview.

89. Thresher interview.

90. Ibid.

91. Ibid.

92. Smart interview, MacDonald interview.

93. Thresher interview.

94. *American Military History Volume II,* 397.

95. *American Military History Volume II,* 397, Carnazza interview.

96. Ginn, 425.

97. *American Military History Volume II,* 398.

98. Jacobs, Lt. Col. Bill M. "Winged Warriors' in Central America," *U.S. Army Aviation Digest,* November/December 1993, 34, Carnazza interview.

99. Carnazza interview.

100. 214th Medical Detachment (RG) Presentation to AMEC 27 Feb, 90, NARA RG 334, File 870-5b-6/40aaa, Carnazza interview.

101. Carnazza interview.

102. 214th Medical Detachment (RG) Presentation to AMEC 27 February 90, NARA RG 334, File 870-5b-6/40aaa.

103. Carnazza interview.

104. *American Military History Volume II,* 402.

105. 214th Medical Detachment (RG) Presentation to AMEC 27 February 1990, NARA RG 334, File 870-5b-6/40aaa.

106. 214th Medical Detachment (RG) Presentation to AMEC 27 February, 90, NARA RG 334, File 870-5b-6/40aaa; Memorandum, Subject: Operation JUST CAUSE Lessons Learned Report, Academy of Health Sciences, Fort Sam Houston, TX, 1 June 1990.

107. Carnazza interview.

108. Fontenot, Col. (ret) Gregory, Degen, Lt. Col. E.J., and Tohn, Lt. Col. David. *On Point: The United States Army in Operation IRAQI FREEDOM,* Naval Institute Press, Annapolis, MD, 2005, 4.

109. Smith, Barry D. "Desert Dust Off: Medevac with the 247th," *Rotor & Wing International,* January 1991, 38.

110. "Commander's CASEVAC System," Report #89-5, CALL, November 1989, 3–4.

111. MEDICAL SYSTEM PROGRESS REVIEW, Army Medical Department, January 31, 1989, Academy of Health Sciences, Fort Sam Houston, TX; White Paper, Health Services Support futures, Final Draft, Academy of Health Sciences, Fort Sam Houston, TX, March 1989.

112. Anderson, Capt. Randall G. *The Dustoff Report.* The Dustoff Association, San Antonio, TX, 1992, 2. *(The Dustoff Report)*

113. Ibid., 20.

114. *American Military History Volume II,* 409.

Chapter Five
Desert Shield/Desert Storm, 1990–1991

1. Ginn, 428.

2. *American Military History Volume II,* 412.

3. Ibid., 413.

4. Doubler, Col. Michael D. *I am the Guard: A History of the Army National Guard, 1636–2000,* Department of the Army, Washington, DC, 2001, 306; Truscott interview.

5. *American Military History Volume II,* 413.

6. Ibid., 414.

7. Ginn, 427.

8. *American Military History Volume II,* 414.

9. Ginn, 428; Foust interview.

10. Ledford, Lt. Gen. Frank F. MC. "Medical Support for Operation DESERT STORM," *The Journal of the U.S. Army Medical Department,* January/February 1992, 3.

11. *American Military History Volume II,* 425.

12. Ginn, 429.

13. Hough 30; Heintz, Maj. David S. *Operations DESERT SHIELD and STORM After Action Review, Delta Company, 326 Medical Battalion "Eagle Dustoff,"* 15 March 1991; Heintz interview.

14. Lt. Col. Brad Pecor interview, 13 February 2007.

15. Lt. Col. (ret) Tommy Mayes interview, 21 February 2007; Ginn, 432; expansive comments by Col. (ret) Scott Heintz to author by email, 17 December 2008.

16. Email to author from Sgt. Maj. (ret) Jeff Mankoff to author, 1 April 2008.

17. "Darmstadt to Dhahran: MEDEVAC Self-Deployment to DESERT SHIELD," *The Journal of the U.S. Army Medical Department,* September/October 1992, 51; personal log of M.Sgt. Mike Craven, 45th Med Co (AA), undated, sent to author.

18. Smart interview.

19. *The Dustoff Report,* 13, Hough, 58, 90, 125.

20. Lt. Col. Jon Fristoe interview, 5 June 2007.

21. Hough, 77.

22. Hough, 131; Carnazza interview.

23. Hough, 92; Griffin, Col. Greg, *Lonestar DUSTOFF in DESERT SHIELD/STORM,* Personal Experience Monograph, U.S. Army War College, undated.

24. Hough, 235, "Technical Report of U.S. Army Aircraft Accident," Case number 1991-05-13-001, procured from the U.S. Army Combat Readiness Center, Fort Rucker, AL.

25. *United States Army Reserve in Operation DESERT STORM*, Washington, DC: Department of the Army, September 1993, 26; Hough, 224, 226, 237; *The Dustoff Report,* 33, 46, 47, 49; Jeffer, Col. Edward K., MC. "The Medical Units of the Army National Guard (ARNG) and Operation DESERT SHIELD/DESERT STORM," *Journal of the U.S. Army Medical Department,* March/April 1992, 20.

26. Veit, Lt. Col. Christoph. "German Medical Assistance for U.S. Forces During the Gulf Crisis: A Stock-taking of Lessons Learned," *The Journal of the U.S. Army Medical Department,* January/February 1992, 58.

27. Hough, 205–224.

28. AAR: 44th Medical Brigade Operations DESERT SHIELD and DESERT STORM, Office of Medical History, Falls Church, VA, DESERT STORM Collection, Box 29; *United States Army Reserve in Operation DESERT STORM,* 89–95; Hough, 6, 215, 220.

29. *The Dustoff Report,* 28.

30. Scales, Maj. Gen. Robert H. *Certain Victory: The U.S. Army in the Gulf War,* 157.

31. Ginn, 428.

32. Novier interview.

33. Carnazza interview.

34. Ibid.

35. Hough, 131, Carnazza interview.

36. Lt. Col. Scott Drennon interview, 20 February 2007.

37. Carnazza interview.

38. *The Dustoff Report,* 21.

39. Carnazza interview.

40. Ibid.

41. Ibid.

42. *The Dustoff Report,* 7; Hough 58.

43. Hough, 220.

44. *The Dustoff Report,* 11; Hough, 77.

45. *The Dustoff Report,* 2; Hough, 6.

46. Lt. Col. Randal Schwallie, *DESERT Dustoff,* Personal Experience Monograph, Army War College, April 25, 2002.

47. Ibid.

48. Ibid.

49. Ibid.

50. Ibid.

51. Ibid.

52. Ibid.

53. Ibid.

54. Ibid., *The Dustoff Report,* 39; Hough, 215.

55. Schwallie, *DESERT Dustoff.*

56. Hough, 228.

57. Hough, 90.
58. Hough, 125; Fristoe interview.
59. Howard, Maj. William. "History of the 50th Medical Company (AA)," undated, 5, procured from author; Heintz, Maj. David S. *Operations DESERT SHIELD and STORM After Action Review, Delta Company, 326 Medical Battalion "Eagle Dustoff,"* 15 March 1991; MacDonald interview.
60. Heintz, Maj. David S. *Operations DESERT SHIELD and STORM After Action Review, Delta Company, 326 Medical Battalion "Eagle Dustoff,"* 15 March 1991; expansive comments by Col. (ret) Scott Heintz to author by email, 17 December 2008.
61. Griffin, *Lonestar DUSTOFF in DESERT SHIELD/STORM.*
62. Ibid.
63. Ibid.
64. Whitcomb, Darrel D., *Combat Search and Rescue in Desert Storm.* Maxwell Air Force Base, AL: Air University Press, 2006, 223; Griffin, Col. Greg, *Lonestar DUSTOFF in DESERT SHIELD/STORM.*
65. Hough, 135.
66. Griffin, *Lonestar DUSTOFF in DESERT SHIELD/STORM.*
67. *The Dustoff Report,* 34; Hough, 207.
68. Hough, 209; Currie, *Twice the Citizen: A History of the USAR, 1908–1995,* 464.
69. *The Dustoff Report,* 37; Hough, 211.
70. *The Dustoff Report,* 51; Hough, 259.
71. *The Dustoff Report,* Hough, 240.
72. *The Dustoff Report,* 58; Hough, 269.
73. Hough, 93.
74. Hough, 252; Carlin, CW2 Victor E. "Operations in the DESERT: A Postscript, *U.S. Army Aviation Digest,* November/December 1992, 26.
75. Hough, 257.
76. *The Dustoff Report,* 38; Hough, 214.
77. AAR, 108 Med Bn Command Report for Operation DESERT STORM, Office of Medical History, Falls Church, VA, DESERT STORM Collection, Box 30.
78. *The Dustoff Report,* 38; Hough, 212.
79. Maj. (ret) Pete Webb interview, 26 September 2006.
80. Hough, 317; Webb interview.
81. Hough, 223.
82. Smart interview.
83. *The Dustoff Report,* 4; Hough, 16, 84; Email from Sgt. Maj. (ret) Jeff Mankoff to author, 1 April 2008.
84. *The Dustoff Report,* 25.
85. MacDonald interview.
86. Heintz interview; MacDonald interview.
87. Smart interview.
88. *The Dustoff Report,* various unit sections.

Chapter Six
Force Reductions, 1992–1995

1. Schwallie, *DESERT Dustoff,* 116.
2. MEMORANDUM FOR Director for Operational Plans and Interoperability, J7 Joint Staff, Washington, DC, 20318, 29 Jan 1992, SUBJECT: USCINCEUR After Action Report on Operation PROVIDE COMFORT, AMEDD C&S MCCS-FD Historical Files, Fort Sam Houston, TX.
3. Lockard interview; Note, at the time, her married name was Pauline Knapp.
4. MEMORANDUM FOR Director for Operational Plans and Interoperability, J7 Joint Staff, Washington, DC, 20318, 29 January 1992, SUBJECT: USCINCEUR After Action Report on Operation PROVIDE COMFORT, AMEDD C&S MCCS-FD Historical Files, Fort Sam Houston, TX, 14.
5. Foust interview.
6. Ibid.
7. *Operation DESERT STORM – Full Army Medical Capability Not Achieved,* GAO/NSIAD-92-175, Government Accounting Office, August 1992, 3–5, Office of Medical History, Falls Church, VA, DESERT STORM File.
8. Ibid., 14, 45.
9. Ibid., 45–48.
10. Ibid., 49.
11. Donnelly, William M., *Transforming an Army at War, Designing the Modular Force, 1991–2005.* Washington, DC: Center for Military History, 2007, 5–8.
12. http://www.nhc.noaa.gov/1992andrew.html.
13. JOINT TASK FORCE ANDREW AFTER ACTION REPORT, Enclosure 7 (AVIATION) to Tab J (J3), Army Aviation Museum Archives, Fort Rucker, AL, 071830ROCT92, File 87020A, 3.
14. Webb interview.
15. MEMORANDUM FOR JTF Andrew Aviation, October 12, 1992, Army Aviation Museum Archives, Fort Rucker, AL, File 870.20A, JOINT TASK FORCE ANDREW AVIATION AFTER ACTION REPORT (TAB R) 090730ROCT92, U.S. Army Aviation Museum, Fort Rucker, AL, File 870.20A.
16. Carroll, Col. Dale A., "The Role of the U.S. Army Medical Department in Domestic Disaster Assistance Operations – Lessons Learned from Hurricane Andrew," Carlisle, PA: U.S. Army War College, 1996, 25.
17. *The Story of JTF Hawaii,* Public Affairs Office, U.S. Army, Pacific, undated.
18. Field Manual 8-10, 1 March 1991, 1-1, 2-9.
19. Ibid., 2-9.
20. Field Manual 8-10-6, 31 October 1991, x.
21. Ibid., 3-1, 3-2.
22. Ibid., 3-8, 3-11.
23. Ibid., 3-11.
24. Ibid., 4-11.
25. Lt. Col. (ret) Van Joy interview, 5 December 2007.
26. Ibid.
27. Ibid.
28. *The U.S. Army in Bosnia and Herzegovina,* AE Pamphlet 525-100, 7 October 2003, 4.

29. *American Military History Volume II*, 424.
30. *The U.S. Army in Bosnia and Herzegovina*, AE Pamphlet 525-100, 7 October 2003, 6.
31. Doubler, *I am the Guard*, 345–346; Currie, *Twice the Citizen: A History of the USAR, 1908–1995*, 521–522.
32. Doubler, *I am the Guard*, 345–346.
33. Currie, *Twice the Citizen: A History of the USAR, 1908–1995*, 537.
34. Schwallie, *DESERT Dustoff*, 116.
35. Lt. Col. Bill LaChance interview, 14 February 2007.
36. MSG dtg 071800Z APR 92, from FORSCOM to numerous addressees, MAST File, Office of Medical History, Falls Church, VA.
37. Department of the Army Force Accounting System Active Army Troop List, December 1992, Hough, 142.
38. Lugo, Lt. Col. Angel L., "The Army's MRI," http://www.military-medical-technology.com/article.cfm?DocID=481.
39. Hough, 30; Quarterly History of the 326th Medical Bn, 1 October 1991 to 30 September 1992, 31 October 1992; MacDonald interview; Truscott interview.
40. Fix, Capt. Gregory D., "The New UH-60Q Black Hawk MEDEVAC Helicopter," *U.S. Army Aviation Digest*, January/February 1993, 43.
41. Novier interview.
42. Ibid.
43. Ginn, 490; Foust interview.
44. *American Military History Volume II*, 429.
45. Kirkpatrick, Charles E., *Ruck it Up! The Post Cold-War Transformation of V Corps, 1990–2000*, Department of the Army, Washington, DC, 20006, 239; Lockard interview.
46. Smart interview.
47. Ibid.
48. Ingram, Sandra, *Somalia Medical Operations*, Camber Corporation, 9 September 1996, 22.
49. Ibid., 67.
50. Ibid., 76.
51. *American Military History Volume II*, 431.
52. Ingram, *Somalia Medical Operations*, 131.
53. Field Manual 100-5, 14 June 1993, vi, 2-7.
54. Ibid., 2-17, 2-24.
55. Ibid., 4-5.
56. Ibid., 5-1.
57. Ibid., 12-12.
58. Ibid., 13-5.
59. Field Manual 8-55, 9 September 1994, 1-2.
60. Ibid., 2-29.
61. Ibid., 4-17.
62. Joint Publication 1, 11 November 1991, iv, 6.
63. Joint Publication 4-02, 26 April 1995, v.
64. Ibid., ix.
65. Ibid., II-1, 5, 6.
66. Condon-Rall, Mary Ellen, *Disaster on Green Ramp: The Army's Response*, Washington, DC, Center for Military History, 1996, 19.
67. Ibid., 21.

68. *American Military History Volume II*, 433–434.
69. Medical Support for Operation UPHOLD DEMOCRACY, HCO Files, Box, 204, Office of Medical History, Falls Church, VA.
70. Lt. Col. Greg Gentry interview, 29 September 2006.
71. Mitchell interview.
72. *American Military History Volume II*, 436; "Task Force Bandit Aids Division in Aviation Missions," *Hawaii Army Weekly*, 9 March 1995, A-6; "President Clinton visits Tropic Lightening Soldiers in Haiti," *Hawaii Army Weekly*, 6 April 1995, A-5; Smart interview.
73. Webb interview.
74. Smart interview.
75. MacDonald interview.
76. MAST Files, Office of Medical History, Falls Church, VA.
77. Simon, Kimberly. "54th Med Honored for MAST Mission," *NW Guardian*, 5 May 1993, 1.
78. Lt. Col. Matt Brady interview, 7 August 2007; Hough, 260.
79. *American Military History Volume II*, 439.
80. Hough, 138; Permanent Orders 102-1, HQ Eighth United States Army, 12 April 1995, Historical Files, 542d Med Co (AA), Fort Campbell, KY.
81. Heintz interview; expansive comments by Col. (ret) Scott Heintz to author by email, 17 December 2008.
82. List: U.S. Army MEDEVAC Units February 1996, MAST file, Office of Medical History, Falls Church, VA.
83. Donnelly, William M. *Transforming an Army at War, Designing the Modular Force, 1991–2005*, Washington, DC: Center for Military History, 2007, 9–10.

Chapter Seven
The Balkans, 1992–Ongoing

1. TRADOC Pam 525-50, 1 October 1996, 2.
2. *The U.S. Army in Bosnia and Herzegovina,* AE Pamphlet 525-100, Washington, DC: Center for Military History, 7 October 2003, 5.
3. *American Military History Volume II*, 440.
4. *The U.S. Army in Bosnia and Herzegovina*, 8.
5. Ibid., 11.
6. *American Military History Volume II*, 441.
7. *The U.S. Army in Bosnia and Herzegovina*, 14.
8. Ibid., 25.
9. Lamoureux interview.
10. Ibid.
11. Ibid.
12. Gouge, Col. Steven F., *Commanding the 212th MASH in Bosnia*, Personal Experience Monogram, U.S. Army War College, 2001, 9–10; Troth, S.Sgt. Jeff, "Medics Pull Soldiers from Bosnia Minefield," *The Mercury*, September 1996, 8.
13. *American Military History Volume II*, 443.

14. TRADOC Pam 525-50, 1 October 1996, 2.
15. Ibid., 3.
16. Ibid., 10.
17. Ibid., 11.
18. Joint Publication 4-02.2, 30 December 1996, i.
19. Joint Publication 4-02.2, 30 December 1996, II-1.
20. Joint Publication 4-02.2, 30 December 1996, III-1, 4, B-B-1.
21. Hough, 16; Novier interview.
22. Hough, 132, 252; MEMORANDUM FOR Record 832d Med Co (AA) Unit History, Maj. Robert Carty, 5 September 2002, MEDEVAC File, Office of Medical History, Falls Church, VA.
23. Hough, 84.
24. Hough, 93; Bosnia Deployment AAR (SFOR4), Bosnia File, Office of Medical History, Falls Church, VA.
25. Hough, 235; *DUSTOFF Association Newsletter*, Summer 1999, 7.
26. Hough, 228.
27. Matt Brady interview.
28. Ibid.
29. Ibid.
30. Lockard interview.
31. "57th Med Co Helps USAF Airlift Sailor from Croatia to Germany," *Dustoff Association Newsletter*, Summer 2001, 6.
32. Dynamic Response Mass Casualty (MASCAL) Exercise AAR, 7 May 2001, Bosnia File, Office of Medical History, Falls Church, VA.
33. Gentry interview.
34. Pouncey, Maj. Michael, 498th Med Co (AA) AAR, 10 April 2002, 498th Med Co, MEDEVAC Files, Office of Medical History, Falls Church, VA; Gentry interview.
35. Task Force 1-25 Aviation SFOR AAR, undated, 25th Infantry Division Museum, Schofield Barracks, HI.
36. Email to author from Col. Frank Leith, New Hampshire ARNG, 27 September 2007.
37. Email to author from Capt. Roger Drury, Vermont ARNG, 21 August 2007.
38. Pamphlet *Task Force Eagle Disestablishment Ceremony, 24 November 2004*, courtesy of C/2d/238th Med Co, Indiana ARNG; *Bosnia-Herzegovina: The U.S. Army's Role in Peace Enforcement Operations 1995–2004*, CMH Pub 70-97-1, Washington, DC: Center for Military History, 2005, 38; various interviews. All from chapters 5–8.
39. Department of the Army Force Accounting System Active Army Troop List, January 1998.
40. Unit History, Capt. Jason Hauk, Commander, USAAAD Honduras.
41. *DUSTOFF Association Newsletter*, Winter/Fall 2000, 8; Drennon interview.
42. *American Military History Volume II*, 446.
43. Ibid., 447.
44. Ibid., 446.
45. TTP From Task Force Hawk Deep Operations, Volume I, Box 157, Office of Medical History, Falls Church, VA.
46. Maher, Lt. Col. Joseph E., "V Corps in the Balkans: The History of Task Force 12," *Army Aviation*, 31 December 1999, 18.
47. Email to author from Maj. Charles Zimmerman, 25 March 2008.
48. Maher, Lt. Col. Joseph E., "V Corps in the Balkans: The History of Task Force 12," *Army Aviation*, 31 December 1999, 20, 22.

49. Lt. Col. (ret) Mike Avila interview, 28 September 2007.
50. *American Military History Volume II*, 449.
51. Phillips, R. Cody, *Operation Joint Guardian, the U.S. Army in Kosovo*, CMH Publication 70-109-1, Washington, DC: Center for Military History, 2007, 22, 27.
52. TFMF Information Paper, 6 October 2000, Box 197, Office of Medical History, Falls Church, VA.
53. Avila interview.
54. Maher, Lt. Col. Joseph E., "V Corps in the Balkans: The History of Task Force 12," *Army Aviation*, 31 December 1999, 22; Avila interview.
55. TTP From Task Force Hawk Deep Operations, Volume II, Combat Health Support, Box 157, Office of Medical History, Falls Church, VA; also reflected in "TF Hawk CAAT Initial Impressions Report (IIR) Final AAR, Chapter 11, Topic C: Evacuation, Box 157, Office of Medical History, Falls Church, VA, and CALLCOMS File number 10004-39128.
56. Interview – Lt. Col. Alan Moloff, Commander 212th CMF, TF Hawk, 17 May 1999, Box 157, Office of Medical History, Falls Church, VA.
57. Interview – Lt. Col. James Bruckart, TF Hawk Surgeon, undated, Box 157, Office of Medical History, Falls Church, VA.
58. *American Military History Volume II*, 451; Smart interview.
59. Fristoe interview.
60. Fristoe, Maj. Jon, "Dustoff in Kosovo," *Dustoff Association Newsletter*, Summer 2000, 10; Fristoe interview.
61. Email from Lt. Col. Jon Fristoe, 5 August 2007; MEDEVAC Kosovo File, Office of Medical History, Falls Church, VA.
62. Email to author from Lt. Col. Jon Fristoe, 5 August 2007; Smart interview; Email to author from Maj. Bill Howard, 22 October 2007.
63. Briefing: Army Medical Department in Support of Peacekeeping Operations in Kosovo, undated, Office of Medical History, Falls Church, VA, Box 190.
64. Briefing: Dustoff Kosovo, 50th Medical Company (AA), undated, MEDEVAC File, Office of Medical History, Falls Church, VA; Phonecon author and CW4 Andrew Feris, 17 September 2007.
65. Email to author from Maj. John Fishburn, 717th Med Co (AA), 5 September 2007.
66. Email to author from Maj. John Fishburn, 717th Med Co (AA) New Mexico ARNG, to author, 6 Sep 2007
67. Phillips, R. Cody, *Operation JOINT GUARDIAN, the U.S. Army in Kosovo*, CMH Publication 70-109-1, Washington, DC: Center for Military History, 2007, 50; Email to author from Mr. Rick Deitz, FORSCOM G3/5/7, 18 October 2007.
68. http://www.nato.int/kfor/chronicle/2003/chronicle_07/11.htm (accessed 18 September 2007); Email to author from Mark Hough, 18 September 2007.
69. Email to author from Mr. Rick Deitz, FORSCOM G3/5/7, 18 October 2007; http://www.nato.int/kfor/chronicle/2004/chronicle_07/12.htm (accessed 18 September 2007).
70. Email to author from Mr. Rick Deitz, FORSCOM G3/5/7, 18 October 2007; Email to author from Maj. John Fishburn, 717th Med Co (AA), 5 Sep 2007. All in chapters 5–8.
71. Operation FOCUS RELIEF, 30th Med Brigade AAR, MEDEVAC Lessons Learned File, Office of Medical History, Falls Church, VA.
72. Bakutis, Bunky, "For Army, a Proud Record," *Honolulu Advertiser*, 3 January 1999, 1.
73. Field Manual 8-10-26, 16 February 1999, vi.

74. Field Manual 8-10-26, 16 February 1999, 1-4.
75. Field Manual 8-10-26, 16 February 1999, 1-5.
76. Field Manual 8-10-26, 16 February 1999, 2-1, 3-1.
77. Field Manual 8-10-6, 14 April 2000, 1-1, O-1.

Chapter Eight
To 9/11, 2000–2001

1. Fontenot, Col. (ret) Gregory. *On Point: The United States Army in Operation IRAQI FREEDOM,* 22.
2. *American Military History Volume II,* 451; Fontenot, *On Point: The United States Army in Operation IRAQI FREEDOM,* 20; Email to author from Maj. Andrew Risio, 19 February 2009.
3. MacDonald interview.
4. MacDonald interview; Email to author from Maj. Andrew Risio, 19 February 2009.
5. Ibid.
6. Lamoureux interview.
7. Heintz interview.
8. Anderson, Lt. Col. Randall G., *CONUS Installation Medical Evacuation (MEDEVAC) Analysis,* Office of The Surgeon General, Department of the Army, Washington, DC, May 2002, unpublished, Office of Medical History, Falls Church, VA, 11-12; Heintz interview.
9. *Jane's All the World's Aircraft, 2006/07,* Coulsdon, England, 2007, 874–881; Smart interview.
10. Air Force Joint Instruction 16-401, Army Regulation 70-50, 1 September 1997, Attachment 3-1; Smart interview; Lamoureux interview.
11. Field Manual 3.0, 1-2, 9-11, 10-1.
12. Joint Publication 4-02, 30 July 2001, v, II-6.
13. Ibid., II-4-7.
14. Ibid., E-1.
15. Change 1, Field Manual 8-10-26, 30 May 2002, 3-5, B-8.
16. Change 1, Field Manual 8-10-26, I-1–5.
17. Field Manual 4-02, 13 February 2003, 1-1.
18. Ibid., 2-1.
19. Ibid., 5-3.
20. Ibid., 6-1 through 10, 7-1 through 5, 8-1 through 8-3.
21. Lawson, Sfc. Rhonda. "Aviators Honored for Sinai Actions," *Army Aviation,* 29 February 2004, 32.
22. Lumbaca, Capt. Sonise. "Black Hawks Replace Hueys for Sinai Mission," *Army Aviation,* 31 July 2006, 40.
23. *The 9/11 Commission Report: Final Report of the National Commission on Terrorist Attacks upon the United States,* New York, NY: W.W. Norton & Company, 2005, 326.
24. Avila interview.
25. *The 9/11 Commission Report: Final Report of the National Commission on Terrorist Attacks upon the United States,* 326.

26. Ibid., 314; Hirrel, Leo P. Ph.D. *Response to Terrorism,* U.S. Joint Forces Command, Norfolk, VA: Office of the Command Historian, 2003, 17.

27. Author phonecon with Lt. Col. Maureen Bellamy, State Army Aviation Officer, 9 October 2007.

28. Email to author from Col. (ret) Scott Heintz, 11 October 2007; expansive comments by Col. (ret) Scott Heintz to author by email, 17 December 2008.

29. Lockard interview: Email to author from Col. (ret) Pauline Lockard, 17 October 2007.

30. Email to author from Maj. Michael Charnley, 10 October 2007. At the time, he was the Battalion S2.

31. *American Military History Volume II,* 461.

32. Email to author from Col. Frank Leith, New Hampshire State Army Aviation Officer, ARNG, 9 October 2007.

33. Matt Brady interview.

34. Avila interview.

35. Mitchell interview.

36. Email to author from Lt. Col. John Lamoureux, 11 October 2007.

37. Email to author from Maj. John Fishburn, 717th Med Co (AA), 10 October 2007.

38. Email to author from Maj. Mike Pouncey, 9 October 2007.

39. Fontenot, Col. (ret) Gregory. *On Point: The United States Army in Operation IRAQI FREEDOM,* 22.

40. Ibid., 23.

41. Briscoe, Dr. Charles H., Kiper, Dr. Richard L., Sepp, Dr. Kalev I., and Schroder, James A. *Weapon of Choice, ARSOF in Afghanistan,* Combat Studies Institute, Fort Leavenworth, KS, 2003, 1.

Chapter Nine
Again, Into Battle, 2001–2003

1. Lt. Col. Art Jackson interview, 12 February 2007.

2. Ibid., 33.

3. *American Military History Volume II,* 465.

4. Ibid., 466.

5. Ibid., 466.

6. Ibid., 469–470.

7. Interview with Brig. Gen. William Fox, by Maj. Robert Glisson, 23 October 2002, OEF Oral History File, Box 28, Office of Medical History, Falls Church, VA.

8. Stewart, Dr. Richard. *The United States Army in Afghanistan: Operation ENDURING FREEDOM,* Washington, DC: Center for Military History, 2003, 32–-45.

9. "Crewmember of the Year" Award Citation, *Dustoff Association Newsletter,* Fall-Winter 2002, 3.

10. XVIII Airborne Corps Annual Historical Review, 2002, History Office, Fort Bragg, NC: 235; "Rescue of the Year" Award Citation, *Dustoff Association Newsletter,* Fall-Winter 2002, 3.

11. 50th Medical Company (AA) Detachment AAR for Operation ENDURING FREE-DOM, 13 September 2002, Capt. James Stanley, Unit historical file, Office of Medical History, Falls Church, VA.

12. Presentation by Col. Scott Heintz to Directorate of Health Care Operations, 25 October 2002, Office of The Surgeon General, OEF Oral History File Box 29, Office of Medical History, Falls Church, VA.

13. XVIII Airborne Corps Annual Historical Review, 2002, History Office, Fort Bragg, NC, 245; Matt Brady interview.

14. Matt Brady interview.

15. Ibid.

16. *American Military History Volume II*, 476.

17. http://www.whitehouse.gov/news/releases/2002/06/20020601-3.html (accessed 19 December 2007).

18. *American Military History Volume II*, 477.

19. Fontenot, Col. (ret) Gregory. *On Point: The United States Army in Operation IRAQI FREEDOM*, 448–480.

20. Maj. Gen. George Weightman interview, 26 November 2007.

21. Ibid.

22. Fontenot, Col. (ret) Gregory. *On Point: The United States Army in Operation IRAQI FREEDOM*, 482–494; 3d MEDCOM EAC OIF AAR, undated, OIF MEDEVAC File, Office of Medical History, Falls Church, VA.

23. Fontenot, Col. (ret) Gregory. *On Point: The United States Army in Operation IRAQI FREEDOM*, 469.

24. Weightman interview.

25. *American Military History Volume II*, 477.

26. Fontenot, Col. (ret) Gregory. *On Point: The United States Army in Operation IRAQI FREEDOM*, 47; *American Military History Volume II*, 478–479.

27. Atkinson, Rick. *In the Company of Soldiers*, New York, NY: Henry Holt and Company, 2005, 93.

28. Gordon, Michael R., and Trainor, Lt. Gen. Bernard E. *Cobra II, The Inside Story of the Invasion and Occupation of Iraq*, Pantheon Books, New York, NY: 2006, 175, 178.

29. Groen, Lt. Col. Michael S. *With the 1st Marine Division in Iraq, 2003, Quantico, Virginia*, History Division, Marine Corps University, 2006, 153.

30. *American Military History Volume II*, 482.

31. Groen, Lt. Col. Michael S. *With the 1st Marine Division in Iraq, 2003*, 247.

32. Atkinson, Rick. *In the Company of Soldiers*, 154.

33. Ibid., 164.

34. Fontenot, Col. (ret) Gregory. *On Point: The United States Army in Operation IRAQI FREEDOM*, 194.

35. *American Military History Volume II*, 483.

36. Ibid., 485.

37. Ibid., 485.

38. Groen, Lt. Col. Michael S. *With the 1st Marine Division in Iraq, 2003*, 349.

39. Atkinson, Rick. *In the Company of Soldiers*, 462.

40. *American Military History Volume II*, 486–490.

41. Matt Brady interview.

42. Weightman interview.

43. Lt. Col. Art Jackson interview, 12 February 2007; email to author from Capt. Anthony Borowski, 10 March 2008.

44. Lt. Col. Judith Robinson, interview with Lt. Col. Bryant Harp, 21 May 2003, OEF Oral History File, Office of Medical History, Falls Church, VA. (Harp/Robinson).

45. Jackson interview, Drennon interview.
46. *Black Jack Journal,* Issue 1, December 2007, MEDEVAC File, Office of Medical History, Falls Church, VA, 4; author phonecon with Sfc. Tomas Ortiz, 9 January 2008.
47. Harp/Robinson interview.
48. Ibid.
49. Maj. William "Casey" Clyde interview, 16 February 2007; Gentry interview.
50. Gentry interview; Salvetti/Ginn interview.
51. Gentry interview.
52. Clyde interview.
53. Gentry interview; Clyde interview.
54. Salvetti/Ginn interview.
55. Gentry interview.
56. Kennedy, Maj. Christopher M. *U. S. Marines in Iraq, 2003: Anthology and Annotated Bibliography,* Washington, DC: History Division, U.S. Marine Corps, 2006, 7; Clyde interview.
57. Clyde interview; Gentry interview.
58. Salvetti/Ginn interview.
59. Clyde interview.
60. Gentry interview.
61. Email to author from Adrian Salvetti, 8 January 2008.
62. North, Lt. Col. (ret) Oliver L. *War Stories: Operation IRAQI FREEDOM*, Regnery Publishing, Inc., Washington, DC., 2003, 99–101. 63. Givings/Ginn interview.
64. Ibid
65. Dahlen/Ginn interview.
66. Mallory/Ginn interview.
67. Clyde interview.
68. Clyde interview; Gentry interview.
69. Salvetti/Ginn interview.
70. Phonecon with Maj. Brian Veneziano, commander Charlie Company, 1st Battalion, 126th Aviation Regiment, Maine ARNG, 7 January 2008; 112th Med Co (AA) Unit History provided by 2d Lt. Jasmine Chase, Unit Historian, Maine ARNG.
71. Schwartz/Barger interview; Ortiz/Barger interview.
72. Ibid.
73. Email to author from Capt. Justin Avery, 20 March 2008.
74. Schwartz/Barger interview.
75. S.Sgt. Dan Ledbetter, 82d Med Co crewmember/Barger interview.
76. Personnel Recovery Team/Barger interview.
77. Email to author form Capt. Jason Avery, 20 March 2008.
78. CW2 Scott Van Hoagland, 82d Med Co crewmember/Barger interview.
79. S.Sgt. Dan Ledbetter, 82d Med Co crewmember/Barger interview.
80. Schwartz/Barger interview.
81. Schwartz/Barger interview; Ortiz/Barger interview.
82. Schwartz/Barger interview.
83. Barger/Personnel Recovery Team interview; email to author from Capt. Jason Avery, 20 March 2008.
84. Schwartz/Barger interview; Ortiz/Barger interview; email to author from Capt. Jason Avery, 20 March 2008.
85. Ortiz/Barger interview.
86. Schwartz/Barger interview.

87. Jackson interview.
88. Ibid.
89. Ibid.
90. Ibid.
91. Ibid.
92. Ibid.
93. Capt. Tom Powell interview, 13 February 2007.
94. Ibid.
95. Jackson interview; Howe, Maj. Robert F. "Soldiers of the 159th Maintain the DUSTOFF Legacy," *U.S. Army Medical Department Journal,* October–December 2005, 18.
96. Drennon interview.
97. Ibid.
98. Ibid.
99. Ibid.
100. Ibid.
101. Drennon, Maj. Scott, 507th Med Co (AA) OIF-AAR, undated, 507th Med Co, MEDEVAC File, Office of Medical History, Falls Church, VA.
102. Ibid.
103. Ibid.
104. Contemporary Operations Study Team, "Interview with Col. Curtis Potts," Combat Studies Institute, Fort Leavenworth, KS, 13 December 2005.
105. Drennon interview.
106. Lamoureux/Barger interview.
107. Ibid.
108. Ibid.
109. Ibid.
110. Ibid.
111. Lamoureux interview.
112. LaChance interview.
113. Ibid.
114. Ibid.
115. Ibid.
116. Ibid.
117. Pecor interview.
118. Ibid.
119. 62d Medical Brigade Annual Historical Reports, 1 January 2003–31 December 2003 and 1 January 2004–31 December 2004, Fort Lewis, WA; MEDEVAC/54th Med Co (AA) File, Office of Medical History, Falls Church, VA; OIF unit History supplied by Lt. Col. Martin Kerkenbush, undated, MEDEVAC Unit Files, Office of Medical History, Falls Church, VA.
120. MacDonald, Lt. Col. David L. *The Joint Patient Movement System, A Solution to Arrest the Erosion of an Efficient and Effective System,* U.S. Army War College, Carlisle Barracks, PA, 2004, 14.
121. MacDonald interview.
122. MacDonald interview; Decision Briefing, 56th Med Bn CDR, MEDEVAC/OIF File, undated, Office of Medical History, Falls Church, VA.
123. OIF External After Action Review (AAR) 56th Medical Battalion (Evacuation), 30 June 2003, MEDEVAC File, Office of Medical History, Falls Church, VA.

124. XVIII Airborne Corps Annual Historical Review, 2003, 219; XVIII Airborne Corps 2004 Annual Historical Summary, 275, both from the Fort Bragg History office; email to author from Maj. Michael Charnley, 249th Med Co (AA), 31 August 2007.

125. Emails to author from 1st Sgt. Greg Patin, 812th Med Co, 24 February 2008, and from CWO4 Michael Knuppel, Flight Operations Officer, 832d Med Co (AA), 10 September 2007.

126. CW4 Jim Brennan interview, 1 April 2007.

127. Ibid.

128. XVIII Airborne Corps Annual Historical Review, 2003, 219; XVIII Airborne Corps 2004 Annual Historical Summary, 275, both from the Fort Bragg History office; email to author from Maj. Michael Charnley, 249th Med Co (AA), 31 August 2007.

Chapter Ten
Aviation Transformation and Domestic Operations, 2002–2005

1. Brady, Maj. Gen. (ret) Patrick. "In Response to MEDEVAC on Track," *Army Aviation Magazine*, 31 March 2004, unk.

2. Lockard interview.

3. Executive Summary, ATI Update, DASGp-HCF, Lt. Col. Anderson, 14 September 2001, MEDEVAC Transformation File, Office of Medical History, Falls Church, VA.

4. Donnelly, William M. *Transforming an Army at War, Designing the Modular Force, 1991–2005,* Washington, DC: Center for Military History, 2007, 20–21.

5. Ibid., 32.

6. Brig. Gen. (ret) Edward Sinclair interview, 5 May 2008.

7. Sinclair interview.

8. Lockard interview.

9. Smart interview.

10. Email to author from Lt. Col. Bill Goforth, 10 March 2008.

11. Fristoe interview.

12. Email to author from Lt. Col. Jon Fristoe, 23 January 2008.

13. Anderson, Lt. Col. Randall G. *CONUS Installation Medical Evacuation (MEDEVAC) Analysis,* Office of The Surgeon General, Department of the Army, Washington, DC, May 2002, unpublished, Office of Medical History, Falls Church, VA, 4–24.

14. Fristoe interview.

15. Executive Summary Subject: MEDEVAC "3 Deep" Aviation Oversight, 6 October 2003, MEDEVAC Transformation File, Office of Medical History, Falls Church, VA.

16. Joy interview.

17. Lockard interview, Joy interview, Sinclair interview.

18. Lockard interview.

19. Heintz interview; expansive comments by Col. (ret) Scott Heintz to author by email, 17 December 2008.

20. Fristoe interview.

21. Ibid., Sinclair interview.
22. Sinclair interview.
23. Fristoe interview.
24. Lockard interview, Fristoe interview, Sinclair interview.
25. Lockard interview.
26. Fristoe interview, Sinclair interview.
27. Lockard interview; Lamoureux interview.
28. Information Paper, Subject: Task Force Aviation, 30 January 2004, Col. Pauline Lockard; Point Paper, Subject: SRC 08 MEDEVAC Discussion, 11 July 2004, Maj. Jon Fristoe; both in MEDEVAC Transformation File, Office of Medical History, Falls Church, VA.
29. Sinclair, Brig. Gen. E.J. "Aviation Transformation: How Far Have We Come?" *Army Aviation,* 3 November 2004, 8.
30. MEMORANDUM FOR MG JAMES D. THURMAN, DIRECTOR, ARMY AVIATION TASK FORCE, 450 ARMY PENTAGON, WASHINGTON DC 20310, 5 January 2004, MEDEVAC Files, Office of Medical History, Falls Church, VA.
31. MEMORANDUM FOR VCSA, SUBJECT: MEDEVAC Force Structure Decisions, 05 February 2004. Office of Medical History, Falls Church, VA, Box 454D.
32. Ibid.
33. Barger, Maj. Lewis, and Greenwood, Dr. John, Interviews with Lt. Gen. James B. Peake, The Surgeon General, U.S. Army, 2d and 7th Sessions, 22 July and 13 August 2004, Oral History Files, Office of Medical History, Falls Church, VA.
34. "Statement by: MG James D. Thurman, Director, Army Aviation Task Force, Office of the Deputy Chief of Staff, G-3 United States Army," before the Tactical Air and Land Forces Subcommittee Committee on the Armed Services United States House of Representatives, on Aviation Industrial Base and Department of Defense Rotorcraft Programs, 4 March 2004. MEDEVAC ATI File, Office of Medical History, Falls Church, VA.
35. Ibid.
36. Briefing: MEDEVAC OVERVIEW: AVN TF Implementation Brief 26 March 2004, Maj. Jon Fristoe, Office of Medical History, Falls Church, VA, Box 454U.
37. Email to author from Lt. Col. Bill Goforth, 10 March 2008.
38. Point Paper, DASG-HCF, Subject: SRC 08 MEDEVAC Discussion, 11 July 2004, MEDEVAC Transformation File, Office of Medical History, Falls Church, VA.
39. MEDEVAC Charter, 1 May 2004, procured from the MEPD Director, Col. Dave MacDonald, Fort Rucker, AL, MEDEVAC ATI File, Office of Medical History, Falls Church, VA.
40. Certificate of Charter SUBJECT: Aeromedical Evacuation, 14 May 2004, MEDEVAC Transformation Files, Office of Medical History, Falls Church, VA.
41. MEMORANDUM FOR ARMY G3, SUBJECT: Request to Retain Unit Designation for Air Ambulance Company, 28 April 2004, Office of Medical History, Falls Church, VA, Box 454D.
42. MacDonald, Lt. Col. David L. "Is MEDEVAC Broke," *Army Aviation Magazine,* 31 October 2004, 14.
43. Ibid.
44. Ibid.
45. Ibid.
46. Forrester, Col. Bill. "MEDEVAC on Track," *Army Aviation Magazine,* 31 January 2005, unk.

47. Brady, Maj. Gen. (ret) Patrick. "In Response to MEDEVAC on Track," *Army Aviation Magazine*, 31 March 2004, unk.
48. Rogers, Sfc. Reginald. "GSAB Brings New Capabilities to the Combat Aviation Brigade," *Army Aviation Magazine,* 30 November 2005, 36.
49. Lockard interview; MacDonald interview; Joy interview.
50. *DUSTOFF Association Newsletter,* Fall/Winter 2003, 6.
51. Total ARMY (Active and Reserve Component) MEDEVAC Sourcing (05-07), Provided by the MEPD, Fort Rucker, AL, MEDEVAC Transformation File, Office of Medical History, Falls Church, VA.
52. Ibid.
53. Ibid.
54. 2003, Current MTOE, data supplied by Lt. Col. Pete Smart, Utility Helicopters Project Office, Redstone Arsenal, AL.
55. Mitchell interview.
56. Fristoe interview; Mitchell interview.
57. Mitchell interview.
58. Ibid.
59. Ibid.
60. Gower Interview, Maj. Ken Koyle interview, 27 September 2006.
61. Kirkland, Richard G. *MASH Angels, Tales of the First Air Evac Helicopters,* Professional Press, Chapel Hill, NC, 2004, 274; http://www.lifeteam.net.
62. Message from: Army Operations Center, DTG: 222251Z FEB 05, MAST Files, Office of Medical History, Falls Church, VA.
63. Ibid; Army Regulation 95-1, para 3-12, HQ DA, Washington, DC, 1 September 1997; Anderson, Lt. Col. Randall G., *CONUS Installation Medical Evacuation (MEDEVAC) Analysis,* Office of The Surgeon General, Department of the Army, Washington, DC, May 2002, unpublished, 10, MEDEVAC Files, Office of Medical History, Falls Church, VA.
64. Reap, Lt. Col. Vincent M. "Winged Warriors in Honduras," *Army Aviation,* 28 February 2005, 28.
65. "NASA Looks Back at Hurricane Katrina One Year Later," *Science Daily*, 28 August 2006; http://www.sciencedaily.com/releases/2006/08/060828074620.htm
66. Louisiana National Guard Timeline of Significant Events Hurricane Katrina: Task Force Pelican, 7 December 2005, 3; procured from Lt. Col. Al Koenig, First Army Historian.
67. http://www.nemaweb.org/?1435 (accessed 20 September 2007).
68. Brunken, S.Sgt., Korey. *The US Army Response to Hurricane Katrina (Draft),* 20 June 2007, 10, MEDEVAC Katrina File, Office of Medical History, Falls Church, VA.
69. Louisiana National Guard Timeline of Significant Events Hurricane Katrina: Task Force Pelican, 7 December 2005, 3.
70. Knabb, Richard D., Tropical Cyclone Report Hurricane Katrina 23–30 August 2005. http://www.nhc.noaa.gov/pdf/TCR-AL122005_Katrina.pdf
71. Barger, Maj. Lewis, Katrina AMEDD Briefing HCO-MH, 13 December 2005, Katrina File, Office of Medical History, Falls Church, VA, Box 181F, slides 108-110. (Barger Katrina Briefing)
72. Ibid., slides 110–112.

73. MFR Nomination for the Army Aviation Association of America Award for Air/Sea Rescue for 2005, from the 812th Med Co (AA) Louisiana ARNG, 29 October 2005, copy received from 1st. Sgt. Greg Patin, MEDEVAC File, Office of Medical History, Falls Church, VA.

74. Haskell, M. Sgt. Robert. "Army Guard Aviators Ramped Up to Meet Katrina's Challenges," *Army Aviation,* 31 October 2005, 44.

75. Louisiana National Guard Timeline of Significant Events Hurricane Katrina: Task Force Pelican, 7 December 2005, 5.

76. Author - Phonecon with Maj. Joseph Brocato, 9 October 2007.

77. Ibid.

78. Louisiana National Guard Timeline of Significant Events Hurricane Katrina: Task Force Pelican, 7 December 2005, 5; author - Phonecon with Maj. Joseph Brocato, 9 October 2007; Brunken, 10–14; Barger Katrina Briefing slide 20.

79. Barger Katrina Briefing, slide 21.

80. McNally, Maj. John, Hurricane Katrina Relief Operations – 498th Medical Company (AA) After Action Report, 23 September 2005, 498th Med Co File, Office of Medical History, Falls Church, VA.

81. Ibid.

82. Ibid.

83. Email to author from Capt. Boudreau to author, 11 December 2007.

84. Barger Katrina Briefing, slide 22; email from Capt. Boudreau to author, 11 December 2007.

85. Email to author from S.Sgt. Steve Vacula, Det 1, C/104th Aviation Battalion (GSAB), Tennessee ARNG [formerly Det 1, 146th Med Co (AA)], 11 October 2007.

86. "Dustoff Gossip," Newspaper of the USAAAD at Fort Polk, LA, 15 April 2006.

87. Ibid.

88. Barger Katrina Briefing, slide 24; Haskell, M. Sgt. Robert, "Army Guard Aviators Ramped Up to Meet Katrina's Challenges," *Army Aviation,* 31 October 2005, 44.

89. Phonecon with Lt. Col. Shon Dermody, CW4 Doug Drost, CW3 Richard Burger, and Sfc. Darwin Kramer, 1022d Med Co (AA) Wyoming ARNG, 4 October 2007.

90. Phonecon with Sgt. Ken Jarrett, 149th Med Co (AA) medic, 5 October 2007.

91. Barger Katrina Briefing slide 28; Author – phonecon with CW3 Jason Graff, 24th Med Co (AA), 5 October 2007.

92. Data supplied by CW4 Michael Knuppel, Flight Operations Officer, 832d Med Co (AA), September 2007.

93. Sommers, Larry. "A Determined Rescue," *At Ease Magazine,* Wisconsin ARNG, undated, received from Lt. Col. Al Koenig, Katrina Historian, First Army Historical Office, Fort Gillem, GA.

94. Emails to author from Maj. Michael Charnley, New York ARNG, 1 August, and 10 October 2007; email to author from 1st Lt. Andy Thaggard, Command Historian, MS, ARNG, 3 October 2007.

95. Email to author from Lt. Col. Paul Frazier, 3 March 2008.

96. Email to author from CW2 Robert Hetrick, 148th Med Co, 29 August 2007, Brennan interview.

97. Barger Katrina Briefing, slide 28; Hosh, Kafia, "D.C. Guard rescues Hurricane Katrina victims," *Belvoir Eagle,* 22 September 2005, A1.

98. Briefing: Fifth US Army, 251639CDT September 2005, Hurricane Katrina/Rita File, Office of Medical History, Falls Church, VA; Phonecon with Sgt. Ken Jarrett, 149th Med Co (AA) flight medic, 5 October 2007.

99. Louisiana National Guard Timeline of Significant Events Hurricane Katrina: Task Force Pelican, 7 December 2005, 11.

100. "Maine Guard Sends Aviation to Support Hurricane Relief Operations," http://www/first.army.mil/pao/2005_Articles/092805 (accessed 17 October 2007).

101. *A Failure of Initiative, Final Report of the Select Bipartisan Committee to Investigate the Preparation for and Response to Hurricane Katrina*, Washington, DC: U.S. Government Printing Office, 2006, 217.

102. Louisiana National Guard Timeline of Significant Events Hurricane Katrina: Task Force Pelican, 7 December 2005, 5–12; email to author from 1st Sgt. Greg Patin, 812th Med Co, 24 February 2008.

103. *A Failure of Initiative, Final Report of the Select Bipartisan Committee to Investigate the Preparation for and Response to Hurricane Katrina*, 230.

104. Ibid., 201, 202, 217.

105. MacDonald interview.

106. MEPD Current Focus Brief 10 August 2005. MEDEVAC MEPD File, Office of Medical History, Falls Church, VA.

Chapter Eleven
Warriors of Compassion

1. Charles Kelly Jr., Remarks at the Inactivation Ceremony for the 57th Med Co, Fort Bragg, NC, recorded by author, 26 January 2007.

2. Neel/Bullard interview, 29.

3. MacDonald interview.

4. Ginn, 322.

5. Thresher interview.

6. Smart interview.

7. Neel, Lt. Col. Spurgeon H. "Medical Considerations in Helicopter Evacuation," *U.S. Armed Forces Medical Journal,* 5(1), February 1954, 220.

8. MacDonald, Lt. Col. David L. *The Joint Patient Movement System, A Solution to Arrest the Erosion of an Efficient and Effective System,* Carlisle, PA: U.S. Army War College, 2004, 16.

9. Ward, Geoffrey C. *The War: an Intimate History 1941–1945,* New York, NY: Alfred A. Knopf Publishers, 2007, 308.

10. Field Manual 1, June 2005, para 1-62.

11. McKiernan, Lt. Gen. David D. "Letters to the Editor," *Army Times,* 28 April 2003, 60.

12. Atkinson, Rick. *In the Company of Soldiers,* 113.

13. Woodward, Robert. *Bush at War,* New York, NY: Simon and Schuster, 2002, 209.

14. Casey, Gen. George W. Jr.. "The Strength of the Nation," *Army Magazine,* October 2007, 19.

15. http://www.louise.house.gov/index.php?option=com_content&task=view&id=781&Itemid (accessed 6 March 2008).

16. Geyer, Georgie Anne. "Challenges for new NATO commander," *Washington Times,* 28 September 2002, A12.

17. *Merriam-Webster's Collegiate Dictionary, Tenth Edition,* Springfield, MA: Merriam-Webster Incorporated, 1999.

18. Cook, 36.
19. Barger/Personnel Recovery Team interview.
20. Email to CW2 Gerald McGowen, given to author 2 April 2007.
21. Thomas Johnson, Dinner Remarks, recorded by author, 25 January 2007.
22. Ceremony remarks recorded by author, 26 January 2007.
23. 57th Medical Company (AA) Inactivation Ceremony, 56th Multifunctional Medical Battalion, Fort Bragg, NC, 26 January 2007.
24. Charles Kelly, Jr., Inactivation of the 57th Med Co (AA) Fort Bragg, NC, 26 Jan 2007, remarks recorded by author.
25. Ibid.

Bibliography

Books

A Failure of Initiative, Final Report of the Select Bipartisan Committee to Investigate the Preparation for and Response to Hurricane Katrina. Washington, DC: U.S. Government Printing Office, 2006.

Annual Report - The Surgeon General of the United States Army. Washington, DC: Historical Unit, U.S. Army Medical Department, 1972.

_____, 1973.

_____, 1974.

_____, 1975.

_____, 1976–1980.

Atkinson, Rick. *In the Company of Soldiers*. New York, NY: Henry Holt and Company, 2005.

Briscoe, Dr. Charles H., Kiper, Dr. Richard L., Sepp, Dr. Kalev I., and Schroder, James A. *Weapon of Choice, ARSOF in Afghanistan*. Fort Leavenworth, KS: Combat Studies Institute, 2003.

Condon-Rall, Mary E. *Disaster on the Green Ramp*. Washington, DC: Center of Military History, United States Army, 1996.

Cook, John L. *Rescue Under Fire: The Story of Dust Off in Vietnam*. Atglen, PA: Schiffer Military/Aviation History, 1998.

Cosmas, Graham A. *MACV The Joint Command in the Years of Escalation 1962–1967*. Washington, DC: Center for Military History, United States Army, 2006.

Cowdrey, Albert E. *The Medics' War.* Washington, DC: Center for Military History United States Army, 1987.

Currie, Col. James T., and Crossland, Col. Richard B. *Twice the Citizen: A History of the United States Army Reserve, 1908–1995.* Washington, DC: Office of the Chief, Army Reserve, 1997.

Donnelly, William M. *Transforming an Army at War, Designing the Modular Force, 1991–2005.* Washington, DC: Center for Military History, 2007.

Dorland, Peter, and Nanney, James. *Dust Off: Army Aeromedical Evacuation in Vietnam.* Washington, DC: Center of Military History, 1982.

Dorr, Robert F. *Chopper: A History of American Military Helicopter Operations from WW II to the War on Terror.* New York, NY: Berkley Books, 2005.

Doubler, Col. Michael D. *I Am the Guard: A History of the Army National Guard, 1636–2000.* Washington, DC: Department of the Army, 2001.

Fontenot, Col. (ret) Gregory, Degen, Lt. Col. E.J., and Tohn, Lt. Col. David. *On Point: The United States Army in Operation Iraqi Freedom.* Annapolis, MD: Naval Institute Press, 2005. *(On Point)*

Futrell, Robert F. *The United States Air Force in Korea 1950–1953.* Washington, DC: Office of Air Force History, United States Air Force, 1983.

Ginn, Richard V.N. Col. (ret). *The History of the U.S. Army Medical Service Corps.* Washington, DC: Office of the Surgeon General and Center of Military History, United States Army, 1997.

Gordon, Michael R., and Trainor, Lt. Gen. Bernard E. *Cobra II, The Inside Story of the Invasion and Occupation of Iraq.* New York, NY: Pantheon Books, 2006.

Greenwood, John T., and Berry, F. Clifton Jr. *Medics at War: Military Medicine from Colonial Times to the 21st Century.* Annapolis, MD: Naval Institute Press, 2005.

Groen, Lt. Col. Michael S. *With the 1st Marine Division in Iraq, 2003.* Quantico, VA: History Division, Marine Corps University, 2006.

Hirrel, Leo P., Ph.D. *Response to Terrorism.* Norfolk, VA: Office of the Command Historian, U.S. Joint Forces Command, 2003.

The History of Aeromedical Evacuation in the Pacific Theater During World War II, document #UH215 L746H, 1945, 40-41.

Holley, Irving B. Jr. *The United States Army in World War II, Special Studies, Buying Aircraft: Materiel Procurement for the Army Air Forces.* Washington, DC: Office of the Chief of Military History, Department of the Army, 1964.

Hough, Mark, M. *United States Army Air Ambulance*. Bellevue, WA: Vedder River Publishing, 1999.

Humes, James C. *Churchill: Speaker of the Century*. New York, NY: Stein & Day Publishers, 1980.

Jane's All the World's Aircraft, 1956/5. London, England, 1957.

_____, *1962/63*. Great Missenden, England, 1963.

_____, *1964/65*. Great Missenden, England, 1965.

_____, *1970/71*. London, England, 1971.

_____, *1982/83*. London, England, 1983.

_____, *1983/84*. London, England, 1984.

_____, *2006/07*. Coulsdon, England, 2007.

Kennedy, Maj. Christopher M. *U.S. Marines in Iraq, 2003: Anthology and Annotated Bibliography*. Washington, DC: History Division, U.S. Marine Corps, 2006.

Kirkland, Richard G. *MASH Angels, Tales of the First Air Evac Helicopters*. Chapel Hill, NC: Professional Press, 2004.

Kirkpatrick, Charles E. *Ruck it Up! The Post Cold-War Transformation of V Corps, 1990–2000*. Washington, DC: Department of the Army, 2006.

Marion, Lt. Col. Forrest L. *That Others May Live: USAF Air Rescue in Korea*, Washington, DC: Air Force History and Museums Program, 2004.

Merriam-Webster's Collegiate Dictionary, Tenth Edition. Springfield, MA: Merriam-Webster Incorporated, 1999.

Neel, Maj. Gen. Spurgeon. *Vietnam Studies: Medical Support 1965–1970*. Washington, DC: Department of the Army, 1991. (Neel, Vietnam Studies)

North, Lt. Col. (ret) Oliver L. *War Stories: Operation Iraqi Freedom*. Washington, DC: Regnery Publishing, Inc., 2003.

The 9/11 Commission Report: Final Report of the National Commission on Terrorist Attacks upon the United States. New York, NY: W.W. Norton & Company, 2005.

Scales, Maj. Gen. Robert H. *Certain Victory: The US Army in the Gulf War*. Washington, DC: Office of the Chief of Staff, United States Army, 1993.

Smith, Robert Ross. *United States Army in World War II, Triumph in the Philippines*. Washington, DC: Office of the Chief of Military History, Department of the Army, 1961.

Stewart, Dr. Richard. *The United States Army in Somalia 1992–1994*. Washington, DC: Center for Military History, 2002.

_____, *The United States Army in Afghanistan: Operation Enduring Freedom*. Washington, DC: Center for Military History, 2003.

_____, *American Military History Volume II, The United States Army in a Global Era, 1917–2003*. Washington, DC: Center for Military History, 2005. (American Military History Vol II)

United States Army Reserve in Operation DESERT STORM. Washington, DC: Department of the Army, 1993.

Van Wagner, Maj. R.D. *1st Air Commando Group: Any Place, Any Time, Anywhere*. Maxwell Air Force Base, AL: Air Command and Staff College, 1986.

Ward, Geoffrey C. *The War: An Intimate History 1941–1945*. New York, NY: Alfred A. Knopf Publishers, 2007.

Weinert, Richard P. Jr. *A History of Army Aviation – 1950–1962*. Fortress Monroe, VA: Office of the Command Historian, United States Army Training and Doctrine Command, 1991.

Whitcomb, Darrel D. *Combat Search and Rescue in Desert Storm*. Maxwell Air Force Base, AL: Air University Press, 2006.

Williams, Glenn M. *So Others Might Live*. Mukilteo, WA: WinePress Publishing, 1998.

Williams, James W. *A History of Army Aviation, From its Beginnings to the War on Terror*. http://www.iuniverse.com/bookstore (accessed 3 January 2007).

Woodward, Robert. *Bush at War*. New York, NY: Simon and Schuster, 2002.

Yearbook, *Stabilization Force 7, Operation Joint Forge Multinational Division-North*. Crystal City, VA: NGB-PA/MTCI Archives, undated.

_____, *Stabilization Force X*. Crystal City, VA: NGB-PA/MTCI Archives, undated.

_____, *Stabilization Force XIII, Multinational Brigade-North Bosnia-Herzegovina*. Crystal City, VA: NGB-PA/MTCI Archives, undated.

_____, *Stabilization Force 14, One Mission – One Team*. Crystal City, VA: NGB-PA/MTCI Archives, undated.

_____, *Stabilization Force 15, Multinational Task Force (North) April 1 to December 1, 2004 Peacekeeping Mission to Bosnia-Herzegovina*. Crystal City, VA: NGB-PA/MTCI Archives, undated.

Articles, Pamphlets, and Studies

"Baby Born During MAST Flight," *U.S. Army Aviation Digest,* September 1976: 22.

Bakutis, Bunky, "For Army, a Proud Record," *Honolulu Advertiser,* 3 January 1999: 1.

Bosnia-Herzegovina: The U.S. Army's Role in Peace Enforcement Operations 1995 – 2004. CMH Pub 70-97-1, Washington, DC: Center for Military History, 2005.

Brady, Maj. Gen. (ret) Patrick, "In Response to MEDEVAC on Track," *Army Aviation Magazine,* 31 March 2004: unk.

Carlin, CW2 Victor E., "Operations in the Desert: A Postscript," *U.S. Army Aviation Digest,* November/December, 1992: 26.

Carr, S.Sgt. Don, "The 507th Has Its 2,000th MAST Patient," *U.S. Army Aviation Digest,* March 1977: 12.

Casey, Gen. George W. Jr., "The Strength of the Nation," *Army Magazine,* October 2007: 19.

"Commander's CASEVAC System," number 89-5, Fort Leavenworth, KS: Center for Army Lessons Learned, November 1989.

Contemporary Operations Study Team, "Interview with Col. Curtis Potts," Fort Leavenworth, KS: Combat Studies Institute, 3 December 2005.

Curtis, Rob. "Letters to the Editor," *Army Times,* 28 April 2003: 60.

"Darmstadt to Dhahran: MEDEVAC Self-Deployment to Desert Shield," *The Journal of the US Army Medical Department,* September/October 1992: 51.

Dell, M.Sgt. Nat, "The Future is Now," *Soldiers,* August 1973: 5–17.

Dell, M.Sgt. Nat, "Toward a Professional Army," *Soldiers,* August 1973: 6–17.

"The Development of the American Helicopter," *AIA Newsletter,* 7(3), August/September 1994: 6.

Driscoll, Col. Robert S., "U.S. Army Medical Helicopters in the Korean War," *Military Medicine,* 166, April 2001: 290–296.

"Dustoff Gossip," Newspaper of the USAAAD at Fort Polk, LA, 15 April 2006.

Fardink, Lt. Col. Paul, "Amazing Men," *Army Aviation Magazine,* 29 February 2000: 27.

Fix, Capt. Gregory D., "The New UH-60Q Black Hawk MEDEVAC Helicopter," *U.S. Army Aviation Digest,* January/February 1993: 43.

Forrester, Col. Bill, "MEDEVAC on Track," *Army Aviation Magazine,* 31 January 2005: unk.

Furbish, Maj. Bruce G., "Dustoff Panama," *U.S. Army Aviation Digest,* November 1982: 38.

"The Gamest Bastards of All," *Time Magazine,* 2 July 1965: 22.

Garrison, Maj. Michael E., "Sinai 'Nomads,'" *Army Aviation,* February 28, 1997: 43.

Geiger, Lt. Col. Victor Geiger, MS, "Views from Readers," *U.S. Army Aviation Digest,* May/June 1991: 51.

Geyer, Georgie Anne, "Challenges for new NATO commander," *Washington Times,* 28 September 2002: A12.

Guilford, Lt. Col. Fredrick R., and Soboroff, Capt. Burton J., "Air Evacuation: An Historical Review," *Journal of Aviation Medicine,* 18, December 1947: 601–616. (Office of Medical History, Falls Church, VA, Archives Box #1).

Halloran, Barney, "Red Hot Mission," *Soldiers Magazine,* January 1973: 17.

Hamner, Capt. Louis, "Helicopters in the Medical Service," *Military Bulletin, U.S. Army Europe,* 11(7), July 1954: 156–158.

Haskell, M. Sgt. Robert, "Army Guard Aviators Ramped Up to Meet Katrina's Challenges," *Army Aviation,* 31 October 2005: 44.

Hosh, Kafia, "D.C. Guard Rescues Hurricane Katrina Victims," *Belvoir Eagle,* 22 September 2005: A1.

Howe, Maj. Robert F., "Soldiers of the 159th Maintain the DUSTOFF Legacy," *U.S. Army Medical Department Journal,* October–December 2005: 18.

Jablecki, Maj. Joseph S., "AMEDD Aviation Update," *U.S. Army Aviation Digest,* July 1988: 6.

Jackson, James O., "West Germany Hellfire from the Heavens," *Time Magazine,* 12 September 1988.

Jacobs, Lt. Col. Bill M., "Winged Warriors in Central America," *U.S. Army Aviation Digest,* November/December 1993: 34.

Jeffer, Col. Edward K., MC, "The Medical Units of the Army National Guard (ARNG) and Operation Desert Shield/Desert Storm," *Journal of the US Army Medical Department,* March/April 1992: 20.

Kitchens, Dr. John W., "Cargo Helicopters in the Korean Conflict, Part 1 of 2," *U.S. Army Aviation Digest,* November/December 1952: 38–44.

_____ "Cargo Helicopters in the Korean Conflict, Part 2 of 2," *U.S. Army Aviation Digest*, January/February 1953: 34–39.

Kruse, Lt. Col. William R., "Separate but not Apart," *U.S. Army Aviation Digest*, September 1985: 38.

Lam, Lt. Col. David M., "From Balloon to Blackhawk, PART I," *U.S. Army Aviation Digest*, June 1981: 41–48.

_____ "From Balloon to Blackhawk, PART II," *U.S. Army Aviation Digest*, July 1981: 44–48.

_____ "From Balloon to Blackhawk, PART III," *U.S. Army Aviation Digest*, August 1981: 44–48.

_____ "From Balloon to Blackhawk, PART IV," *U.S. Army Aviation Digest*, September 1981: 45–48.

Lawrence, Lt. Col. G. P. MC., "The Use of Autogiros in the Evacuation of Wounded," *Military Surgeon*, 73(6), December 1933: 314–321. (Office of Medical History, Falls Church, VA, Archives Box #1).

Lawson, Sfc. Rhonda, "Aviators Honored for Sinai Actions," *Army Aviation*, February 29, 2004: 32.

Ledford, Lt. Gen. Frank F. MC, "Medical Support for Operation Desert Storm," *The Journal of the US Army Medical Department*, January/February 1992: 3.

Loeb, Vernon, "Fighting a 'Battle of Perceptions,'" *Washington Post*, 10 November 2003: A20.

Lumbaca, Capt. Sonise, "Black Hawks Replace Hueys for Sinai Mission," *Army Aviation*, 31 July 2006: 40.

MacDonald, Lt. Col. David L., "Is MEDEVAC Broke," *Army Aviation Magazine*, 31 October 2004: 14.

Maddox, Maj. Gen. Bobby J., "Army Aviation Branch Implementation," *U.S. Army Aviation Digest*, August 1983: 2.

Maher, Lt. Col. Joseph E., "V Corps in the Balkans: The History of Task Force 12," *Army Aviation*, 31 December 1999: 18.

"MAST Anniversary," *U.S. Army Aviation Digest*, July 1980: 7.

"The MAST Program," *U.S. Army Aviation Digest*, October 1976: 8.

McAndrews, Kevin, "Helicopter Crew Seeks Gubernatorial Rider," *The Prairie Rider*, June 1986: 1. NGB/PA-MTCI Archives, Alexandria, VA.

McKiernan, Lt. Gen. David D. "Letters to the Editor," *Army Times*, 28 April 2003: 60.

Neel, Lt. Col. Spurgeon H., "Helicopter Evacuation in Korea," *U.S. Armed Forces Medical Journal*, VI(5), May 1955: 691–703. (Neel, Helicopter Evacuation)

Neel, Lt. Col. Spurgeon H., "Aeromedical Evacuation," *Army Magazine*, April 1956: 30–33. (Neel, Aeromedical Evacuation)

Neel, Col. Spurgeon H., "Army Aeromedical Evacuation Procedures in Vietnam," *Journal of the American Medical Association*, 204(4), 22 April 1968: 99–103.

Neel, Lt. Col. Spurgeon H., "Medical Considerations in Helicopter Evacuation," *U.S. Armed Forces Medical Journal*, 5(1), February 1954: 220.

Pratt, Capt. Bob, "USAR Unit Aids in D.C. Aircraft Recovery Operations," *Army Reserve Magazine*, Spring 1982: unk.

Pecoraro, Maj. Richard, "Dustoff Europe," *Medical Bulletin of the U.S. Army, Europe*, July 1984: 23.

Phillips, R. Cody, *Operation Joint Guardian, the U.S. Army in Kosovo*, CMH Publication 70-109-1, Washington, DC: Center for Military History, 2007.

"President Clinton Visits Tropic Lightening Soldiers in Haiti," *Hawaii Army Weekly*, 6 April 1995: A-5.

Reap, Lt. Col. Vincent M., "Winged Warriors in Honduras," *Army Aviation*, 28 February 2005: 28.

Risio, Maj. Andrew, "421st Medical Evacuation Battalion History and Accolades," *Army Medical Department Journal*, October/November/December 2005: 9.

Simon, Kimberly, "54th Med Honored for MAST Mission," *NW Guardian*, 5 May 1993: 1.

Sinclair, Brig. Gen. E.J., "Aviation Transformation: How Far Have We Come?" *Army Aviation*, 3 November 2004: 8.

Smith, Col. Allen D., "Air Evacuation – Medical Obligation and Military Necessity," Maxwell AFB, AL: Air University Quarterly Review, Summer 1953: 98.

Smith, Barry D., "Desert Dust Off: Medevac with the 247th," *Rotor & Wing International*, January 1991: 38.

Sommers, Larry, "A Determined Rescue," *At Ease Magazine*, Wisconsin ARNG, undated, received from Lt. Col. Al Koenig, Katrina Historian, First Army Historical Office, Fort Gillem, GA.

Story, Maj. Dennis C., "Aviation Medicine, Its Origins and a Training perspective," *U.S. Army Aviation Digest*, July 1988: 2–5.

"Task Force Bandit Aids Division in Aviation Missions," *Hawaii Army Weekly,* 9 March 1995: A-6.

The U.S. Army in Bosnia and Herzegovina, AE Pamphlet 525-100, Washington, DC: Center for Military History, 7 October 2003.

Thompson, Loren, "Army XXI Aviation: Time for the V-22," *Army Magazine,* 1 November 1999: unk.

Troth, S.Sgt. Jeff, "Medics Pull Soldiers from Bosnia Minefield," *The Mercury,* September 1996: 8.

United States General Accounting Office, Report to the Chairman, Subcommittee on Military Personnel and Compensation, Committee on Armed Services, House of Representatives, OPERATION DESERT STORM Full Army Medical Capability Not Achieved. GAO/NSIAD-92-175, August 1992.

Veit, Lt. Col. Christoph, "German Medical Assistance for US Forces During the Gulf Crisis: A Stock-taking of Lessons Learned," *The Journal of the US Army Medical Department,* January/February 1992: 58.

Wells, Christina, "Dustoff: Med Choppers Ready Anytime," *Medical Bulletin of the U.S. Army, Europe,* January 1976: 25.

Wells, Maj. Kristin L., "Luck of the Irish," *The Retired Officer Magazine,* October 1986: 36.

Whitcomb, Darrel D., "Combat Search and Rescue: A Longer Look," *Aerospace Power Journal,* Maxwell AFB, AL: Summer 2000: 39.

Wood, Maj. William C., "MEDEVAC on the European Battlefield," *U.S. Army Aviation Digest,* August 1977: 5.

Archival Material

Air University Library, Maxwell AFB, Alabama

United States Army Medical Service Combat Development Group Project NR AMSCD 56-6, Aeromedical Evacuation Final Report, December 1959. M-41566-NC (AMSCD 56-6)

Office of Medical History, Falls Church, Virginia

After Action Report: AHUAS TARA II, Box 157E.

After Action Report: 44th Medical Brigade Operations DESERT SHIELD and DESERT STORM, undated, DESERT STORM Collection, Box 29.

After Action Report: 108 Medical Battalion Command Report for Operation DESERT STORM, undated, Desert Storm Collection, Box 30.

Anderson, Lt. Col. Randall G., *CONUS Installation Medical Evacuation (MEDEVAC) Analysis,* OTSG, Department of the Army, Washington, DC, May 2002, unpublished, MEDEVAC File.

Army Aviation Plan 2004 [ATP-04], undated, procured from the MEPD Office, Fort Rucker, AL, Transformation File.

ARNORTH AAR Briefing, 8 December 2006.

Barger, Maj. Lewis, Katrina AMEDD Briefing HCO-MH, 12 December 2005, Katrina File.

Black Jack Journal, Issue 1, December 2007, MEDEVAC File, Evacuation Battalions.

Briefing: Army Medical Department in Support of Peacekeeping Operations in Kosovo, undated, AMEDD History Office, Box 190.

Briefing: Dustoff Kosovo, 50th Medical Company (Air Ambulance), undated, Box 452H.

Briefing: Fifth US Army, 251639CDT September 2005, Hurricane Katrina/Rita.

Certificate of Charter SUBJECT: Aeromedical Evacuation, 14 May 2004, MEDEVAC Transformation Files.

Decision Briefing, 56th Medical Battalion, CDR, MEDEVAC/OIF File, undated.

Drennon, Maj. Scott, 507th Med Co (AA) OIF-AAR, undated, 507th Med Co, MEDEVAC File, Office of Medical History, Falls Church, VA.

Executive Summary, ATI Update, DASGp-HCF, Lt. Col. Anderson, 14 September 2001, MEDEVAC Transformation File, Office of Medical History, Falls Church, VA.

Heintz, Col. Scott, Presentation to Directorate of Health Care Operations, OTSG, 25 October 2002, OEF Oral History File Box 29.

Interview – Lt. Col. James Bruckart TF Hawk Surgeon, undated, Box 157.

Interview – Lt. Col. Alan Moloff, Commander 212th CMF, TF Hawk 17 May, 1999, Box 157.

"Joint Services Operational Requirement for the Advanced Vertical Lift Aircraft (JSX JSOR)," April 1985, Box HCO-FD (AVN).

Katrina AMEDD Briefing prepared by Maj. Lew Barger, HCO-MH, 12 December 2005, Box 181F. (Barger Katrina Briefing)

MAST Military Assistance to Safety and Traffic, Appendices to Report of Test Program by the Interagency Study Group, March 1971, Box HCO-FD (AVN).

McNally, Maj. John, Hurricane Katrina Relief Operations – 498th Medical Company (AA) After Action Report, 23 September 2005.

MEDEVAC Charter, 1 May 2004, MEDEVAC ATI File.

Medical Support for Operation RESTORE DEMOCRACY, HCO Files, Box 204.

Memorandum for Army G3, Subject: Request to Retain Unit Designation for Air Ambulance Company, 28 April 2004, Box 454D.

Memorandum For Record, Subject: V-22 Joint Working Group Meeting, 4 March 1986, MEDEVAC Files, Box HCO-FD (AVN).

Memorandum for Deputy Chief of Staff for Personnel, Subject: Inclusion of Medical Service Corps (67J) Aviators in the Aviation Branch, 7 April 1983, MEDEVAC File, Notebook AVN BR vs 67J.

Memorandum For Mg James D. Thurman, Director, Army Aviation Task Force, 450 Army Pentagon, Washington, DC 20310, 5 January 2004, MEDEVAC Files.

Memorandum For Record, Subject: General Officer Aviation Branch Composition Meeting, 7 April 1983. MEDEVAC File, Notebook AVN BR vs 67J.

Memorandum for Deputy Chief of Staff for Operations and Plans, Subject: TRADOC Proposal to Centralize Aviation Proponency and Form an Aviation Branch, 8 April 1983, MEDEVAC File, Notebook AVN BR vs 67J.

Memorandum for the Chief of Staff, Army, Subject: Aviation Branch Composition – Action Memorandum, 13 April 1983, MEDEVAC File, Notebook AVN BR vs 67J.

MEPD Current Focus Brief 10 August 2005. MEDEVAC MEPD File.

Message from: Army Operations Center, DTG: 222251Z FEB 05. MAST Files.

Newsletter – The American Helicopter Society, July 1961, 57th Med Co (AA) File.

Nomination Package for Mr. Craig Honaman to the DUSTOFF Association Hall of Fame, 16 April 2007, Box HCO-FD (AVN).

Operation DESERT STORM – Full Army Medical Capability Not Achieved, GAO/NSI-AD-92-175, Government Accounting Office, August 1992. DESERT STORM File.

OIF External After Action Review (AAR) 56th Medical Battalion (Evacuation), 30 June 2003. MEDEVAC/Battalion File.

"Over Two Decades of Service: An Update on MAST," no author, 1987, Box HCO-FD (AVN).

Point Paper, DASG-HCF, Subject: SRC 08 MEDEVAC Discussion, 11 July 2004, MEDEVAC Transformation File.

Pouncey, Maj. Michael, 498th Med Co (AA) AAR, 10 April 2002, 498th Med Co, MEDE-VAC Files, Office of Medical History, Falls Church, VA.

62d Medical Brigade Annual Historical Reports, 1 January 2003 – 31 December 2003 and 1 January 2004 – 31 December 2004, Fort Lewis, WA, MEDEVAC/54th Med Co (AA) File.

Somalia Medical Operations, Ingram, Sandra, Camber Corporation, 9 September 1996, Box 185.

Stanley, Capt. James, "50th Medical Company (AA) Detachment AAR for Operation Enduring Freedom," 13 September 2002. OEF File.

TF Hawk CAAT Initial Impressions Report (IIR) Final AAR, Chapter 11, Topic C: Evacuation, Box 157.

TF Medical Falcon Information Paper, 6 October 2000, Box 197.

Transformation Briefing, MEPD, Fort Rucker, AL, undated, MEDEVAC Transformation File.

TTP From Task Force Hawk Deep Operations, Vol I, Box 157.

TTP From Task Force Hawk Deep Operations, Vol II, Combat Health Support, Box 157.

U.S. Army Center for Military History, Washington, DC

Directory and Station List of the United States Army, U11.U58A7; January 1951, July 1951, January 1952, August 1952, October 1952, June 1953, June 1954, December 1954, April 1955, December 1955, April 1956, December 1956, June 1957, December 1957, April 1958, October 1958, June 1959, December 1959, April 1969, October 1969, June 1961, December 1961, June 1962, December 1962, June 1963, December 1963, June 1964, December 1964, June 1965, December 1965, June 1966, December 1966, June 1967, December 1967, June 1968, April 1969, December 1969, April 1970, December 1970, October 1971, May 1972, September 1972, September 1973. Force Structure and Unit History Branch.

Department of the Army Force Accounting System Active Army Troop List U11.U58A7; June 1974, December 1974, June 1975, December 1975, June 1976, March 1977, September 1977, April 1978, October 1978, June 1979, March 1980, December 1980, June 1981, December 1981, June 1982, December 1982, June 1983, December 1983, June 1984, December 1984, June 1985, December 1985, June 1986, December 1986, June 1987, December 1987, June 1988, December 1988, June 1989, June 1990, December 1992, August 1996, January 1998, July 1999, February 2000, April 2001, February 2002, January 2003. Force Structure and Unit History Branch.

U.S. Army Military History Institute, Carlisle Barracks, PA

Carroll, Col. Dale A., "The Role of the U.S. Army Medical Department in Domestic Disaster Assistance Operations – Lessons Learned from Hurricane Andrew," U.S. Army War College, April 1996.

Gouge, Col. Steven F., "Commanding the 212th MASH in Bosnia," Personal Experience Monogram, U.S. Army War College, 2001.

Griffin, Col. Greg, "Lonestar DUSTOFF in Desert Shield/Storm," Personal Experience Monograph, U.S. Army War College, undated.

Knisely, Lt. Col. Benjamin M., "Army Medical Department Aviation and Its Relationship to the New Army Aviation Branch," U.S. Army War College, April 1985.

MacDonald, Lt. Col. David L., "The Joint Patient Movement System, A Solution to Arrest the Erosion of an Efficient and Effective System, " U.S. Army War College, April 2004.

Palmer, Lt. Col. Gerald A., "Army Medical Department Issues from Operation Desert Shield," U.S. Army War College, June 1991.

Peake, Col. James B., "Message to Warfighters: Historical Perspective on Combat Medicine," U.S. Army War College, 17 March 1988.

Richards, Lt. Col. Donn R., "Medical Trends: An Evaluation of Medical Care Given in Vietnam, Grenada, Panama, and Desert Storm," U.S. Army War College, April 1999.

Schwallie, Lt. Col. Randal A., "Desert DUSTOFF," Personal Experience Monograph, U.S. Army War College, 25 April 2002.

"USARV Aviation Operational Procedures Guide, 1 June 1970," MACV Command Historian's Collection.

National Archives and Records Administration (NARA)

Annual Historical Review, 1-228th Aviation Battalion, Fort Kobbe, Panama, 1 October 1988–30 September 1989, Record Group 338, file 870-5c-57/4.

214th Medical Detachment (RG) Presentation to AMEC 27 February 90, Record Group 334, File 870-5b-6/40aaa.

History, Headquarters 1st Helicopter Ambulance Company, Command Report for June 1953. Record Group 407, Stack 270, Box 23.

History, Headquarters 1st Helicopter Ambulance Company, Command Report for July, 1953. Record Group 407, Stack 270, Box 23

History, Headquarters 8055th MASH, APO 301, 1 October–31 October 1950. NARA, Record Group 407, Stack 270, Box 23.

History, Aeromedical Units, NARA, Record Group 112 Stack 390, 57th Medical Detachment.

History, Headquarters 15th Medical Battalion, 1st Cavalry Division, 1 January–31 December 1968, 10 January 1969. NARA Record Group 112, Stack 390, Aeronautical Units, 15th Medical Battalion, Box 1.

History of JTF-Bravo, NARA, Record Group 338, file 870-5b-6/36.

Wagner, Donald, O., *The System of Field Medical Service in Theaters of Operations: Its Principles ands the Types of Units Authorized.* Unpublished manuscript, September, 1959. NARA, Record Group 112, Stack 390, Box 287, HU 314.7.

Tropic Lightening Museum, Schofield Barracks, HI

Task Force 1-25 Aviation SFOR AAR, undated.

The Story of JTF Hawaii, Public Affairs Office, U.S. Army, Pacific, undated.

Uniformed Services University of the Health Sciences, James A. Zimble Learning Resource Center, Bethesda, MD

Anderson, Capt. Randall G., *The Dustoff Report*. The Dustoff Association, San Antonio, Texas, 1992. USUHS/LRC call # UH503D974.

U. S. Army Aviation Museum Archives, Fort Rucker, AL

"Fact Sheet" Subject: V-22 (Osprey) Program, Purpose: To Inform the CG TRADOC about the rationale of the SECDEF and HQDA in their decision to cancel the V-22 Program. 11 May 1989. From Historian, U.S. Army Aviation Center, Fort Rucker, AL.

JOINT TASK FORCE ANDREW AVIATION AFTER ACTION REPORT (TAB R) 090730ROCT92, File 870.20A.

_____ Enclosure 7 (AVIATION) to Tab J (J3), 071830ROCT92 , File 87020A.

Letter from Maj. Gen. (ret) George Putnam, 4 March 2004, Aviation Branch Implementation File.

MAST: Military Assistance to Safety and Traffic, Book 2 of 2

Item 1. Sears, Lt. Col. Robert L., "An Air Medical Evacuation System for Highway Accident Victims," Arizona State University, Tempe, AZ, June 1968. Unpublished.

Item 3. Letters, Subject: Review of Proposal for Military Support of Air Medical Evacuation Systems (AMES) to Aid Highway Accident Victims, 20 August 1969.

Item 5. MEMORANDUM SUBJECT: Project MAST, several documents and memoranda.

Item 7. MAST, Military Assistance To Safety and Traffic, Report of Test Program by the Intragency Study Group, July–December 1970.

MEMORANDUM for JTF Andrew Aviation, 12 October 1992, File 870.20A.

MSG from HQDA Washington, DC, dtg 132225Z Apr 79, Subject: Commissioned Officer Aviation Management, Aviation Branch Implementation File.

Pettyjohn, Lt. Col. Frank S., M.D. *Review of the U.S. Army Aeromedical Research Laboratory Conference on Aeromedical Evacuation, 15–16 January 1974.* Fort Rucker, AL: U.S. Army Aeromedical Research Laboratory, August 1974. (AD/A-001544)

Army Medical Department Museum Archives, Fort Sam Houston, TX

Pamphlet. *421st Medical Company*, March 1966.

Pamphlet. *Dustoff Europe, 421st Med Co, 15th Med Det, 63rd Med Det*, 1969.

Army Medical Department Center and School, Fort Sam Houston, TX

MEDICAL SYSTEM PROGRESS REVIEW, Army Medical Department, January 31, 1989, Academy of Health Sciences, Fort Sam Houston, TX.

MEMORANDUM FOR: Director for Operational Plans and Interoperability, J7 Joint Staff, Washington, DC, 29 Jan 1992, SUBJECT: USCINCEUR After Action Report on Operation PROVIDE COMFORT, AMEDD C&S MCCS-FD Historical Files, Fort Sam Houston, TX.

MEMORANDUM, SUBJECT: Operation JUST CAUSE Lessons Learned Report, Academy of Health Sciences, Fort Sam Houston, TX, 1 June 1990.

White Paper, Health Services Support Futures, Final Draft, Academy of Health Sciences, Fort Sam Houston, TX, March 1989.

Historian's Office, Fort Bragg, NC

XVIII Airborne Corps Annual Historical Review, 2002, History Office.

XVIII Airborne Corps Annual Historical Review, 2003, History Office.

XVIII Airborne Corps Annual Historical Summary, 2004, History Office.

Historian's Office, Fort Campbell, KY

Historical Files of the 101st Airborne Division (Airmobile).

Historical Files of the 50th Medical Co (AA).

Historical Files of the 542nd Medical Co (AA).

Historian's Office, Fort Gillem, GA

Brunken, S.Sgt., Korey, *The U.S. Army Response to Hurricane Katrina (Draft),* 20 June 2007, JTF-Katrina History Group (Provisional), First Army.

Louisiana National Guard Timeline of Significant Events Hurricane Katrina: Task Force Pelican, 7 December 2005, from Lt. Col. Al Koenig.

Interviews

By author:
Col. Dave MacDonald, Fort Rucker, AL, 14 September 2006.
2d Lt. Andrew Russ, Fort Rucker, AL, 24 September 2006.
Capt. Jason Richards, Fort Rucker, AL, 25 September 2006.
Maj. (ret) Peter Webb, Fort Rucker, AL, 26 September 2006.
Maj. Brian Almquist, Fort Rucker, AL, 26 September 2006.
Sfc. Jim Burbach, Fort Rucker, AL, 26 September 2006.
Maj. Ken Koyle, Fort Rucker, AL, 27 September 2006.
S.Sgt. Lee Bucklin, Fort Rucker, AL, 27 September 2006.
Lt. Col. Vinny Carnazza, Fort Rucker, AL, 27 September 2006.
S.Sgt. George Hildebrandt, Fort Rucker, AL, 28 September 2006.
Lt. Col. Greg Gentry, FortMcPherson, GA, 29 September 2006.
Col. (ret) Doug Moore, Arlington, VA, 31 October 2006.
Col. (ret) Jim Truscott, OTSG, Arlington, VA, 5 January 2007.
1st Lt. Rebecca Joseph, Fort Bragg, NC, 24 January 2007
S.Sgt. Joseph Lemons, Fort Bragg, NC, 25 January 2007.
S.Sgt. Shawn McNabb, Fort Bragg, NC, 25 January 2007.
CW4 Scott Markgraf, Fort Bragg, NC, 25 January 2007.
Maj. Brady Rose, Fort Bragg, NC, 26 January 2007.
Lt. Col. Art Jackson, Fort Sam Houston, TX, 12 February 2007.
Col. Randy Schwallie, Fort Sam Houston, TX, 12 February 2007.
Capt. Thomas Powell, Fort Sam Houston, TX, 13 February 2007.
Lt. Col. Brad Pecor, Fort Sam Houston, TX, 13 February 2007.
Lt. Col. William LaChance, Fort Sam Houston, TX, 14 February 2007.

Col. (ret) Randy Maschek, Fort Sam Houston, TX, 15 February 2007.
Maj. Gen. (ret) Patrick Brady, Cibolo, TX, 15 February 2007.
Maj. William "Casey" Clyde, Fort Sam Houston, TX, 16 February 2007.
Col. (ret) Frank Novier, San Antonio, TX, 18 February 2007.
Sfc. Christopher Downey, Fort Hood, TX, 20 February 2007.
CW3 Leroy Thompson, Fort Hood, TX, 20 February 2007.
S.Sgt. Brandon Coughlin, Fort Hood, TX, 20 February 2007.
Lt. Col. Scott Drennon, Fort Hood, TX, 20 February 2007.
M.Sgt. Kevin Gillin, Fort Sam Houston, TX, 21 February 2007.
Col. (ret) Dan Gower, Fort Sam Houston, TX, 21 February 2007.
Brig. Gen. (ret) Jerome Foust, Fort Sam Houston, TX, 21 February 2007.
Lt. Col. (ret) Tommy Mayes, San Antonio, TX, 21 February 2007.
Col. Pat Hastings and Lt. Col. Brian Kueter, Fort Sam Houston, TX, 23 February 2007.
Cmd. Sgt. Maj. Alfred Rodriguez, Fort Sam Houston, TX, 23 February 2007.
Lt. Col. Pete Smart, Atlanta, GA, 6 March 2007.
Maj. Tanya Peacock, Atlanta, GA, 7 March 2007.
1st Sgt. Tim Barr, Indiana ARNG, Shelbyville, IN, 9 March 2007.
S.Sgt. Derrick Kuhns, Indiana ARNG, Shelbyville, IN, 9 March 2007.
CW2 Scott Osborne, Indiana ARNG, Shelbyville, IN, 9 March 2007.
Sgt. Terry Hansome, Indiana ARNG, Shelbyville, IN, 9 March 2007.
Col. (ret) Pauline Lockard, Chevy Chase, MD, 14 March 2007.
Lt. Col. Bob Mitchell, Carlisle Barracks, PA, 19 March 2007.
Col. (ret) Art Hapner, Fairfax, VA, 23 March 2007.
Col. (ret) Tom Scofield, Lake Ridge, VA, 30 March 2007.
CW4 Jim Brennan, Georgia ARNG, Atlanta, GA, 1 April 2007.
S.Sgt. Andrew Quen, Fort Campbell, KY, 2 April 2007.
SPC Aaron Tuten, Fort Campbell, KY, 2 April 2007.
CW3 James Van Meter, Fort Campbell, KY, 2 April 2007.
CW2 Gerald McGowen, Fort Campbell, KY, 2 April 2007.
Sgt. Michael Bishop, Fort Campbell, KY, 2 April 2007.
S.Sgt. Thomas Harris, Fort Campbell, KY, 3 April 2007.
S.Sgt. Will Kosnitch, Fort Campbell, KY, 3 April 2007.
Lt. Col. John Lamoureux, Arlington, VA, 24 May 2007.
CW2 Michael Espinoza, Wiesbaden Airbase, Germany, 4 June 2007.
CW3 Travis Workman, Wiesbaden Airbase, Germany, 4 June 2007.
Sgt. Boyd Smith, Wiesbaden Airbase, Germany, 4 June 2007.
S.Sgt. Luis Ramirez, Wiesbaden Airbase, Germany, 5 June 2007.
Lt. Col. Jon Fristoe, Wiesbaden Airbase, Germany, 5 June 2007.
Maj. Robert Howe, Wiesbaden Airbase, Germany, 5 June 2007.
Sfc. James Gambill, Landstuhl, Germany, 6 June 2007.
S.Sgt. Rusty Borders, Landstuhl, Germany, 6 June 2007.
CW4 Mike Carson, Landstuhl, Germany, 6 June 2007.
Maj. Andrew Risio, Landstuhl, Germany, 6 June 2007.
1st Sgt. Eric Blaine, Landstuhl, Germany, 6 June 2007.
Maj. Anthony Meador, Ketterbach, Germany, 8 June 2007.
CW2 Jason LaCrosse, Ketterbach, Germany, 8 June 2007.
Sfc. James Carwell, Ketterbach, Germany, 8 June 2007.
Sgt. Robert Reavis, Sacramento, CA, 14 July 2007.
Sfc. James Moore, Sacramento, CA, 14 July 2007.
1st Sgt. Gary Volkman, Sacramento, CA, 16 July 2007.

CW4 Rick Lynn, Sacramento, CA, 16 July 2007.
CW4 Barry Brown, Salem, OR, 18 July 2007.
1st Sgt. Kevin Hoggard, Salem, OR, 18 July 2007.
S.Sgt. Jason Johnson, Salem, OR, 18 July 2007.
Maj. David Strayer, Salem, OR, 18 July 2007.
Lt. Col. Mathew Brady, Alexandria, VA, 7 August 2007.
Col. (ret) Scott Heintz, by telephone, 16 September 2007.
Lt. Col. (ret) Mike Avila, Arlington, VA, 28 September 2007.
Col. (ret) William Thresher, Lansdowne, VA, 23 October 2007.
Maj. Gen. George Weightman, Fort Meade, MD, 26 November 2007.
Lt. Col. (ret) Van Joy, by telephone, 5 December 2007.
Brig. Gen. (ret) Edward J. Sinclair, by telephone, 5 May 2008.

Other Interviews

Barger, Maj. Lewis, and Greenwood, Dr. John, Interviews with Lt. Gen. James B. Peake, The Surgeon General, U.S. Army, 2d through 7th Session, 22 July and 13 August 2004, Oral History Files, Office of Medical History, Falls Church, VA.

Barger, Maj. Lewis, OIF Oral History File, Office of Medical History, Falls Church, VA. With:

  Maj. James Schwartz, 82d Med Co (AA), 19 May 2003. (Schwartz/Barger)
  Capt. Enrique Ortiz, 82d Med Co (AA), 19 May 2003. (Ortiz/Barger)
  Several crewmembers of the 82d Med Co (AA), 19 May 2003. (crewmember name/
     Barger)
  Personnel Recovery Team, 19 May 2003 (Personnel Recovery Team/Barger)
  Maj. John Lamoureux, 50th Med Co (AA), 1 October 2003. (Lamoureux/Barger)

Ginn, Col. (ret) Richard V., *In Their Own Words: The 498th in Iraq 2003*, Office of Medical History, Army Medical Command, Falls Church, VA, undated. With:

  Maj. Greg Gentry   (Gentry/Ginn)
  Capt. Jeremy McKenzie   (McKenzie/Ginn)
  Capt. Adrian Salvetti   (Salvetti/Ginn)
  Capt. Thomas Mallory   (Mallory/Ginn)
  CW2 Paul Bryant   (Bryant/Ginn)
  CW2 Al Hill   (Hill/Ginn)
  CW2 Jason Wright   (Wright/Ginn)
  S.Sgt. Gregory Givings   (Givings/Ginn)
  S.Sgt. Bryant Williams   (Williams/Ginn)
  Spc. Robert Dahlen   (Dahlen/Ginn)
  Spc. Michael Tilley   (Tilley/Ginn)

Glisson, Maj. Robert, interview with Brig. Gen. William Fox, 23 October 2002, OEF Oral History File, Box 28, Office of Medical History, Falls Church, VA.

Maj. Gen. (ret) Spurgeon Neel, U.S. Air Force Oral History interview by John Bullard, 3 March 1977, Brooks AFB, TX. (Neel/Bullard)

Maj. Gen. (ret) Spurgeon Neel, Senior Officers Oral History Program interview by Lt. Col. Anthony Gaudiano, Carlisle Barracks, PA, 1985. (Neel/Gaudiano)

Lt. Col. Judith Robinson, interview with Lt. Col. Bryant Harp, 21 May 2003, OEF Oral History File, Office of Medical History, Falls Church, VA. (Harp/Robinson)

Recorded Remarks by Author

Charley Kelly, Jr., Inactivation of the 57th Med Co (AA) Fort Bragg, NC, 26 January 2007.

Thomas "Egor" Johnson, Inactivation Dinner of the 57th Med Co (AA) Fort Bragg, NC, 25 January 2007.

Public Law

Title 10, U.S.C., Section 2635, Section 814, Public Law 93-155.

Joint Publications

JP 1, *Joint Warfare of the US Armed Forces*, 11 November 1991.
JP 4-02, *Doctrine for Health Service Support in Joint Operations*, 26 April 1995.
JP 4-02, *Doctrine for Health Service Support in Joint Operations*, 30 July 2001
JP 4-02.2, *Joint Tactics, Techniques, and Procedures for Patient Movement in Joint Operations*, 30 December 1996.

U.S. Army Field Circulars, Manuals, Pamphlets, Regulations

Air Force Joint Instruction 16-401, Army Regulation 70-50, 1 September 1997.
Army Regulation 95-1, HQ DA, Washington, DC, 1 September 1997.
Army Regulation 500-4, HQ DA, Washington, DC, 15 January 1982.

FC 8-45, *Medical Evacuation in the Combat Zone*, October 1986.
FM 1, *The Army*, June 2005.
FM 3.0, *Operations*, 14 June 2001.
FM 4-02, *Force Health Protection in a Global Environment*, 13 February 2003.
FM 8-8 / NAVMED P-5047 / AFM 160-20, *Medical Support in Joint Operations*, 1 June 1972.

FM 8-10, *Medical Support Theater of Operations*, 10 April 1970.

FM 8-10, *Health Service Support in a Theater of Operations*, October 1978.

FM 8-10, *Health Service Support in a Theater of Operations*, 1 March 1991.

FM 8-10-6, *Medical Evacuation in a Theater of Operations, Tactics, Techniques, and Procedures*, 31 October 1991.

FM 8-10-6, *Medical Evacuation in a Theater of Operations, Tactics, Techniques, and Procedures*, 14 April 2000.

FM 8-10-26, *Employment of the Medical Company (Air Ambulance)*, 16 February 1999.-Change 1, 30 May 2002.

FM 8-15, *Medical Support in Divisions, Separate Brigades, and the Armored Cavalry Regiment*, September 1972.

FM 8-35, *Transportation of the Sick and Wounded*, December 1970.

FM 8-35, *Evacuation of the Sick and Wounded*, January 1977.

FM 8-35, *Evacuation of the Sick and Wounded*, 22 December 1983.

FM 8-55, *Army Medical Service Planning Guide*, 23 October 1960.

FM 8-55, *Planning for Health Service Support*, 15 February 1985.

FM 8-55, *Planning for Health Service Support*, 9 September 1994.

FM 100-5 *Operations*, 20 August 1982.

FM 100-5 *Operations*, 5 May 1986.

FM 100-5 *Operations*, 14 June 1993.

TRADOC Pamphlet 525-50, 1 October 1996.

TRADOC Pamphlet 525-72, 1 June 1996.

Newsletters

DUSTOFF Association Newsletter, November, 1995. (DAN)

_____, June 1996.

_____, Fall 1996.

_____, Summer 1997.

_____, Fall 1997.

_____, Spring 1998.

_____, Fall 1998.

_____, Summer 1999.

_____, Spring/Summer 2000.

_____, Fall/Winter 2000.

_____, Spring/Summer 2001.

_____, Fall/Winter 2001.

_____, Spring/Summer 2002.

_____, Fall/Winter 2002.

_____, Spring/Summer 2003.

_____, Fall/Winter 2004.

_____, Spring/Summer 2005.

_____, Fall/Winter 2005.

_____, Spring/Summer 2006.

_____, Fall/Winter 2006.

On-line Research

http://www.lifeteam.net/ (accessed 6 August 2007).

http://www.centenialofflight.gov/essay/Rotary/MASH/HE12G7.htm (accessed 14 March 2007).

http://.allexperts.com/e/1983_beirut_barracks_bombing.httm (accessed 19 April 2007).

http://www.nhc.noaa.gov/1992andrew.html (accessed 24 May 2007).

http://www.military-medical-technology.com/article.cfm?DocID=481 (accessed 9 May 2007).

http://www.nemaweb.org/?1435 (accessed 20 September 2007).

http://www/first.army.mil/pao/2005_Articles/092805 (accessed 5 November 2007).

http://www.transchool.eustis.army.mil/lic/documents/OCOT_Interviews/klingenhagen.htm (accessed 5 November 2007).

http://www.whitehouse.gov/news/releases/2002/06/20020601-3.html (accessed 19 December 2007).

http://www.nhc.noaa.gov/pdf/TCR-AL122005_Katrina.pdf (accessed 18 September 2008).

http://www.sciencedaily.com/releases/2006/08/060828074620.htm (accessed 18 September 2008).

Unpublished Documents

Dustoff Follies Notebook, unpublished, in six volumes and still being used, Hohenfels Dustoff Alert Facility, Germany.

Heintz, Maj. David S., *Operations Desert Shield and Storm After Action Review, Delta Company, 326 Medical Battalion "Eagle Dustoff,"* 15 March 1991. Procured from author.

Howard, Maj. William, "History of the 50th Medical Company (AA)," undated. Procured from author.

Moore, Lt. Col. Douglas, "Air Ambulance Support for the Combat Division," Fort Leavenworth, KS: Command and General Staff College, June 1974. Procured from author.

Moore, Douglas E., Col. (ret), "The Mount Saint Helens Search and Rescue Effort May 18-29, 1980," procured from author.

Pamphlet *Task Force Eagle Disestablishment Ceremony, 24 November 2004,* courtesy of Charlie Company, 2d Battalion, 238th Aviation Regiment, Indiana ARNG.

57th Medical Company (AA) Inactivation Ceremony, 56th Multifunctional Medical Battalion (P), Fort Bragg, NC, 24 January 2007. Procured from Lt. Col. Scott Putzier.

Unit History, Capt. Jason Hauk, Commander, USAAAD Honduras, undated. Emailed to author, 19 April 2007.

Index

A

Abrams, Gen. Creighton
    reorganization of the Army, 225
    tribute to MEDEVAC units, 54
    views on the use of the Reserve Component in the Vietnam War, 67
Abrams, Gen. John, Aviation Restructuring Initiative and, 231
Afghanistan, Operation ENDURING FREEDOM and, 245–252
Agosta, Lt. Col. Rick, career and MEDEVAC role, 194
AH-64 Apache helicopters
    Operation DESERT SHIELD and, 149
    Operation ENDURING FREEDOM and, 247, 251
    Operation IRAQI FREEDOM and, 258, 275
    Task Force Hawk and, 213–214
    upgrades to, 121
AH-1 Cobra helicopters, MAST duties and, 300
Aideed, Muhammed, ambush of United Nations troops and, 183–184
"Air Ambulance Support for the Combat Division" (Moore), 63
Air Florida crash, rescue efforts after, 99
AirLand Battle concept
    description, 79
    doctrinal crystallization of, 117–120, 173, 225
    MEDEVAC support for, 104, 105
    Medical Force 2000 and, 141
    reorganization of the air ambulance MEDEVAC assets and, 117–120, 124
    UH-60 Black Hawk helicopter support for, 85
Al Qaeda, September 11, 2001 terrorist attacks and, 245–252
Albania
    Operation SHINING HOPE and, 215
    operations in, 211–215
Alison, Col. John, Project 9 role, 7–8

D

H

I

K

M

N

O

Q

R

V

W